# Register Now for Online Access to Your Book!

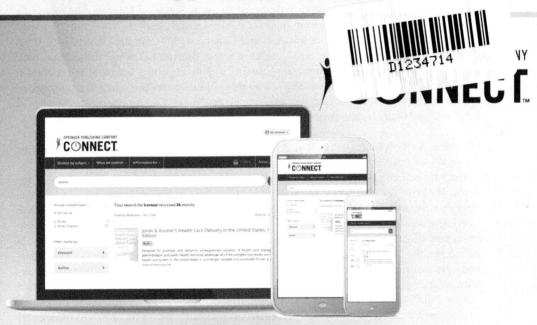

Your print purchase of *Evaluation of Health Care Quality for DNPs, Second Edition,* **includes online access to the contents of your book**—increasing accessibility, portability, and searchability!

**Access today at:**
**http://connect.springerpub.com/ content/book/978-0-8261-3158-4 or scan the QR code at the right with your smartphone and enter the access code below.**

*Scan here for quick access.*

**1J28KK7XR**

SPC

**SPRINGER PUBLISHING COMPANY**
View all our products at springerpub.com

**Joanne V. Hickey, PhD, RN, FAAN, FCCM,** holds of the Patricia L. Starck/PARTNERS Professorship in Nursing and the Coordinator of the Doctor of Nursing Practice program at the University of Texas Health Science Center at Houston, School of Nursing. She received a baccalaureate degree in nursing from Boston College, an MSN from the University of Rhode Island, an MA in counseling from Rhode Island College, a PhD from the University of Texas at Austin, and a post-master's certificate as a nurse practitioner from Duke University. Dr. Hickey is a fellow of the American Academy of Nursing and a fellow of the American College of Critical Care Medicine. She is a member of numerous professional organizations including the American Nurses Association, Sigma Theta Tau International, Society of Critical Care Medicine, and American Association of Neuroscience Nursing.

**Christine A. Brosnan, DrPH, RN,** recently retired as an associate professor from the University of Texas Health Science Center at Houston, School of Nursing, where in addition to teaching and clinical research, she held a number of administrative positions, including Track Director for the MSN in Education Program, Assistant Dean for Professional Development, and Associate Dean for Academic Affairs. She received a BSN from Georgetown University, an MSN from the University of Texas Medical Branch in Galveston, and a doctorate in public health from the University of Texas Health Science Center at Houston School of Public Health. The major area of study in her doctoral work was health services organizations. Dr. Brosnan has collaborated in research studies on the cost and effectiveness of newborn screening, screening for hypertension and obesity in children, and the early detection of type 2 diabetes. She has over 35 published articles, abstracts, chapters, proceedings, and letters, and has delivered numerous presentations on health care evaluation and related topics. Her article "Type 2 Diabetes in Children and Adolescents: An Emerging Disease" received the Excellence in Writing Award from the *Journal of Pediatric Health Care*.

# Evaluation of Health Care Quality for DNPs

## Second Edition

Joanne V. Hickey, PhD, RN, FAAN, FCCM

Christine A. Brosnan, DrPH, RN

*Editors*

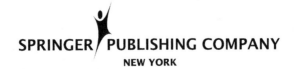

SPRINGER PUBLISHING COMPANY
NEW YORK

Springer Publishing Company, LLC
11 West 42nd Street
New York, NY 10036
www.springerpub.com

*Acquisitions Editor*: Margaret Zuccarini
*Senior Production Editor*: Kris Parrish
*Composition*: diacriTech

*ISBN*: 978-0-8261-3157-7
*e-book ISBN*: 978-0-8261-3158-4

18 19 20 / 5 4 3 2

The author and the publisher of this Work have made every effort to use sources believed to be reliable to provide information that is accurate and compatible with the standards generally accepted at the time of publication. Because medical science is continually advancing, our knowledge base continues to expand. Therefore, as new information becomes available, changes in procedures become necessary. We recommend that the reader always consult current research and specific institutional policies before performing any clinical procedure. The author and publisher shall not be liable for any special, consequential, or exemplary damages resulting, in whole or in part, from the readers' use of, or reliance on, the information contained in this book. The publisher has no responsibility for the persistence or accuracy of URLs for external or third-party Internet websites referred to in this publication and does not guarantee that any content on such websites is, or will remain, accurate or appropriate.

**Library of Congress Cataloging-in-Publication Data**

Names: Hickey, Joanne V., editor. | Brosnan, Christine A., editor.
Title: Evaluation of health care quality for DNPs / Joanne V. Hickey, PhD,
  RN, FAAN, FCCM Christine A. Brosnan, DrPH, RN, editors.
Other titles: Evaluation of health care quality in advanced practice nursing
Description: Second edition. | New York, NY: Springer Publishing Company,
  LLC, 2017. | Revision of: Evaluation of health care quality in advanced
  practice nursing / [edited by] Joanne V. Hickey, Christine A. Brosnan.
  c2012. | Includes bibliographical references and index.
Identifiers: LCCN 2016015496 | ISBN 9780826131577
Subjects: LCSH: Nursing audit. | Medical care—Evaluation.
Classification: LCC RT85.5 .E82 2017 | DDC 610.73068—dc23 LC record available at
https://lccn.loc.gov/2016015496.

Special discounts on bulk quantities of our books are available to corporations, professional associations, pharmaceutical companies, health care organizations, and other qualifying groups. If you are interested in a custom book, including chapters from more than one of our titles, we can provide that service as well.
**For details, please contact:**
Special Sales Department, Springer Publishing Company, LLC
11 West 42nd Street, 15th Floor, New York, NY 10036-8002
Phone: 877-687-7476 or 212-431-4370; Fax: 212-941-7842
E-mail: sales@springerpub.com

Printed in the United States of America by Gasch Printing.

We dedicate this book to:

- *Pioneers and thought leaders . . . the pioneers in the field of evaluation, including Florence Nightingale, Ernest Codman, Avedis Donabedian, and Lu Ann Aday, who have elevated evaluation into a science-based process; and the thought leaders who are demanding that a solid evaluation must be an integral part in all health care endeavors.*

- *Students and colleagues (current and future) . . . and particularly advanced practice nurses, who have an unprecedented opportunity to impact new models of health care quality that will influence health policy for an ultimate transformation of the health care system.*

- *Our contributing authors . . . recognized experts in their disciplines, these leaders are much sought after for their expertise in practice, education, research, and consultation. Our request to share their knowledge through writing was met with gracious acceptance and production of excellent manuscripts. Their passion for quality health care and especially the role of evaluation in achieving quality health care is the heart and soul of this book.*

- *Our husbands . . . who supported our passion for creating this book even though it took considerable time away from other home and family-based activities. Jim Hickey and Pat Brosnan served as in-house editors and wise listeners and counsels as we grappled with the best ways to organize ideas and find the right words to illuminate the work of evaluation.*

# CONTENTS

# CONTRIBUTORS

**Juliana J. Brixey, PhD, MPH, RN**   Associate Professor of Biomedical Informatics and Nursing, Department of Family Health, University of Texas Health Science Center at Houston, School of Nursing and School of Biomedical Informatics, Houston, Texas

**Christine A. Brosnan, DrPH, RN**   Associate Professor, retired, University of Texas Health Science Center at Houston, School of Nursing, Houston, Texas

**Patrick G. Brosnan, MD**   Professor of Pediatrics, retired, Department of Pediatrics, University of Texas Health Science Center at Houston, School of Medicine, Houston, Texas

**Nancy Manning Crider, DrPH, MS, RN, NEA-BC**   Assistant Professor, Department of Family Health, University of Texas Health Science Center at Houston, School of Nursing, Houston, Texas

**Eileen R. Giardino, PhD, RN, APRN, NP-C, ANP-C**   Associate Professor, Department of Family Health, University of Texas Health Science Center at Houston, School of Nursing, Houston, Texas

**Deanna E. Grimes, DrPH, RN, FAAN**   Professor, Division Head, Community Health Nursing Director, MSN/MPH Program, University of Texas School of Public Health, University of Texas Health Science Center at Houston, School of Nursing, Houston, Texas

**Richard M. Grimes, PhD, MBA**   Adjunct Professor, University of Texas Health Science Center at Houston, Medical School, Houston, Texas

**Joanne V. Hickey, PhD, RN, FAAN, FCCM**   Patricia L. Starck/PARTNERS Professor of Nursing, University of Texas Health Science Center at Houston, School of Nursing, Department of Family Health, Houston, Texas

**Ronda G. Hughes, PhD, MHS, RN, FAAN**   Associate Professor, Marquette University, College of Nursing, Milwaukee, Wisconsin

**Sharon McLane, PhD, MBA, RN-BC**   Retired informatician and nursing services administrator, Lakeland, Florida

**J. Michael Swint, PhD**   Professor of Health Economics, George McMillan Fleming Professor, Director, Division of Management, Policy, and Community Health, University of Texas Health Science Center at Houston, School of Public Health, Houston, Texas

**Elizabeth Ulrich, EdD, RN, FACHE, FAAN**   Professor, Department of Family Health, University of Texas Health Science Center at Houston, School of Nursing, Houston, Texas; Editor, *Nephrology Nursing Journal*

**Nancy F. Weller, DrPh, MPH, MS, RN**   Assistant Professor, Department of Nursing Systems, University of Texas Health Science Center at Houston, School of Nursing, Houston, Texas

# PREFACE

Although evaluation is not a new concept to nurses, it is most often associated with the nursing process designed to evaluate the outcomes of health care for an individual patient. Competency in evaluation of patient outcomes is an expectation of all professional nurses. However, what is new is the expectation of high-level competency for doctor of nursing practice (DNP) graduates in evaluating health care, including health professional groups, patient populations, organizations, systems, programs, health informatics, practice guidelines/protocols, health policy, and other health-related entities, from a systematic and comprehensive evaluation perspective. The bar for evaluation has been raised for DNPs. Along with the higher expectations comes a new opportunity to influence high-level decision making in health care.

Recognizing the need for DNPs to be prepared in evaluation beyond individual patients, we searched for textbooks and other resources that would be helpful for DNPs as they conducted their work. Surprisingly, little was found beyond case studies and general principles, although there were several books on program evaluation. Although helpful, these resources did not address the full scope of evaluation required in DNP advanced practice. With this background, we began planning the second edition of this text, guided with a focus on DNPs with the assistance of input from our colleagues, students, and practicing DNPs. Some of our esteemed colleagues graciously agreed to share their expertise through the written word and have contributed chapters to this book.

The intended audiences are students enrolled in advanced practice nursing programs, especially DNP programs; DNPs and other advanced practice nurses at the master and doctoral levels; nurse administrators; directors of quality improvement; faculty teaching evaluators; and others interested in evaluation of health care from a practice and clinical perspective. In selecting content, it was our intention to provide an overview of the state of the science of evaluation and what is known about evaluation and its application to common practice issues in which DNPs will lead or participate. As we reviewed the literature, it became clear that evaluation as applied to health care is underdeveloped and evolving. It is a nonlinear and messy process; there is no one right way to conduct an evaluation. The form of an evaluation is based on its intended purpose and use. The clear and urgent message is that all aspects of health care entities must be evaluated systematically for effectiveness and to guide and inform decision making. DNPs can contribute to developing the science, processes, and uses of evaluation in health care. Although the consensus is in agreement with a national call to action, the processes and timelines for evaluation are poorly established. The intent of this book is to lay a foundation for DNPs to assume their important role in evaluation.

Section I addresses the underpinnings of evaluation. Chapter 1 elaborates on the role of DNPs in evaluation. Through a brief history, overview, mandate, and other aspects of high-level evaluation, the DNP is brought to the table of evaluation. Chapter 2 addresses the nature of evidence, the basic building block of evaluation, and provides a critical review of characteristics, sources, and quality of evidence as it applies to rigorous evaluation. The conceptual foundations for evaluation are discussed in Chapter 3. A number of frameworks are described to provide the reader with different models for addressing evaluation. Chapter 4 is new to this edition and addresses evaluation and outcomes. The national imperative for cost effectiveness is addressed in Chapter 5 through an overview of economic evaluation.

Evaluation of organizations, systems, and standards for practice is the focus of Section II. Chapter 6 examines the evaluation of organizations and systems, while Chapter 7 addresses health care informatics and patient care technology within health care. With the redesign of health care delivery, organizations and systems are being restructured and redesigned to be more responsive to patient–family-centered care models. An integral part of health care is health informatics, as well as patient care technology integration and evaluation. The current national trend toward electronic medical records is creating challenges because of the far reaching impact on organizations, systems, and individual patients. Chapter 8 is new and addresses program evaluation, a common focus for DNP professional work. Chapter 9, another new chapter, focuses on quality improvement as a developing science and important work in all health care delivery. Chapter 10 discusses the important area of patient care standards, guidelines, and protocols from the perspective of how they are developed, implemented, and evaluated. Finally, Chapter 11 examines the critical role of teams as instrumental in the delivery of high quality and safe care.

Section III addresses the evaluation of population health, health policies, and the future. From a lens of populations, Chapter 12 addresses characteristics, risk factors, determinants, and the evaluation of population health. Chapter 13 discusses the important step of translating outcomes from evaluation into health policy. DNPs are encouraged to seek opportunities for advocacy and leadership in influencing health policy development, implementation, and evaluation. Chapter 14 examines challenges and trends for the future, including the increased demand for comprehensive high-level evaluation by DNPs and related competencies.

The content from the first edition has been updated and chapters added as previously described. Some of the unique features of the book are key definitions of terms, examples to illustrate a point, and case studies to provide exemplars of comprehensive evaluations, including clinical applications and recommended resources for perusal and reference. As educators and practitioners, we were keenly aware of the multiple definitions of key terms. Unless evaluators and users of evaluations are clear about terminology, confusion and misunderstandings abound, leading to underutilized or misdirected evaluations. The examples in the book come from a variety of practice settings and foci to provide the reader with an appreciation of the multiple uses of evaluation. This is also true of the case studies, which provide a more comprehensive overview of the evaluation process, outcomes, and uses. Readers may wish to explore other resources to augment their understanding and broaden their perspective of aspects of evaluation. Selected resources are thus provided for these purposes.

Our sincere hope is that this book will meet our primary aim of providing a useful and helpful resource to assist DNPs in assuming responsibility and accountability for competency in the conduct of high-level evaluation that will inform decision making for those engaged in health care delivery and practice. It speaks loudly to the recommendation outlined in the Institute of Medicine's report *The Future of Nursing: Leading Change, Advancing Health* that nurses should be full partners with other health professionals in redesigning health care.

*Joanne V. Hickey*
*Christine A. Brosnan*

# ACKNOWLEDGMENTS

We are indebted to many wonderful people who helped make this book possible. We especially wish to acknowledge Dr. Janet C. Meininger, PhD, RN, FAAN, Lee and J.D. Jamail Distinguished Professor in the UT Health School of Nursing, for her helpful review of evaluation and outcomes discussed in Chapter 4.

# UNDERPINNINGS OF EVALUATION

# CHAPTER ONE

# EVALUATION AND DNPS: THE MANDATE FOR EVALUATION

Joanne V. Hickey and Christine A. Brosnan

*What we call the beginning is often the end.*
*And to make an end is to make a beginning.*
*The end is where we start from.*
*—T. S. Eliot*

According to Scriven (1991), a noted expert in evaluation, evaluation is the systematic determination of the quality or value of something. The doctor of nursing practice (DNP) role includes multiple facets of evaluation in health care which are discussed in this chapter along with major health care issues driving the mandate for enhanced evaluation.

## EVALUATION AND PROFESSIONAL NURSING PRACTICE

All professional registered nurses evaluate care provided to individual patients as part of the nursing process. The American Nurses Association (ANA, 2010, p. 63) defines *evaluation* as the process of determining the progress toward attainment of expected outcomes including the effectiveness of care. The ANA's definition of evaluation is a *discipline-focused* description of the patient's responses to interventions and specific outcomes, as well as the care provided by the professional nurse. However, this definition is focused primarily on the patient–nurse relationship. The emergence of the DNP degree in the last decade has expanded the scope of evaluation for the graduates of these programs. The following briefly describes the background and expected competencies of DNP graduates in evaluation.

## HEALTH CARE ISSUES INFLUENCING GRADUATE NURSING EDUCATION

Graduate nursing education occurs within the context of societal demands and needs as well as the interprofessional work environment (American Association of Colleges of Nursing [AACN], 2011, p. 5). The seminal report, *To Err Is Human,* published by the Institute of Medicine (IOM, 1999), focused national attention on the state of patient safety, noting that between 44,000 and 98,000 people die each year from medical errors. A current report suggests that these numbers were grossly underestimated. In a review of four studies published between 2006 and 2012 that used the Global Trigger Tool, between 210,000 and 400,000 preventable deaths per year were reported (James, 2013). In 2001, *Crossing the Quality Chasm: A New Health System for the 21st Century* (IOM, 2001) addressed the problematic state of the health care system and leadership for nursing practice. These reports highlight the human errors and financial burden caused by fragmentation and system failures in health care. Among the recommendations resulting from these reports are that health care organizations and groups should promote health care that is safe, effective, patient-centered, timely, efficient, and equitable. These six elements have become a framework for judging quality in health care.

The *Health Professions Education: A Bridge to Quality* report from the IOM (2003) and the National Research Council of the National Academies (2005, p. 74) identified competencies that all health professionals must have for practice in the 21st century. Included are competencies to provide patient-centered care, work in interdisciplinary teams, employ evidence-based practice, utilize quality improvement methodologies, and integrate informatics in providing care. The IOM called for dramatic restructuring of all health professionals' education and, noted that the best prepared senior level nurses should be in key leadership positions and participate in executive decisions. These reports and others were very influential in promoting a call to action by the nursing profession.

In July 2015, the IOM turned over some of its responsibilities to the National Academy of Medicine, which became part of the National Academy of Sciences. We will continue to cite the IOM because, as a unit of the Academies, it retains responsibility for consensus studies (National Academy of Medicine, 2016).

## BACKGROUND FOR THE DEVELOPMENT OF THE DNP DEGREE

The AACN established the AACN Task Force on the Practice Doctorate in Nursing in 2002 to examine trends in practice-focused doctoral education and to make recommendations about the need for and the nature of a practice doctorate in nursing. The group recommended moving forward with the establishment of the degree in nursing, which was approved in 2004. The 2004 DNP position statement calls for a transformational change in the education required for professional nurses who will practice at the most advanced level of nursing. The recommendation underscored that nurses practicing at the highest level should receive doctoral level preparation. The recommendation emerged from multiple factors including the expansion of scientific knowledge required for safe nursing practice and growing concerns regarding the quality of patient care delivery and outcomes within an increasingly complex health care system. An important product of the Task Force was a definition of advanced nursing practice. Advanced nursing practice is broadly defined by AACN (2004) as:

> any form of nursing intervention that influences health care outcomes for individuals or populations, including the direct care of individual patients,

management of care for individuals and populations, administration of nursing and health care organizations, and the development and implementation of health policy. (p. 2)

The recommendation that the nursing profession establish the DNP as its highest practice degree was approved, and the DNP Essentials Task Force was established. The Task Force was charged with developing the curricular expectations to guide and shape DNP education. The work of the Task Force resulted in the approval of the *Essentials of Doctoral Education for Advanced Nursing Practice* in 2006, which is now the foundational framework for all DNP programs.

## DNP ESSENTIALS

The obligation for evaluation is integral to professional nursing practice and health care delivery. *The Essentials of Doctoral Education for Advanced Nursing Practice*, published by the AACN (2006), outlines expectations for DNP graduates including evaluation and expected competencies. The document is organized around specific areas of practice called "Essentials." Each Essential includes a description of the area of practice and related expected competencies. The *DNP Essentials* (Exhibit 1.1) serves as the blueprint for DNP education and its expected outcome competencies. All but DNP Essential VI include the words *evaluate* or *evaluation* in their description. However, it implies that interprofessional teams must be evaluated to determine performance standards.

---

**EXHIBIT 1.1**

**Doctor of Nursing Practice (DNP) Essentials**

A number of *The Essentials of Doctoral Education for Advanced Nursing Practice* (2006), henceforth referred to as *DNP Essentials*, address evaluation. The following lists expectations for evaluation by DNP-prepared nurses as addressed in the specific DNP Essential.

*Essential I: Scientific Underpinnings for Practice*

- Use science-based theories and concepts to *evaluate* outcomes.
- Develop and *evaluate* new practice approaches based on nursing theories and theories from other disciplines.

*Essential II: Organizational and Systems Leadership for Quality Improvement and Systems Thinking*

- *Evaluate* the cost effectiveness of care, and use principles of economics and finance to redesign effective and realistic care delivery strategies.
- Develop and *evaluate* care delivery approaches that meet current and future needs of patient populations based on scientific findings in nursing and other clinical sciences, as well as organizational, political, and economic sciences.
- Develop and/or *evaluate* effective strategies for managing the ethical dilemmas inherent in patient care, the health care organization, and research.
- Design, direct, and *evaluate* quality improvement methodologies to promote safe, timely, effective, efficient, equitable, and patient-centered care.

---

*(continued)*

---

**EXHIBIT 1.1**

**Doctor of Nursing Practice (DNP) Essentials (continued)**

---

*Essential III: Clinical Scholarship and Analytical Methods for Evidence-Based Practice*

- Design and implement processes to *evaluate* outcomes of practice, practice patterns, and systems of care within a practice setting, health care organization, or community against national benchmarks to determine variances in practice outcomes and population trends.
- Design, direct, and *evaluate* quality improvement methodologies to promote safe, timely, effective, efficient, equitable, and patient-centered care.

*Essential IV: Information Systems/Technology and Patient Care Technology for the Improvement and Transformation of Health Care*

- Design, select, and use information systems/technology to *evaluate* programs of care, outcomes of care, and care systems.
- Design, select, use, and *evaluate* programs that *evaluate* and monitor outcomes of care, care systems, and quality improvement including consumer use of health care information systems.
- *Evaluate* consumer health information sources for accuracy, timeliness, and appropriateness.

*Essential V: Health Care Policy for Advocacy in Health Care*

- Develop, *evaluate*, and provide leadership for health care policy that shapes health care financing, regulation, and delivery.

*Essential VII: Clinical Prevention and Population Health for Improving the Nation's Health*

- *Evaluate* care delivery models and/or strategies using concepts related to community, environmental and occupational health, and cultural and socioeconomic dimensions of health.

*Essential VIII: Advanced Nursing Practice*

- Design, implement, and *evaluate* therapeutic interventions based on nursing science and other sciences.

*Source:* AACN (2006).

---

## IMPACT OF DNP GRADUATES

The emergence of the DNP degree in the last decade as the terminal practice degree in nursing has caused nursing leaders to rethink the education of nurses and the optimal utilization of the growing number of DNP graduates. Graduates of DNP programs not only represent the traditional advanced practice nursing roles of nurse practitioner, clinical nurse specialist, nurse anesthetist, and nurse midwife, but also include nurse executives and nurse informaticists.

The scope of evaluation has expanded with the advent of the DNP degree. The DNP graduate moves beyond the single patient/client and discipline-specific focus to also address evaluation at a population, organizational, and systems level. With this perspective, the DNP expands the depth and scope of evaluation to include the theoretical and scientific approaches utilized by behavioral, social, and organizational scientists to evaluate more complex multidisciplinary questions. The theoretical foundation of evaluation is grounded in science and the rigorous methodologies used to conduct systematic evaluations of phenomena of interest to those engaged in the delivery and utilization of health care services. In order for any evaluation to have credibility, it must be based on the best practices of evaluation science and methodologies considered to be valid and reliable by industry standards.

The DNP graduate must engage in evaluation at this level of expertise to be viewed as a credible health professional by health and other professionals, administrators, legislators, insurers, and leaders who have expertise in evaluation science and methodology. The results of evaluations provide information to inform decision makers whose decisions affect the health care system.

The focus of an evaluation can be broad and comprehensive and may include quality indicators, clinical outcomes, and the risks–benefits of health care for a population, an organization, or a system. Table 1.1 provides examples of the scope of evaluation possibilities in which DNPs might engage. The contributions of DNPs are integral to achieving a high-quality health care system for the nation, and thus DNPs must develop the competencies to engage in high-level evaluation processes both independently and as members of an interprofessional team. Only then will the full potential of DNP graduates to achieve high quality and safe outcomes be realized.

It is, therefore, the primary purpose of this book to assist DNP students and graduates to understand evaluation as an integral component of their practice and to master the theoretical and scientific underpinnings of evaluation in the health care system. In *The Future of Nursing: Leading Change, Advancing Health* report (IOM, 2010), Dr. Harvey Fineberg, president of the IOM, said, "achieving a successful healthcare system in the future rests upon the future of nursing." If nurses are going to lead the transformation of health care, as *The Future of Nursing* report suggests, then that transformation must be based on credible evaluation data. DNP graduates have the knowledge and competencies to assume a leadership role in evaluation of the current and future health care delivery system and its components.

**TABLE 1.1  Examples of Evaluations by DNPs**

| Focus | Description | Example |
|---|---|---|
| *Patient/client or groups/populations* | | |
| Groups of patients/ clients | • A group may be defined as a set of patients who have in common a provider(s), disease, or receive care in a particular setting.<br>• Focus of patient-centered evaluation is usually directed at response to care and health outcomes. | • In a diabetic group within a practice, how do the patients/ clients' outcomes compare with national, evidence-based guidelines such as targeted HbA1c, weight, and blood pressure levels? |
| Populations | • A set of persons having a common personal or environmental characteristic.<br>• The common characteristic may be anything that influences health such as age, diagnosis, level of disability, etc. (Maurer & Smith, 2004). | • The outcomes of patients with ischemic stroke in a multifacility health care system as compared with national guidelines.<br>• Patient satisfaction with care and with his or her encounter with the health care system. |

(continued)

**TABLE 1.1   Examples of Evaluations by DNPs (*continued*)**

| Focus | Description | Example |
|---|---|---|
| ***Organization*** | | |
| Models of care | • A conceptual model or diagram that broadly defines the way health services are delivered. | • The effectiveness of models of practice such as interprofessional teams or solo practice in decreasing length of stay. |
| Evidence-based practice | • The integration of best research evidence, expert opinion, and patient values in making decisions about the care of individual patients (IOM, 2003). | • The adherence to evidence-based guidelines for myocardial infarction as patients move from one unit to another along the continuum of care. |
| Quality improvement | • A formal approach to the analysis of performance and systematic efforts for improvement through a planned program within an organization. | • Integration of health care technology and information systems into point of service care for a particular diagnosis or condition. |
| ***Systems*** | | |
| Cost effectiveness analysis (CEA) | • A comparative evaluation of two or more interventions in which costs are calculated in dollars (or the local currency) and end points are calculated in health-related units (Drummond, Sculpher, Torrance, O'Briend, & Stoddart, 2005). | • Assists health professionals in making decisions about equipment purchases or establishing new programs or services. |
| Responsiveness to community needs | • The ability of a person, unit, or organization to address the expressed needs of a community.<br>• The community is usually described as external to the health care organization or system and may be people living in the same area as the facility, a facility such as a housing project, or an ethnic group with ties to the health care facility. | • Develops programs based on expressed needs of the community of interest through a partnership with that community so that the community partners are stakeholders in the program.<br>• Examples of such programs are starting a Saturday clinic for immunization at the local school, a prenatal clinic for high-risk mothers in a community with a high incidence of premature deliveries, or a hypertension clinic at a local industrial plant for workers. |

## THE AFFORDABLE CARE ACT

## Background

The Patient Protection and Affordable Care Act (P.L. 111–148), also known as the Affordable Care Act (ACA), had a profound impact on the quality of health care in the United States and on millions of individuals who can now obtain health insurance coverage. It is also a challenge and an opportunity for DNPs to change the face of health care in America.

For decades, Americans debated the need for universal health care. Supporters of the existing health care system argued that the United States had the best and most innovative care in the world, especially in the treatment of colorectal cancer, breast cancer, acute myocardial infarctions, and ischemic strokes (Oberlander, 2012; Rice et al., 2014). They noted that in countries with national health care systems, patients often had to wait for weeks and even months for needed surgery or medical care. They cited the lack of physicians available to meet the needs of the newly insured and the cost to the taxpayer for individuals who could not afford insurance (Auerbach et al., 2013). In the background was an undercurrent of mistrust in the competence of the federal government to manage a large complicated health care system. A majority of Americans had health insurance and although they knew their premiums frequently increased, they feared a change would be even more disruptive than the status quo (Aaron, 2014).

Proponents of change argued that Americans needed a universal comprehensive health care system that was effective, efficient, and equitable. Although the United States spent more than any other developed country on health care, the outcomes for many individuals and for the population as a whole did not reflect the enormous cost (Muennig & Glied, 2010; Rice et al., 2014). Millions of citizens had little or no access to health care because they did not have the resources to pay for it. Finding health insurance at a reasonable price could be daunting. Those who did have insurance and went on to develop a chronic illness, such as diabetes mellitus, were at risk for losing their policies because insurers increased premiums to the point that some consumers could no longer afford them (Oberlander, 2012; Rice et al., 2014; Stevenson, 2015).

Many children and adolescents were eligible for Medicaid or the Children's Health Insurance Program, and most persons over 65 years of age were eligible for Medicare. However, access to care among adults 18 to 64 varied widely across the country. Radley and Schoen (2012) reported that during 2009 to 2010, 95% of those living in hospital referral regions in Massachusetts were likely to have insurance compared with only 50% in some regions in Texas. Adults without insurance were less likely to have consistent health care.

Several barriers prevented a comprehensive and systematic evaluation of health care quality (Provonost & Lilford, 2011). There was no standardized method that reliably compared the effectiveness of interventions across geographic regions of the country. Data were often retrieved from paper records, making it hard to decipher and lacking in the specific information needed to measure outcomes. Data collected electronically frequently focused on information more related to business performance than to patient outcomes (Lee, 2010; Sadeghi, Barzi, Mikhail, & Shabot, 2013).

The Affordable Care Act (ACA), signed into law by President Barack Obama on March 23, 2010, was an attempt to overhaul the United States' health care system in order to provide quality care to all Americans. Implementation of the two major components of the ACA is being phased in over several years. The first component expanded insurance coverage. The second component addressed the need to improve health care quality (Blumenthal & Collins, 2014; Vincent & Reed, 2014).

## Major Components

### Coverage

It was anticipated that the ACA would eventually increase health care access for about 30 million individuals who, prior to the law, could not afford care (Oberlander, 2012). It was hoped that the ACA could accomplish this through a combination of individual and employer insurance requirements and adjustments to public health programs.

The ACA used a variety of methods to increase the number of Americans eligible for health insurance. In 2010, the law mandated that young adults up to 26 years of age may be covered by their parents' insurance policies. Insurance companies could no longer deny policies to individuals with preexisting conditions such as cancer or diabetes, and the individual cap on lifetime spending was removed (Blumenthal & Collins, 2014). The law also required that insurance companies cover a number of screening and prevention services without a copayment from participants (Jost, 2014; Rice et al., 2014; Vincent & Reed, 2014).

Another method used to increase coverage was the individual mandate that required nearly all U.S. citizens to obtain health insurance policies meeting at least minimal coverage standards. Those not complying risked penalties. Depending on their income, individuals unable to afford premiums received subsidies (Rice et al., 2014; Vincent & Reed, 2014). The ACA encouraged states to set up health insurance exchanges beginning in 2014. These exchanges offered a selection of private insurance policies designed to meet the economic and health needs of individuals and families. Persons in states that chose not to set up the exchanges could purchase insurance from the exchanges provided by the federal government (Rice et al., 2014). Americans with incomes between 100% and 400% of the federal poverty level were declared eligible for federal tax credits that they could use to purchase health coverage through insurance exchanges (Ho & Marks, 2015).

The ACA increased the number of Americans eligible for Medicaid. In 1965, Medicaid was authorized to provide health coverage to the disabled, pregnant women and children who met state poverty guidelines (Rudowitz, Artiga, & Arguello, 2014). Under the ACA, individuals with incomes up to 138% of the federal poverty level are eligible for coverage by state Medicaid programs (Blumenthal & Collins, 2014; Jost, 2014; Rice et al., 2014). In 2015, the federal poverty level for a family of four was $24,250 but state guidelines vary widely (Wachino, 2015). Although the federal government initially covered the entire cost of the expansion, the states' contribution will gradually increase. After 2020, states will assume 10% of the increased Medicaid cost (Blumenthal & Collins, 2014; Jost, 2014).

The ACA also expanded the Children's Health Insurance Program (CHIP). Enacted under the Balanced Budget Act of 1997, CHIP was designed to provide health insurance coverage for low-income children whose families are above Medicaid limits. Both Medicaid and CHIP are administered by the states with the federal government and states sharing the cost. However, there are important differences in the structure of the two programs. CHIP may be organized separately or as a Medicaid expansion. Under CHIP, states have greater autonomy in determining eligibility and in collecting copayments and premiums based on family income. States are also able to offer benefits independent of Medicaid requirements. The federal government provides a higher contribution to the states for CHIP than it does for Medicaid (an estimated average of 70% versus 57%). However, there is a federal cap on expenditures for CHIP that does not apply to Medicaid; and states can stop enrolling altogether if the cap is approached (Rudowitz et al., 2014).

The employer mandate is a critical provision of the ACA which obliges many employers who, in the past, did not offer health insurance to their employees to provide insurance or face penalties. However, full implementation of the mandate was delayed until 2016 (Bagley, 2014).

## Quality of Care

National legislation and public demand have raised the bar on what quality health care means. The second component of the ACA focused on improving the quality of care and reducing unnecessary and ineffective interventions which are estimated to contribute $750 billion annually to health costs in America (Smith, 2012). The ACA authorized changes to Medicare that will result in the development and evaluation of programs to keep high-risk patients out of hospitals, link payment to quality outcomes, and use short-term and long-term indicators to measure outcomes of care. The law also directed the establishment of a national quality improvement strategy with the goal of enhancing the health care of individuals, groups, and populations (Kaiser Family Foundation, 2013).

The ACA encouraged a shift from unbalanced and patchy health care to a comprehensive and accountable system through structural and process changes. The new health care system offers incentives to provide seamless and holistic health care (Ebner, 2010). An important initiative was the formation of Accountable Care Organizations (ACOs) under the Medicare program (McWilliams, Landon, Chernew, & Zaslavsky, 2014). ACOs are composed of groups of health care professionals who collaborate in assessing patient needs, developing and implementing comprehensive and long-term plans of care, and evaluating the effectiveness and efficiency of interventions and programs (Kocher & Sahni, 2010). The goal of these organizations is to increase quality by coordinating primary, secondary, and tertiary health care. Patient care is integrated from acute treatment in a hospital facility to postacute treatment in, for example, a skilled nursing facility, and to in-home support as needed (Ackerly & Grabowski, 2014). The ACO is charged with setting quality goals for patient outcomes and financial goals for treatment that are based on performance standards. Providers and facilities receive financial incentives if the goals are met, and loss of revenue serves as a disincentive if goals are not met (McWilliams et al., 2014).

Bundling is an incentive frequently associated with ACOs that is used to encourage providers to offer coordinated care that is effective and efficient. Bundling refers to a process in which hospitals and providers receive a fixed amount of money for delivering care during an episode that might include acute and postacute hospitalization. Providers may keep the profits if they spend less than anticipated and may lose money if they spend more (Ackerly & Grabowski, 2014; Baicker & Levy, 2013).

Patient-centered medical homes are seen as another way to encourage cooperation among providers (Vincent & Reed, 2014). This model of care places the patient at the center of a designated team of health professionals that may include physicians, nurses, therapists, pharmacists, and other professionals depending on patient needs. The goal is to provide timely access to appropriate care.

The ACA also mandated the creation of systematic and robust methods of evaluation. The nonprofit Patient Centered Outcomes Research Institute (PCORI), established in 2010, was charged with examining the *effectiveness* of health care interventions and programs so that consumers and providers have the evidence needed to select truly useful management plans. In 2012, PCORI began supporting comparative clinical effectiveness research especially for serious medical problems affecting large segments of the population, and for methodological issues that impact research investigations (Newhouse, Barksdale, & Miller, 2015; Patient Centered Outcomes Research Institute, 2014).

## Implementation and Challenges

### Coverage

Americans are enrolling for health insurance coverage through the marketplace at levels close to the predicted numbers. Out of an estimated 14,416,716 individuals who applied and were declared eligible for insurance coverage through the marketplace in April 2015, an estimated 11,688,074 chose a specific plan (Kaiser Family Foundation, 2015a). Among those who enrolled for coverage through the marketplace, 70% rated their plans as good or excellent (Burwell, 2015).

It is anticipated that by 2017 an estimated 37 million Americans will have health coverage as a result of the ACA. This includes adult children under 26 who can now be covered under their parents' insurance and Americans who obtained coverage through Medicaid expansion, CHIP, direct enrollment, state or federal marketplaces, or their employers (Aaron, 2014; Blumenthal & Collins, 2014). Annual growth in health spending per capita has fallen from an estimated 5.6% between 2000 and 2009 to 3.0% between 2010 and 2012. The decrease is noteworthy because during the past 40 years, the growth of health care spending was consistently higher than the growth of the gross domestic product. The reduction in health spending may signal a reversal in that trend (Claxton, 2015).

The Health Insurance Marketplace and Medicaid expansion component of the ACA was implemented in 2014 (Ho & Marks, 2015). Medicaid expansion, a key component of the ACA, was challenged by a number of states that, for a variety of reasons, did not want to participate in the program. In 2012, the Supreme Court ruled that although Medicaid expansion was acceptable, the states could not be forced to participate. Among most states that chose not to expand Medicaid, adults without children are not eligible to receive benefits (Kaiser Family Foundation, 2015b). To lessen the impact of the Supreme Court decision on individual coverage, the federal government permitted states to offer private health insurance with Medicaid dollars (Jost, 2014; Rosenbaum & Sommers, 2013).

The ACA faced a major test in 2015 when the Supreme Court agreed to hear *King v. Burwell* (2015), which questioned the legality of providing tax credit subsidies to persons purchasing health insurance coverage in nonparticipating states through exchanges set up by the federal government. In a major victory, the Supreme Court ruled in June 2015 that it was legal for the government to provide these subsidies (Hall, 2015; Shear, 2015).

### Quality of Care

Researchers have begun to examine the benefit of the quality improvement initiatives to patient well-being. For example, McWilliams et al. (2014) compared 32,334 patients (the ACO group) with 251,593 patients who received care from other providers (the control group). The study surveyed both groups to determine their experiences over a 4-year period that began 3 years prior to ACOs initiation and ended 1 year after. The average age of patients in each group was 74.8 years. While there were no significant differences in the two groups prior to ACO contracts, patients in the ACO group compared with the control group reported significant improvement in prompt access to care and perceived improved communication between their primary physicians and specialists after the ACOs were implemented. These early indications of better patient experiences may indicate greater satisfaction with the coordinated care that ACOs provide.

Sylvia Burwell, U.S. Secretary of Health and Human Services (Burwell, 2015), described the pursuit of quality as an essential and consistent goal of the ACA. She noted that many Medicare services are linking pay to performance, and by 2018, an estimated 90% of fee-for-service payments will be connected to quality performance indicators. There is strong support for the Partnership for Patients, an alliance with hospitals to improve patient safety and reduce readmissions for patients who have been discharged within the prior 30 days. The electronic health record (EHR) is facilitating the collection of valid and reliable data that can be used to measure outcomes and determine the effectiveness of patient care. An estimated 73% of doctors used EHRs in 2013, up from 18% in 2001 (Burwell, 2015).

Perhaps the biggest challenge facing the ACA in the future is its complexity, which resulted from efforts to bridge Americans' deep philosophical divisions concerning government and health care. Many citizens against the ACA were generally satisfied with their health insurance coverage and distrustful of government interference. On the other extreme, some support national health insurance through an extension of Medicare and feel the ACA is insufficient. The law was created as a complicated compromise placed atop an expensive and elaborate health care structure that was never an organized system. There is a general assumption that the ACA will benefit from amendments that will ultimately simplify the program (Aaron, 2014).

## Impact on Nurses

The ACA offers DNPs an opportunity to help change the way health care is practiced in the United States. The patient-centered coordinated team approach that nurses have always provided is congruent with the call for medical homes that serve populations of patients across the life span. Nurse-managed health clinics have provided quality care to individuals and communities for decades.

Currently, these clinics are gaining greater prominence because of the recognition they received from the federal government (Burwell, 2015; Holt, Zabler, & Baisch, 2014). Responding to a physician shortage, DNPs who are advanced practice nurses will increasingly provide efficient and effective primary care to patients. With the skills to assume leadership positions, DNPs are also well situated to take on administrative roles within these new health care models (Auerbach et al., 2013; Vincent & Reed, 2014).

Because of their education, DNPs are uniquely qualified to collaborate with other health professionals in examining the effectiveness of primary care models and in evaluating the quality of care provided to populations (American Association of Colleges of Nursing, 2006). There are many opportunities. For example, 800 million dollars were made available through the Transforming Clinical Practice Initiative to health professionals who assume a greater role in using innovative modes of care (Burwell, 2015). In the coming years, the evaluation of access to care, health care outcomes, cost of care, quality indicators, and standards will become even more important (Vincent & Reed, 2014). Implementing the ACA will be challenging, but it affords the DNP an historic opportunity to assume a major role in advancing the health of all Americans (IOM, 2010).

## TRENDS AND HEALTH CARE PRIORITIES

The current transformation of the U.S. health care system has led to a realignment of the key priorities that are shaping the transformation. There is new consideration of determinants of health, prevention, population health, patient/community engagement, quality and safety, a value-based health care system, and system performance. These trends are briefly addressed in the following text.

## Determinants of Health

Although the current understanding of health and illness is multifactorial, 40 years ago this approach was new and innovative. Engel (1977) published an article in *Science* suggesting that health and illness were actually the products of a complex interaction among biological, psychological, and social factors. This idea was a major shift in thinking and reflected a gradual move in science away from a reductionist world view of a simple cause–effect relationship toward a systems orientation view. Engel proposed the development of a more holistic approach to understanding and treating patients by both researchers and practitioners; his idea was termed the *biopsychosocial model*. This idea was transformational in its conceptualization of health and illness and was a paradigm shift in thinking about the interaction of health and illness. Current concepts around "patient centeredness" evolved from this model (Burke, 2013, p. 137). Patient-centered care is an approach to care that relies on a partnership between the provider and patient based on a comprehensive view of the patient and his or her values and goals. It is based on effective communication, respect, and empathy, with the goals of improving patient care outcomes and reducing unnecessary costs (Rickert, 2012).

Several national and international organizations have embraced a determinant of health framework to address current and future population health initiatives. For example, *Healthy People 2020* describes the determinants of health as the range of personal, social, economic, and environmental factors that influence health status. The interrelationships among these factors determine individual and population health. This framework suggests that interventions that target multiple determinants of health are most likely to be effective. In addition, the determinants of health reach beyond the boundaries of traditional health care and public health sectors; sectors such as education, housing, transportation, agriculture, and environment can be important allies in improving population health (www .healthypeople.gov/2020/about/foundation-health-measures/Determinants-of-Health). *Healthy People 2020* is exploring these questions by:

- Developing objectives that address the relationship between health status and biology, individual behavior, health services, social factors, and policies.
- Emphasizing an ecological approach to disease prevention and health promotion. An ecological approach focuses on both individual-level and population-level determinants of health and interventions (see Figure 1.1).

The World Health Organization (WHO) also addressed determinants of health. According to WHO, the determinants of health include the social and economic environment, the physical environment, and the person's individual characteristics and behavior. They underscore that many factors interact to affect the health of individuals and communities. Whether people are healthy or not is determined by their circumstance and environment (http://www.who.int/hia/evidence/doh/en/#). Income and social status, education, physical environment, social support networks, genetics, and health services are all components of the

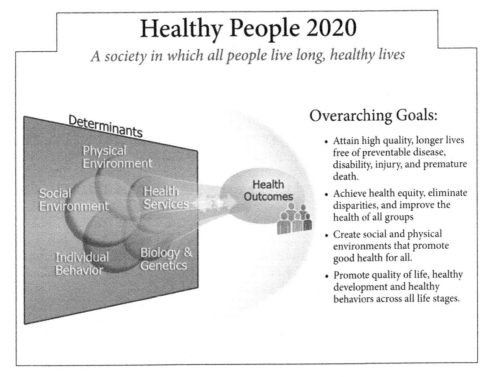

**Figure 1.1** Goals of Healthy People 2020.
*Source:* Healthy People 2020 (2015).

determinants of health. Recognition of the complexity of health and illness is important for anyone wishing to evaluate health-related attributes of populations, communities, organizations, or systems.

## Prevention

To prevent literally means to keep something from happening. In clinical practice, the term *prevention* is used for those interventions that occur before the initial onset of disorder. A common classification of prevention includes the following:

- *Primary prevention*—to promote health prior to the development of disease or injuries through institution of interventions designed to avoid occurrence of disease either through eliminating disease agents or increasing resistance to disease.
- *Secondary prevention*—to detect disease in the early stages prior to the development of symptoms.
- *Tertiary prevention*—to reverse, arrest, or delay progression of disease through rehabilitation or treatment.

Interestingly, the scope of prevention has changed over time from what was once the domain of public health to a current major focus on prevention in clinical practice. Concurrently, clinical care is increasingly moving toward population-based care. As clinical practices become larger, with defined populations, these large practices are dealing with the realities of a transition from individual-based care to population-based care (Starfield, Hyde, Gervas, & Heath, 2008). The redefining of public health and population health has been stimulated by the development of patient-centered medical homes. As a result, the previous boundaries of public health and population-based care are changing.

## Population Health

To understand the concept of population health, we begin with the basic concept of health. The World Health Organization (WHO, 2000) published the most commonly cited definition of health: "Health is the state of well-being and not merely the absence of disease or infirmity." This definition suggests dimensions of health beyond those related to the presence or absence of disease. *Population health* is defined as "the health outcomes of a group of individuals, including the distribution of such outcomes within the group" (Kindig & Stoddart, 2003). The groups may be based on geographic populations such as countries or communities, but can also be other groups such as patients, patients with particular health problems, organizations, or any other defined group (Kindig & Stoddart, 2003). The health outcomes of such groups or institutions are of relevance to policy makers in both the public and private sectors as well as to evaluators.

Confusion often exists between the concepts of population health and public health. The traditional view of public health has been that it provides the critical functions of local and state health departments such as prevention of epidemics, control of environmental hazards, and the encouragement of healthy behaviors. The new and broader definition of the public health system offered by *The Future of the Public's Health in the 21st Century* (IOM, 2002) calls for "building a new generation of intersectoral partnerships that draw on the perspectives and resources of diverse communities and actively engage them in health action" (IOM, 2002) for the population.

## Patient/Community Engagement

The IOM (2001) defines *patient-centered care* as: "Providing care that is respectful of and responsive to individual patient preferences, needs, and values, and ensuring that patient values guide all clinical decisions." This definition implies a goal of advocacy for the patient. Patient-centered care is one of six interrelated elements constituting high-quality health care that the IOM (2001) report identified. The term *patient-centered* means considering patients' cultural traditions, personal preferences, values, family situations, social circumstances, and lifestyles. It supports active involvement of patients and their families in the design of new care models and in decision making about individual options for treatment (IOM, 2001).

The Centers for Disease Control and Prevention (CDC) defines *community engagement* as "the process of working collaboratively with groups of people who are affiliated by geographic proximity, special interests or similar situations with respect to issues affecting their well-being" (CDC, 2011). Community engagement is a fundamental value of public health based on the belief that the public has a right to participate. The public health community believes that by using the "collective intelligence" and working together, problems will be more accurately identified and more effective solutions developed. Through this process, people have an opportunity to understand and to engage collaboratively in the processes of change.

Both patient-centeredness and community engagement are critical elements in the design of a health care system for the 21st century. The question is how to measure and evaluate these lofty concepts. Work is underway to develop effective tools for these purposes.

## Quality and Safety

Within the current national imperatives for health care quality and safety, the mandate for evaluation of care has never been more vital to meeting societal needs. Quality care is safe care, and safe care is a hallmark of quality. Evaluating the quality of care delivered to clients/patients is a necessity that emerges from the social contract between health professionals and society. Implicit in this social contract is the accountability of all health professionals to their clients/patients for the quality and safety of the services they render and for the expectation of care with predictable outcomes (Sidani & Braden, 1998).

Although there is a clear mandate for providing high quality in health care, the ambiguity associated with defining quality is surprising. How the word *quality* is defined depends on the context and perspective of the stakeholder such as the patient, family member, provider, program, insurer, accreditor, evaluator, institution, or system. For example, quality can be *outcomes* in which quality is defined as meeting the overall clinical results reasonably expected by a patient. Quality can be viewed from the lens of *interpersonal engagement* of the patient and provider. Another major definition of quality may be *satisfaction* by the consumer with providers and payers. *Efficiency* of health care delivery is another dimension of quality, while *utilization*, which refers to underuse, overuse, or misuse of medical services, may be a focus of interest. Finally, *safety* is often considered synonymous with quality and may be defined as avoidance of medical error. The IOM (2001) defines *quality in health care* as: "The degree to which health services for individuals and populations increase the likelihood of desired health outcomes and are consistent with current professional knowledge." This definition is from a national population perspective for the goal of health care in the United States. A clear operational definition of quality, reflective of focus, along with the metrics for measurement is important for evaluation.

Quality is often viewed as a surrogate for value, another word with multiple meanings. It will be discussed from the perspective of system level changes in the U.S. health care system.

## Value-Based Health Care System

The U.S. health care system is moving from a volume and fee-for-service model to one using value-based payment (quality/outcomes and cost/price). A core issue in health care is the value of health care delivered. *Value* is defined as patient health outcomes per dollar spent or cost of delivering desired outcomes (Porter, 2010). Porter (2010) described *outcomes* as the health results that matter for a patient's condition over the care cycle, and *costs* as the total expense of care for a patient's condition over the care cycle. A full care cycle includes outpatient, inpatient, rehabilitative care, and support services such as social work and nutrition.

According to Porter (2010), the transition to a value-based health care system will take fundamental changes that include: organizing care into integrated practice units around patients' medical conditions (e.g., organizing primary and preventive care to serve distinct patient groups); measurement of outcomes and related cost for every patient; bundled price reimbursement for a care cycle; integration of care delivery across separate facilities; and building and enabling an information technology platform to support access to and integration of information.

At a time when it is clear that the high cost of U.S. health care is unsustainable, especially in light of poor outcomes, a new way of financing health care concurrent with better outcomes is needed. It is possible, say many noted experts (Berwick, Nolan, & Whittington, 2008; Porter, 2010), to have better outcomes and lower cost simultaneously. Cost is the actual expense of patient care; thus, cost must be measured around the patient and the full cycle of care. That means the cost of all resources used in providing care, including out-of-pocket expenses incurred by the patient, must be included. Tools such as detailed process maps help to graphically display the steps in the process of care provided, and offer an opportunity for a team to analyze and recommend revisions to the process that improve value and decrease costs. This may be done by addressing fragmentation of care, inefficiencies in delivery, and underuse and overuse of services that do not contribute to improved outcomes and value for the patient.

Bundled reimbursement rather than fee-for-service can be based on a *single payment* for a full cycle of care for an acute medical problem, or on *time-based reimbursement* for the overall care of a chronic condition or for primary/preventative care for a defined patient population (Porter, 2010). This approach discourages unnecessary use of resources, and encourages efficient and effective use of resources and processes of care that result in good outcomes at reasonable costs.

From this brief overview of a few key points of value-based health care, it is clear that health informatics will play a major role in the future. Health informatics is much more than the electronic medical record. It is technology that integrates various forms of data that will support data-based decision making and the integration of services across settings and cycles of care. It is evident that systems level evaluation by knowledgeable health professionals such as DNPs is needed to guide the transformation of health care.

## Performance of Health Care Systems

Significant effort has been directed at optimizing the performance of health care systems to achieve improved organizational and patient outcomes. One framework that has been used to guide organization and systems performance is the Triple Aim initiative. The IHI Triple Aim is a framework developed by the Institute of Healthcare Improvement (IHI) that describes an approach to optimizing health system performance. The underlying premise is that new designs must be developed to simultaneously augment the three dimensions that are referred to as the "Triple Aim": improving the patient experience of care (including quality and satisfaction); improving the health of populations; and reducing the per capita cost of health care (Berwick et al., 2008; IHI, 2012).

According to the Commonwealth Fund and other reputable sources, the U.S. health care system is the most expensive in the world, with over 17% of the gross domestic product currently devoted to health care. However, the United States ranks low on many indicators of health compared with other countries that spend far less on health care (Commonwealth Fund, 2015). The idea that spending alone will equal better health care performance and outcomes is just not true. The Triple Aim is focused not only on better experiences for patients and a healthier population, but is also based on the assumption that these goals can be accomplished at less cost than our current financial investment in health care. The Triple Aim provides a broad and comprehensive framework for evaluation of health care. Both the IHI and Commonwealth Fund have indicators that demonstrate achievement of objectives that are helpful for evaluation purposes.

The previous section has addressed major trends and priorities in health care at the level of the current health care delivery system. The next section examines systems for a three level approach at the micro-, meso-, and macrolevels.

## A SYSTEMS PERSPECTIVE: MICROSYSTEMS, MESOSYSTEMS, AND MACROSYSTEMS

The differentiation of microsystem, mesosystem, and macrosystem influences evaluation. A *health care clinical microsystem* refers to the small, functional frontline units that provide most health care to most people (Nelson, Batalden, Godfrey, & Lazar, 2011, p. 3). A *health care clinical microsystem* is a "small group of people including health professionals and patients and their families who work together in a defined setting on a regular basis to create care for discrete subpopulations of patients" (Nelson et al., 2011, p. 2). A *mesosystem* is a larger unit in which midlevel leaders are responsible for large clinical programs, clinical support services, and administrative services (Nelson et al., 2011, p. 7). The mesosystem is composed of linked clinical and supporting microsystems and is part of the embedded systems within larger organizations (Nelson et al., 2011, p. 7). It is the layer between the microsystem and the macrosystem, and is often the interface between the two. A *macrosystem* refers to broader, overarching sectors such as large corporate, state, or national organizations or systems. Its leaders are responsible for organization-wide performance (Nelson et al., 2011).

When planning an evaluation, the DNP must consider its purpose. The evaluation can focus on a single level (e.g., microsystem, mesosystem, or macrosystem), or it can include all three levels. At the micro level, the emphasis is on evaluating the quality of a particular intervention or program, and often involves examining its effectiveness in achieving expected outcomes (Sidani & Braden, 1998). An evaluation addressing a problem at the mesosystem level may focus on a division, such as surgical services, in which multiple units that provide clinical care to surgical patients are included. An example of a possible evaluation focus might be policies and procedures for one particular clinical service. At the macro level, the emphasis shifts to a broad and comprehensive focus in which evaluation of the quality of programs or initiatives at the organization or systems level is addressed. For example, an evaluation might investigate the organizational policies on drug reconciliation as patients transition from one unit to another.

## EVALUATION AND RELATED TERMS AND CONCEPTS

There are many definitions of evaluation, and some are reflective of a specific type of evaluation. As noted previously, evaluation is the systematic determination of the quality or value of something (Scriven, 1993). Other generic and broad definitions of evaluation include: a process that requires judgments to be made about the extent to which something satisfies a criterion or criteria; the systematic application of scientific and statistical procedures for measuring program conceptualization, design, implementation, and utility; making comparisons based on these measurements; and the use of the resulting information to optimize program outcomes (Centers for Disease Control and Prevention [CDC], 1999). Other related terms and concepts often used in evaluation have some commonalities as well as differences with evaluation. They include program evaluation, quality assurance, quality improvement, and outcomes research. Table 1.2 includes terms commonly referred to in evaluation.

**TABLE 1.2  Definitions of Frequently Used Terms in Evaluation of Health Care**

| Term | Definitions |
|---|---|
| Accountability | The obligation to demonstrate and take responsibility for performance in light of agreed expectations. |
| Analysis | An investigation of the component parts of a whole and their relationships in making up the whole; the process of breaking a complex topic or substance into smaller parts to gain a better understanding of it. |

*(continued)*

**TABLE 1.2 Definitions of Frequently Used Terms in Evaluation of Health Care (*continued*)**

| Term | Definitions |
| --- | --- |
| Assessment | The evaluation or estimation of the nature, quality, or ability of someone or something; the act of making a judgment about something; appraisal. |
| Benchmarking | The process of comparing one's processes and performance metrics to industry bests and/or best practices from other industries. |
| Best practices | The most up-to-date patient care interventions, which result in the best patient outcomes and minimal patient risk of complications or death (Robert Wood Johnson Foundation [RWJF], 2013). |
| Criterion | ". . . an attribute of structure, process, or outcome that is used to draw an inference about quality" (Donabedian, 2003, p. 60). |
| Critique | A critical review of an object, process, literature, or performance; a critical examination or estimate of a thing or situation in order to determine its nature and limitations or its conformity to standards or criteria. |
| Effectiveness | • The extent to which planned outcomes, goals, or objectives are achieved as a result of an activity, strategy, intervention, or initiative intended to achieve the desired effect, under ordinary circumstances (not controlled circumstances such as in a laboratory).<br>• A measure of the accuracy or success of a diagnostic or therapeutic technique that occurs in an average clinical environment.<br>• The extent to which a treatment achieves its intended purpose. |
| Efficacy | • The extent to which a specific intervention, procedure, or service produces the desired effect, under ideal conditions (controlled environment, lab circumstances). |
| Efficiency | • The ratio of the output to the inputs of any system.<br>• An efficient system or person is one who achieves higher levels of performance (outcome, output) relative to the inputs (resources, time, money) consumed. |
| Evaluation | • The process of determining progress toward attainment of expected outcomes including the effectiveness of care (ANA, 2010, p. 63).<br>• "The systematic application of scientific and statistical procedures for measuring program conceptualization, design, implementation, and utility; making comparisons based on these measurements; and the use of the resulting information to optimize program outcome" (CDC, 1999). |
| Formative evaluation | • An appraisal occurring during the implementation of an intervention (such as a program or patient interaction) often designed to make course corrections, if necessary. |
| Indicators | • A quantitative or qualitative variable that provides simple and reliable means to measure achievement, monitor performance, or to reflect changes. |
| Monitor | • The process of observing and checking the progress in quality of specific characteristics over a period of time. |

(*continued*)

**TABLE 1.2   Definitions of Frequently Used Terms in Evaluation of Health Care (*continued*)**

| Term | Definitions |
|---|---|
| Quality | • Medical quality is the degree to which health care systems, services, and supplies for individuals and populations increase the likelihood for positive health outcomes and are consistent with current professional knowledge (IOM, 1990). |
| Quality assurance | • Quality assurance is an older term that is still used in the literature, although quality improvement is the term seen more frequently.<br>• A program for the systematic monitoring and evaluation of the various aspects of a project, service, or facility to ensure that standards of quality are being met.<br>• "All actions taken to establish, protect, promote, and improve the quality of health care" (Donabedian, 2003, p. xxiv). |
| Quality of care | • A measure of the ability of the provider, health care facility, or health plan to provide services for individuals and populations that increase the likelihood of desired health outcomes and are consistent with current professional knowledge (RWJF, 2011). |
| Quality improvement | • An assessment process examining a patient's care or an organizational or systems problem for the purpose of improving processes or outcomes.<br>• Initiatives with a goal to improve the processes or outcomes of the care being delivered.<br>• *Clinical quality improvement* is an interdisciplinary process designed to raise the standards for the delivery of preventive, diagnostic, therapeutic, and rehabilitative measures in order to maintain, restore, or improve health outcomes of individuals and populations (IOM, 1990). |
| Standard | • Authoritative statement established and promulgated by credible professional sources through which the quality of a practice, service, or education can be judged (ANA, 2010). |
| Summative evaluation | • An appraisal or evaluation that occurs at the end of an intervention or program. |
| Synthesis | • The composition or combination of parts or elements so as to form a whole; the combining of often diverse conceptions into a coherent whole. |
| Transparency | • "The process of collecting and reporting health care cost, performance, and quality data in a format that can be accessed by the public and is intended to improve the delivery of service and ultimately improve the health care system" (RWJF, 2011).<br>• Ensuring openness in the delivery of services and practices with particular emphasis on valid, reliable, accessible, timely, and meaningful data that are readily available to stakeholders, including the public. |

## A BRIEF HISTORY OF HEALTH CARE EVALUATION

Individuals change history, and the modern history of health care evaluation was particularly influenced by three visionaries: Florence Nightingale, Ernest Codman, and Avedis Donabedian. Each brought to health care the idea that interventions should be more than worthy efforts and should produce real benefit to patients.

It is said that Florence Nightingale not only took care of patients, she also counted them. Born in 1820, she was drawn to mathematics, nursing, and public health, none of which was considered a desirable career for a wealthy woman living in 19th century England (Spiegelhalter, 1999). As a professional nurse, she had the vision to integrate her keen observational skills with her knowledge of statistics and public health to improve patient care. Nightingale is a recognized pioneer in the evaluation of health care outcomes because she clearly understood the goal of care. She said, "In dwelling upon the vital importance of *sound* observation, it must never be lost sight of what observation is for. It is not for the sake of piling up miscellaneous information or curious facts, but for the sake of saving life and increasing health and comfort" (Nightingale, 1859, p. 70).

Born in 1869 into a prominent family, Ernest Codman was a Harvard-educated physician who accepted a position at Massachusetts General Hospital (MGH) soon after completing his medical education. He seemed to be following the path of a successful physician of his day (American College of Surgeons, 2010; Donabedian, 1989). However, he began to wonder if the prevailing medical interventions actually improved patient health and soon focused on the idea of measuring end results, an idea that was not well received by colleagues or hospital administrators. Without the necessary support to proceed, he left MGH and founded his own hospital in which he put his theories about evaluation into practice. In 1924, he described his concept of "end result": "It is that every hospital should track each patient with the object of ascertaining whether the maximum benefit has been obtained and to find out if not, why not" (Codman, 2009, pp. 2766–2770).

Dr. Codman kept cards on each of his patients in his newly established hospital. On each card he wrote how he had treated the patient and whether his treatment helped or hurt. Patients with similar conditions were placed on the same wards, and he suggested that they should be under the care of a physician with specialized knowledge about the condition. Codman collected patient information during a hospital stay and analyzed it to determine the success or failure of medical care. He encouraged his colleagues to do as he did, but very few shared his enthusiasm or curiosity. The more he exhorted members of the medical community to examine the results of their interventions, the more they distanced themselves from him. The preoccupation with using patient outcomes to learn about improving care changed the course of his life and resulted in some success. Codman integrated his ideas into projects and published works, which received acclaim during his lifetime. However, he was never able to convince his colleagues that evaluating medical care would lead to improved patient health (Donabedian, 1989).

A more recent physician leader in quality improvement was Avedis Donabedian, who developed a model for health care evaluation that is still widely used today. Born in 1919, Dr. Donabedian spent a major portion of his professional career teaching and writing at the University of Michigan (Suñol, 2000). He discerned that health care outcomes could not be measured in isolation (Mulley, 1989); rather, they must be viewed within the context of the quality of care (Donabedian, 1980). He understood that methodologies must differ based on the perspective of the evaluation. That is, the methods used to evaluate the quality of care to an individual patient are different from the methods used to evaluate system or population outcomes (Donabedian, 1980).

Donabedian (1980) defined *quality* as "a judgment concerning the process of care, based on the extent to which care contributes to valued outcomes." He outlined indicators of *structure, process*, and *outcome* as pathways to evaluating quality of care. He described *structure* as "the relatively stable characteristics of the providers of care, of the tools and resources they have at their disposal and of the physical and organizational settings in which they work" (Donabedian, 1980). He described *process* as "a set of activities that go on within and between practitioners and patients," and *outcomes* as "a change in a patient's current and future health status that can be attributed to antecedent health care" (Donabedian, 1980).

Each of these leaders had an unswerving dedication to improving patient health. They had the clarity of vision to see the link between practitioner–patient interactions and health status, and the perseverance to continue their work regardless of the obstacles. Their influence continues to impact health care evaluation and quality improvement science today.

## NEGLECT OF EVALUATION

There are a number of reasons why so many resources are spent on developing new interventions and programs while comparatively little time is spent on evaluating them. First, the concept of evaluation itself is threatening. Most practitioners follow care protocols they believe will produce good outcomes if applied competently. Evaluating care can be seen as questioning the practitioners' personal dedication, knowledge, and skills.

Second, the available evidence may be insufficient to determine if a treatment or program is really effective. Practitioners may follow protocols and still have poor outcomes because they are doing the wrong thing right. The standard of care is only as good as the evidence supporting it.

Third, evaluation is difficult and complex (Mulley, 1989). For example, in the intensive care unit, practitioners must adjust for patient demographic characteristics and prior health status before measuring patient outcomes. Age, gender, socioeconomic status, and severity of illness all factor into developing a case mix. Feasibility must also be considered. Tracking indicators of care over a long period of time may be essential to determine if a program benefits a population, but this may be seen as too costly and impractical.

Fourth, technology keeps changing at a rapid pace. Practitioners may find themselves in the middle of evaluating a program when new information or a new technique makes the current program obsolete. Finally, innovation is exciting and often brings funding and acclaim to a system or institution. Evaluation can seem to be a necessary but tedious process that diverts resources and time away from patient care (Bloom, Fischer, & Orme, 1999).

The case of hormone replacement therapy (HRT) is a good example of the complexities inherent in evaluating interventions. Practitioners had long recognized that HRT provided relief to menopausal women from the effects of vasomotor symptoms such as hot flashes and night sweats. During the 1990s, reviews of mainly observational studies suggested that HRT had additional benefits including a decrease in both cardiovascular disease and hip fractures (Barrett-Connor, Grady, & Stefanick, 2005). HRT treatment for all menopausal women became the standard of care and prescriptions soared, climbing to 91 million in 2001 (Hersch, Stefanick, & Stafford, 2004). Practitioners followed protocols and diligently recommended HRT to their patients because they thought it was the right thing to do. Patients learned about the importance of hormone therapy from newspaper articles, the Internet, and TV, and were glad to take a pill that might prevent serious and debilitating disorders. A few practitioners may have observed adverse events among their patients, but probably not enough to be alarming. An individual practitioner lacked the sample size to detect a significant increase in morbidity or mortality.

Findings from the Women's Health Initiative Estrogen Plus Progestin Trial (WHI-EPT) and the Heart and Estrogen/Progestin Replacement Study (HERS) were released (Hulley et al., 1998; Rossouw et al., 2002). These studies were randomized controlled trials and involved thousands of women. Depending upon the kind of hormone medication prescribed, results indicated that women on HRT had an increased risk for certain cardiovascular diseases and cancers. The number of prescriptions plummeted as the standard of care changed, and practitioners became more cautious in their treatment. This case illustrates that an individual practitioner frequently lacks the resources and expertise to evaluate a new and widely accepted intervention that becomes the standard of care. It is also an example of practitioners unwittingly doing the wrong thing right.

## AN OVERVIEW OF HEALTH CARE EVALUATION

Health care evaluation may be described as a systematic and objective determination of the structure, process, and outcomes of care. The goal of evaluation is to provide the practitioner and other stakeholders with the information needed to make decisions about future actions. Evaluation is most often a collaborative process because the very nature of health care is collaborative. The DNP works with other professional practitioners in providing patient care; similarly, the DNP usually collaborates with other health professionals to arrive at a judgment about the benefits, risks, and cost of care.

The DNP is one member of a team comprising professionals who have the skill and knowledge to contribute their expertise to the endeavor. Depending upon the purpose, perspective, depth, and scope of the evaluation, team members may include stakeholders, economists, administrators, politicians, patients, and other health care professionals. The team leader should be selected based on the unique expertise required for the specific project, and team members should be assigned tasks based on their skills. During the planning phase of the project, the team leader should have frequent discussions with the administrator or sponsor requesting the evaluation. This is to ensure that the goal and purpose of the study are clearly understood, that methods are appropriate to the setting, and that adequate financial and structural support will be provided. Suggested stages in the evaluation process are briefly described in the following text and are examined in greater detail in Chapter 8.

The first stage in *planning* is to discuss the *purpose* of the evaluation (see Table 1.3). The purpose may be to examine only one approach (for example, the outcome of care) or to examine all three approaches to quality assurance

---

**TABLE 1.3  Stages in the Evaluation Process**

Plan the evaluation
- Purpose
- Perspective
- Model or framework
- Design and methodology

Implement the study
- Use a management plan
- Carefully follow protocol

Disseminate the results

---

(the structure, process, and outcome of care). An outcome evaluation may focus on the *effectiveness* of an intervention, program, or policy. *Effectiveness* refers to a change in health status resulting from an intervention provided under usual conditions. Effectiveness differs from *efficacy*, a term frequently used to describe a change in health status resulting from an intervention provided under controlled conditions (Brook & Lohr, 1985; Donabedian, 2003).

The team may choose to conduct a formative evaluation, a summative evaluation, or both. *Formative evaluation* refers to an appraisal occurring during the implementation of a program in which the results are used to revise and improve the rest of the program. *Summative evaluation* refers to an appraisal that occurs at the end of a program in which the results are used to determine the benefit and future use of the program. Formative is often used interchangeably with process evaluation, and summative evaluation is used interchangeably with outcome. They do not always mean the same thing (Fitzpatrick, Sanders, & Worthen, 2004).

For example, as part of a hospital program to prevent nosocomial infections, a practitioner conducts a process evaluation to determine if the correct protocol for hand washing is being used by the staff. The evaluation is formative if data about hand washing methods are collected during the course of the evaluation and used to make adjustments to the current hand washing protocol. The evaluation is summative if data about hand washing methods are collected at the end of the evaluation and used to modify future programs to prevent nosocomial infections. In each case the evaluation focused on a process of care (hand washing) but differed on how the results were used.

Second, the team determines the evaluation's *perspective*. Will the evaluation be viewed from the perspective of an individual, an organization (such as a hospital or clinic facility), or a population (of a city, state, or country)? Methods vary depending upon the perspective of the study.

Third, the team selects a compatible *conceptual model or framework*. The conceptual model provides the framework from which evaluation activities flow. Donabedian's model has been briefly described, and will be further discussed in the next chapter along with other evaluation models.

Fourth, the team chooses an appropriate evaluation *design and methods*. There are several alternatives from which to choose, depending upon the type of evaluation and the resources available. One alternative is to identify the criteria of interest, collect and analyze the data, and compare the findings to a standard that may be internally developed or externally required by an accrediting body or government agency. A *criterion* refers to characteristics used to appraise the quality of care. A *standard* refers to a measurable reference point that is used for comparison. Generally, criteria are expressed in relation to standards (Donabedian, 2003; Fitzpatrick et al., 2004). For example, if an evaluation is focused on diabetes mellitus management, an appropriate criterion could be the level of HbA1c. The standard might be "95% of clinic patients will maintain an HbA1c < 7%."

The team decides on the methods they will use to assess and analyze data collected. In this context, *assessment* is part of the methodology and refers to the collection of data. *Monitoring* refers to a periodically scheduled collection of data. Monitoring may be used to detect trends and to determine compliance with guidelines and protocols (Donabedian, 2003; Fitzpatrick et al., 2004). The team selects the type of data to be collected, the most suitable sources of data, the instruments that will be used to collect data, the time period for data collection, and the personnel responsible for gathering the data. In the preceding example, evaluators could, over the course of a year, retrospectively monitor the medical records of a sample of patients with diabetes.

*Analysis* refers to the procedures and calculations used to describe or make inferences about the data collected. Depending upon the perspective and scope of the appraisal, analysis may be as simple as comparing the results of the evaluation to a standard. For example, data obtained from a retrospective medical record review might be analyzed and the mean value for each patient calculated. The percent of patients who maintained an HbA1c < 7% would then be determined and the results compared with the standard of 95%. In contrast, analysis of complex designs may require application of sophisticated statistical techniques.

During *implementation*, the team conducts the evaluation. The number of personnel and resources needed to implement the study depends upon the complexity and scope of the evaluation. A plan that is clear and understood by everyone involved greatly increases the chance of success.

During the *dissemination* stage, the team submits a report that clearly describes the results, including the strengths and weaknesses of the evaluation, conclusions, recommendations, and implications. The report may be submitted to the administrator or sponsor who requested the evaluation, presented at a professional meeting, or prepared for publication.

## A COMPARISON OF RESEARCH AND QUALITY IMPROVEMENT

Evaluation activities that are categorized as research and activities categorized as quality improvement (QI) share similarities. All evaluations are systematic and objective; they flow from a conceptual framework, make comparisons, and draw conclusions. Most use some sort of patient data. Many, but not all, QI studies fit the definition of research.

### Purpose

The purpose of research is to generate new generalizable knowledge that may or may not directly improve current health practice or patient health status (Bloom et al., 1999). Research as described in 45CFR 46.102(d) is "a systematic investigation, including research development, testing and evaluation designed to develop or contribute to generalizable knowledge" (CDC, 1999; U.S. Department of Health & Human Services [USDHHS], 2009). Whether a QI study examines an intervention, a program, or a policy, the primary purpose is frequently to improve current health practice and patient status. The purpose may or may not be to generate new knowledge. Generally, if the evaluator's purpose is to monitor an accepted and standard practice or to improve health status, QI will likely fall into the category of nonresearch regardless of whether or not new knowledge about that specific practice or population is generated (CDC, 1999; Morris & Dracup, 2007; Newhouse, 2007).

## Study Designs and Methods

Types of research designs and methods may overlap in evaluation, but research studies often apply more rigorous designs, including controls and randomization, than are found in QI studies (McNett & Lawry, 2009). Randomized controlled trials and observational designs are frequently used in research, and data are obtained from a wide variety of sources. By comparison, QI studies are more likely than research studies to monitor structure–process–outcome criteria through medical record review. Findings are frequently compared with an internal or external standard rather than to a similar group of patients.

## Patient Risk

Research often involves a greater potential for harm than QI activities because research places patients at more risk than they would be under standard clinical protocols or care (Reinhardt & Ray, 2003). The testing of a new intervention, a rigorous design, and the desire to generalize findings entails risk and data collection that are not encountered for standard health practice (Casarett, Karlawish, & Sugarman, 2000). Prior to beginning a study that involves human subjects, researchers must submit a study proposal to the institutional review board (IRB) of a hospital or agency. The IRB may decide that the study is exempt from review or that a review is needed before approval can be given, allowing investigators to proceed. Many QI studies are exempt from IRB review (USDHHS, 2009).

Distinguishing evaluation activities that need IRB approval and those that do not can be problematic. Experts in the field continue to debate the attributes of each category (Miller & Emanuel, 2008). One way to address this concern is to appoint an administrator to review QI studies before implementation. This administrator would also liaison with IRB members to confirm that correct procedures were being followed (McNett & Lawry, 2009).

## Implementation

In research studies, the principal investigator selects an area of interest, writes a proposal for funding, and assumes leadership of the project (Fitzpatrick et al., 2004). QI activities are frequently made at the request of administrators, policy makers, politicians, or stakeholders. Often, the team member with the greatest expertise in the area assumes leadership. The DNP may be a leader in an evaluation focused on the processes of care or a team member in an evaluation focused on the economic efficiency of care.

## Dissemination

There is an expectation in research that the findings are generalizable and that results will be published in order to expand scientific knowledge (CDC, 1999). Results from QI studies may or may not be generalizable. If they are not, a report is often presented internally to the administrator who requested the study. Decision makers within the organization will then determine whether to implement the recommendations in order to change health care practice, revise an existing program, or modify policy. During the last few years, the need to share findings from rigorously conducted QI studies has grown. The science of QI is also developing rapidly and gaining increased credibility as an effective approach to improving health care delivery. As a consequence, more of these studies are being published. Intent to publish does not by itself make the evaluation subject to IRB review, although some journal editors require at least an IRB letter stating that the study is exempt before acceptance for publication.

## THE RELATIONSHIP OF POLICY AND ADVANCED PRACTICE

A policy refers to a plan of action that incorporates goals and procedures (Guralnik, 1979; "Policy," 2016). Health care policies may be at the organizational, local, or national level. They evolve from scientific evidence, cultural values, and political influence. The development of rules for patient visitation provides an example of the factors impacting policy decisions. Nightingale (1859), among others, discussed the benefits and harms of visitors to patient well-being. There has been a longstanding debate among health care professionals about who should be allowed to visit and the timing of visits in hospital units, particularly in specialty care units. Concerns included increased risk of infection, lack of time available to interact with families, and confidentiality issues (DeLeskey, 2009; Frazier, Frazier, & Warren, 2010; Kamerling, Lawler, Lynch, & Schwartz, 2008; Powazek, Goff, Schyving, & Paulson, 1978).

Changing cultural norms and research affected this debate as patients, along with their families and friends, became vocal about having input into the decision-making process. Policies changed as evidence indicated the benefit to patients when those close to them were allowed to visit (Walls, 2009). At the micro level, individual hospitals developed policies that encouraged family visits. Kamerling et al. (2008) described a quality improvement program designed to increase visitation through an interprofessional collaboration of family and health care professionals, through staff education, and through increased administrative support. Over a 3-year period, visitation increased from 44% to 90%. At the macro level, on April 15, 2010, President Barack Obama (2010) signed a memo directing the Secretary of Health and Human Services "to ensure that hospitals that participate in Medicare or Medicaid respect the rights of patients to designate visitors."

Policy formulation and implementation are iterative processes. DNPs, along with other health care professionals, evaluated the impact of hospital visitation on patient outcomes. The results informed decision makers and were, in part, responsible for a change in local and national policy. In many of the nation's hospitals, therefore, flexible visitation has become the standard of care, and, in many cases, nursing professionals are responsible for quality improvement projects that ensure the standards are implemented.

## THE ROLE OF ETHICS IN EVALUATION

Having a solid ethical framework is basic to the DNP's role of evaluator. Ethical evaluators systematically and objectively analyze *all* of the information, both positive and negative. Threats to conducting an ethical evaluation may be explicit or implicit (Fitzpatrick et al., 2004). Some common threats are reviewed in this section.

First, a DNP may be biased toward an intervention, program, or policy because the DNP developed it. If an evaluator sets out to *prove* that a program works, there is little doubt that the DNP will have a hard time being objective. It may be that the practitioner has put years of labor into implementing a program and believes that it benefits patients. It may be that a great deal of effort has been put into developing these policies, and their implementation has brought professional success. It does not matter. Human nature is such that it is very difficult to be unbiased about one's own accomplishments.

Second, a DNP may find it hard to be objective because there is administrative support for the program the practitioner has been asked to evaluate. For example, suppose a supervisor has developed a lucrative follow-up program for elderly patients hospitalized with pneumonia. The goal of the program is to decrease future hospitalizations by providing periodic home care. After systematically and objectively examining the program, the DNP realizes that the frequency of hospitalizations among these patients has not decreased. In a survey, patients say they are generally satisfied receiving care at home, but find the visits to be inconveniently timed and disruptive to the family routine. Some patients report they even enjoy leaving the home on occasion and do not mind keeping clinic appointments. An evaluator might be concerned about reporting these negative results to the administrator.

A third threat relates to structural deficiencies. In the home care example, the practitioner realizes that while administration is touting the benefits of the program, the resources that the hospital provides are inadequate. In order to keep expenses down, the hospital has hired nurses who are not sufficiently qualified and has failed to provide adequate administrative support. Reporting these findings to administration will be a challenge.

There are approaches a practitioner can use when confronted with an explicit or implicit conflict of interest. The DNP can discuss the goals and processes of evaluation with an administrator before beginning the study. While working with a team does not always lead to objectivity, a team that includes a member who does not report to the same hospital administrators may also increase the chances of conducting an objective evaluation (Fitzpatrick et al., 2004).

The American Evaluation Association (2004) developed five principles to facilitate ethical conduct for professionals involved in any type of evaluation regardless of the discipline. The first principle focuses on the importance of an objective and systematic examination. The second principle states that the evaluator must be competent. For example, a DNP must possess not only advanced nursing skills, but also have the appropriate knowledge and skills needed to conduct an evaluation. Third, evaluators should be honest in planning, implementing, and reporting study results. Fourth, evaluators must respect all individuals and groups including those requesting the evaluation, team members, and patients. Fifth, evaluators must be aware that their responsibility extends to the general public. In conducting the evaluation and reporting the results, they should consider its impact on the cultural and political environment of society.

## SUMMARY

This chapter acquainted DNPs with the basic concepts and definitions related to evaluation, and highlighted the expectation to evaluate within the Essentials documents for doctor of nursing practice education. The message is clear that DNPs are responsible and accountable to conduct evaluations. The fundamental purpose of evaluation is to provide information for decision making. Within the backdrop of a developing body of knowledge about evaluation, the DNP must understand what is possible methodologically and what outcomes one can expect.

There are many ways to conduct evaluations, and professional evaluators tend to agree that there is no "one best way" to do any evaluation. Instead, good evaluation requires carefully thinking through the questions that need to be answered, what is being evaluated, and the way in which the information generated will be used. Subsequent chapters will lead the DNP down a path to an increased understanding of evaluations in specific areas of interest in health care.

## REFERENCES

Aaron, H. J. (2014). Here to stay—Beyond the rough launch of the ACA. *New England Journal of Medicine, 370*(24), 2257–2259.

Ackerly, D. C., & Grabowski, D. C. (2014). Post-acute care reform—Beyond the ACA. *New England Journal of Medicine, 370*(8), 689–691.

American Association of Colleges of Nursing. (2004). *AACN position statement on the practice doctorate in nursing.* Washington, DC: Author.

American Association of Colleges of Nursing. (2006). *The essentials of doctoral education for advanced nursing practice.* Washington, DC: Author.

American Association of Colleges of Nursing. (2011). *The essentials of master's education in nursing.* Washington, DC: Author.

American College of Surgeons. (2010). *History and archives of the American College of Surgeons: Ernest A. Codman.* Retrieved from https://www.facs.org/about%20acs/archives/pasthighlights/codmanhighlight

American Evaluation Association. (2004). *Guiding principles for evaluators.* Fairhaven, MA: American Evaluation Association. Retrieved from http://www.eval.org/p/cm/ld/fid=51

American Nurses Association. (2010). *Nursing: Scope and standards of practice* (2nd ed.). Washington, DC: Author.

Auerbach, D. I., Chen, P. G., Friedberg, M. W., Reid, R., Lau, C., Buerhaus, P. I., & Mehrotra, A. (2013). Nurse-managed health centers and patient-centered medical homes could mitigate expected primary care physician shortage. *Health Affairs, 32*(11), 1933–1941.

Bagley, N. (2014). The legality of delaying key elements of the ACA. *New England Journal of Medicine, 370*(21), 1967–1969.

Baicker, K., & Levy, H. (2013). Coordination versus competition in health care reform. *New England Journal of Medicine, 369*(9), 789–791.

Barrett-Connor, E., Grady, D., & Stefanick, M. L. (2005). The rise and fall of menopausal hormone therapy. *Annual Review of Public Health*, *26*, 115–140. doi:101146/annurev.publhealth.26.021304.144637.

Berwick, D. M., Nolan, T. W., & Whittington, J. (2008). The triple aim: Care, health, and cost. *Health Affairs*, *27*(3), 759–769.

Bloom, M., Fischer, J., & Orme, J. G. (1999). *Evaluating practice-guidelines for the accountable professional*. Needham Heights, MA: Allyn & Bacon.

Blumenthal, D., & Collins, S. R. (2014). Health care coverage under the Affordable Care Act—A progress report. *New England Journal of Medicine*, *371*(3), 275–281.

Brook, R. H., & Lohr, K. N. (1985). Efficacy, effectiveness, variations, and quality. Boundary crossing research. *Medical Care*, *23*(5), 710–722.

Burke, J. (2013). *Health analytics: Gaining the insights to transform health care*. Hoboken, NJ: John Wiley and Sons.

Burwell, S. M. (2015). Setting value-based payment goals—HHS efforts to improve U.S. health care. *New England Journal of Medicine*, *372*(10), 897–899.

Casarett, D., Karlawish, J. H. T., & Sugarman, J. (2000). Determining when quality improvement initiatives should be considered research: Proposed criteria and potential implications. *JAMA*, *282*(17), 2275–2280.

Centers for Disease Control and Prevention. (2010). *Defining public health research and public health non-research*. Retrieved from http://www.cdc.gov/od/science/integrity/docs/defining-public-health-research-non-research-1999.pdf

Centers for Disease Control and Prevention. (2011). *Principles of community engagement* (2nd ed.). Retrieved from http://www.atsdr.cdc.gov/communityengagement/pdf/PCE_Report_508_FINAL.pdf

Claxton, G. (2015). *Health care costs 101*. Retrieved from https://kaiserfamilyfoundation.files.wordpress.com/2015/04/2-garyclaxtonpresentation_pi.pdf

Codman, E. A. (2009). The registry of bone sarcomas as an example of the end-result idea in hospital organization. *Clinical Orthopaedics and Related Research*, *467*, 2766–2770. doi:10.1007/s11999-009-1048-7.

Commonwealth Fund. (2015). *Mirror, mirror on the wall: 2014 update: How the U.S. health care system compares internationally*. Retrieved from http://www.commonwealthfund.org/publications/fund-reports/2014/jun/mirror-mirror

DeLeskey, K. (2009). Family visitation in the PACU: The current state of practice in the United States. *Journal of PeriAnesthesia Nursing*, *24*(2), 81–85.

Donabedian, A. (1980). *Explorations in quality assessment and monitoring. Vol. 1. The definition of quality and approaches to its assessment*. Ann Arbor, MI: Health Administration Press.

Donabedian, A. (1989). The end results of health care: Ernest Codman's contribution to quality assessment and beyond. *Milbank Quarterly*, *67*(2), 233–261.

Donabedian, A. (2003). *An introduction to quality assurance in health care*. New York, NY: Oxford University Press.

Drummond, M. F., Sculpher, M. J., Torrance. G. W., O'Briend, B. J., & Stoddart, G. L. (2005). *Methods for the economic evaluation of health care programmes*. Oxford, UK: Oxford University Press.

Ebner, A. L. (2010). What nurses need to know about health care reform. *Nursing Economics*, *28*(3), 191–194.

Engel, G. (1977). The need for a new medical model: A challenge for biomedicine. *Science*, *196*, 129–136.

Fitzpatrick, J. L., Sanders, J. R., & Worthen, B. R. (2004). *Program evaluation. Alternative approaches and practical guidelines.* Boston, MA: Pearson Education.

Frazier, A., Frazier, H., & Warren, N. A. (2010). A discussion of family-centered care within the pediatric intensive care unit. *Critical Care Nursing Quarterly, 33*(1), 82–86.

Guralnik, D. B. (1979). *Webster's new world dictionary of the American language.* New York, NY: Simon and Schuster.

Hall, M. A. (2015). King v. Burwell—ACA Armageddon averted. *New England Journal of Medicine, 373*(6), 497–499.

Healthy People 2020. (2015). *Determinants of health.* Retrieved from http://www.healthypeople .gov/2020/about/foundation-health-measures/Determinants-of-Health

Hersch, A. L., Stefanick, M. L., & Stafford, R. S. (2004). National use of postmenopausal hormone therapy. *JAMA, 291*(1), 47–53.

Ho, V., & Marks, E. (2015, April). *Effects of the Affordable Care Act on health insurance coverage in Texas as of March 2015 (Issue Brief No 11).* Retrieved from http://bakerinstitute.org/files/9129/

Holt, J., Zabler, B., & Baisch, M. J. (2014). Evidence-based characteristics of nurse-managed health centers for quality and outcomes. *Nursing Outlook, 62,* 428–439.

Hulley, S., Grady, D., Bush, E., Furberg, C., Herrington, D., Riggs, B., & Vittinghoff, E. (1998). Randomized trial of estrogen plus progestin for secondary prevention of coronary heart disease in postmenopausal women. Heart and Estrogen/Progestin Replacement Study (HERS) Research Group. *JAMA, 280*(7), 605–613.

Institute of Healthcare Improvement. (2012). *IHI Triple Aim initiative.* Retrieved from http://www.ihi .org/Engage/Initiatives/TripleAim/pages/default.aspx

Institute of Medicine. (1990). *Medicare: A strategy for quality assurance* (Vol. 1). Washington, DC: National Academies Press.

Institute of Medicine. (1999). *To err is human: Building a safer health system.* Washington, DC: National Academies Press.

Institute of Medicine. (2001). *Crossing the quality chasm: A new health system for the 21st century.* Washington, DC: National Academies Press.

Institute of Medicine. (2002). *The future of the public's health in the 21st century.* Washington, DC: National Academies Press.

Institute of Medicine. (2003). *Health professions education: A bridge to quality.* Washington, DC: National Academies Press.

Institute of Medicine. (2010). *The future of nursing: Leading change, advancing health.* Washington, DC: National Academies Press.

James, J. T. (2013). A new, evidence-based estimate of patient harms associated with hospital care. *Journal of Patient Safety, 9*(3), 122–128.

Jost, R. (2014). How the expansion of healthcare coverage is playing out. *Healthcare Financial Management, 68*(9), 138–140.

Kaiser Family Foundation. (2013). *Focus on health reform.* Retrieved from http://kff.org/health-reform/fact-sheet/summary-of-the-affordable-care-act/

Kaiser Family Foundation. (2015a). *Monthly marketplace statistics.* Retrieved from http://kff.org/ health-reform/state-indicator/state-marketplace-statistics/

Kaiser Family Foundation. (2015b). *Where are states today? Medicaid and eligibility levels for adults, children, and pregnant women.* Retrieved from http://kff.org/medicaid/fact-sheet/where-are-states-today-medicaid-and-chip/

Kamerling, S. N., Lawler, L. C., Lynch, M., & Schwartz, A. J. (2008). Family-centered care in the pediatric post anesthesia care unit: Changing practice to promote parental visitation. *Journal of PeriAnesthesia Nursing, 23*(1), 5–16.

Kindig, D., & Stoddart, G. (2003). What is population health? *American Journal of Public Health, 93*(3), 380–383.

King v. Burwell. 759 F.3d 358. (2015). Retrieved from http://www.supremecourt.gov/opinions/14pdf/14-114_qol1.pdf

Kocher, R., & Sahni, N. R. (2010). Physicians versus hospitals as leaders of accountable care organizations. *New England Journal of Medicine, 363*(27), 2579–2582.

Lee, T. H. (2010). Putting the value framework to work. *New England Journal of Medicine, 363*(26), 2481–2483.

Maurer, F., & Smith, C. M. (2004). *Community/public health nursing.* St Louis, MO: Elsevier.

McNett, M., & Lawry, K. (2009). Research and quality improvement activities: When is institutional review board review needed? *Journal of Neuroscience Nursing, 41*(6), 344–347.

McWilliams, J. M., Landon, B. E., Chernew, M. E., & Zaslavsky, A. M. (2014). Changes in patients' experiences in Medicare accountable care organizations. *New England Journal of Nursing, 371*(18), 1715–1724.

Miller, F. G., & Emanuel, E. J. (2008). Quality-improvement research and informed consent. *New England Journal of Medicine, 358*(8), 765–767.

Morris, P. A., & Dracup, K. (2007). Quality improvement or research? The ethics of hospital project oversight. *American Journal of Critical Care, 16,* 424–426.

Muennig, P. A., & Glied, S. A. (2010). What changes in survival rates tell us about US Health Care. *Health Affairs, 29*(11), 1–9.

Mulley, A. G. (1989). E. A. Codman and the end results idea: A commentary. *Milbank Quarterly, 67*(2), 257–261.

National Academy of Medicine. (2016). *Welcome to NAM.edu.* Retrieved from http://nam.edu

National Research Council of the National Academies. (2005). *Advancing the nation's health needs: NIH research training programs.* Washington, DC: National Academies Press.

Nelson, E. C., Batalden, P. B., Godfrey, M. M., & Lazar, J. D (Eds.). (2011). *Value by design: Developing clinical microsystems to achieve organizational excellence.* San Francisco, CA: Jossey-Bass.

Newhouse, R. P. (2007). Diffusing confusion among evidence-based practice, quality improvement, and research. *JONA, 37*(10), 432–435.

Newhouse, R., Barksdale, D. J., & Miller, J. A. (2015). The Patient-Centered Outcomes Research Institute. *Nursing Research, 64*(1), 72–77.

Nightingale, F. (1859). *Notes on nursing.* USA: ReadaClassic.com. (Reproduced in 2010.)

Obama, B. (2010, April 15). *Presidential memorandum—Hospital visitation.* Washington, DC: The White House. Retrieved from http://www.whitehouse.gov/the-press-office/presidential-memorandum-hospital-visitation

Oberlander, J. (2012). Unfinished journey—A century of health care reform in the United States. *New England Journal of Medicine, 367*(7), 585–590.

Patient-Centered Outcomes Research Institute. (2014). *About us. Why PCORI was created.* Retrieved from http://.pcori.org/about-us/

Policy. (2016). *Merriam-Webster dictionary online.* Retrieved from www.merriam-webster.com/dictionary/policy

Porter, M. E. (2010). What is value in health care? *New England Journal of Medicine, 363,* 2477–2481.

Powazek, M., Goff, J. R., Schyving, J., & Paulson, M. A. (1978). Emotional reactions of children to isolation in a cancer hospital. *Journal of Pediatrics, 92*(5), 834–837.

Provonost, P. J., & Lilford, R. (2011). A road map for improving the performance of performance measures. *Health Affairs, 30*(4), 569–573.

Radley, D. C., & Schoen, C. (2012). Geographic variation in access to care—The relationship with quality. *New England Journal of Medicine, 367*(1), 3–6.

Reinhardt, A. C., & Ray, L. N. (2003). Differentiating quality improvement from research. *Applied Nursing Research, 16*(1), 2–8.

Rice, T., Unruh, L. Y., Rosenau, P., Barnes, A. J., Saltman, R., & vanGnneken, E. (2014). Challenges facing the United States of America in implementing universal coverage. *Bulletin World Health Organization, 92,* 894–902.

Rickert, J. (2012). *Patient-centered care: What it means and how to get there.* Retrieved from http://healthaffairs.org/blog/2012/01/24/patient-centered-care-what-it-means-and-how-to-get-there/

Robert Wood Johnson Foundation. (2013). *Quality/equality glosssary.* Retrieved from http://www.rwjf.org/en/library/research/2013/04/quality-equality-glossary.html

Rosenbaum, S., & Sommers, B. D. (2013). Using Medicaid to buy private health insurance—The great new experiment? *New England Journal of Medicine, 369*(1), 7–9.

Rossouw, J. E., Anderson, G. L., Prentice, R. L., LaCroix, A. Z., Kooperberg, C., Stefanick, M. L., . . . Ockene, J. (2002). Risks and benefits of estrogen plus progestin in healthy postmenopausal women: Principal results from the women's health initiative randomized controlled trial. *JAMA, 288*(3), 321–333.

Rudowitz, R., Artiga, S., & Arguello, R. (2014, March). *Children's health coverage: Medicaid, CHIP and the ACA (Issue Brief).* Retrieved from http://kff.org/health-reform/issue-brief/childrens-health-coverage-medicaid-chip-and-the-aca/

Sadeghi, S., Barzi, A., Mikhail, O., & Shabot, M. M. (2013). *Integrating quality and strategy.* Burlington, MA: Jones & Bartlett Learning.

Scriven., M. (1991). *Evaluation thesaurus* (4th ed.). Newbury Park, CA: Sage, pp. 1, 4–5.

Scriven, M. (1993). *Hard-won lessons in program evaluation* (New Directions for Program Evaluation, No. 58). San Francisco, CA: Jossey-Bass.

Shear, M. D. (2015, June 25). Obama gains vindication and secures legacy with health care ruling. *New York Times.* Retrieved from http://www.nytimes.com/2015/06/26/us/politics/obama-supreme-court-aca-ruling-health-care.html?_r=0

Sidani, S., & Braden, C. J. (1998). *Evaluating nursing interventions: A theory-driven approach.* Thousand Oaks, CA: Sage Publications.

Smith, M. D. (2012). Best care at lower cost. The path to continuously learning health care in America. *Report of the Institute of Medicine.* Retrieved from http://www.iom.edu/Reports/2012/Best-Care-at-Lower-Cost-the-Path-to-Continuously-Learning-health-Care-in-America/Report-Brief.aspx

Spiegelhalter, D. J. (1999). Surgical audit: Statistical lessons from Nightingale and Codman. *Journal of the Royal Statistical Society, A, 162*(Pt. 1), 45–58.

Starfield, B., Hyde, J., Gervas, J., & Heath, I. (2008). The concept of prevention: A good idea gone astray? *Journal of Epidemiology Community Health, 62,* 580–583.

Stevenson, M. B. (2015). The intersection of public health and the Affordable Care Act: The changing role of public health. *Journal of Public Health Management and Practice, 21*(1), 80–82.

Suñol, R. (2000). Avedis Donabedian. *International Journal for Quality in Health Care, 12*(6), 451–454.

U.S. Department of Health & Human Services. (2009, January 5). *Office for Human Research Protections (OHRP). OHRP quality improvement frequently asked questions.* Retrieved from http://archive.hhs.gov/ohrp/qualityfaq.html

Vincent, D., & Reed, P. G. (2014). Affordable Care Act: Overview and implications for advancing nursing. *Nursing Science Quarterly, 27*(3), 254–259.

Wachino, V. (2015, January). *2015 federal poverty level standards (CMCS Information Bulletin).* Retrieved from https://www.medicaid.gov/federal-policy-guidance/downloads/cib-01-29-2015.pdf

Walls, M. (2009). Staff attitudes and beliefs regarding family visitation after implementation of a formal visitation policy in the PACU. *Journal of PeriAnesthesia Nursing, 24*(4), 229–232.

World Health Organization. (2000). WHO definition of health. Retrieved from http://www.who.int/about/definition/en/print.html

# CHAPTER TWO

# THE NATURE OF EVIDENCE AS A BASIS FOR EVALUATION

Joanne V. Hickey

*It ain't so much what you don't know that gets you into trouble, it's what you know for sure that just ain't so.*
—Mark Twain

Evaluation is based on collecting, analyzing, organizing, and critically reviewing evidence to make a judgment or decision about value. This chapter defines evidence from a generic perspective and discusses the sources of evidence in its many forms. It describes how evidence is organized and ranked, addresses evidence integrity, and examines how evidence is used and interpreted for evaluation. This information provides a basis for exploring how doctor of nursing practice (DNP) graduates acquire and use evidence for evaluation. This chapter is organized around a broad discussion of evidence and then focuses on the use of evidence by DNPs. Evidence, within the context of evidence-based practice in patient-centered clinical practice, is discussed in Chapter 10.

## BASIC CONCEPTS FROM EPISTEMOLOGY AND LOGIC

The root of the word *epistemology* comes from the Greek *epistēmē* (knowledge) and *logos* (study of). Epistemology is the branch of philosophy that investigates the origin, nature, methods, validity, and limitations of human knowledge. It also addresses related notions of truth, belief, and justification. Logic is the branch of philosophy that focuses on valid reasoning, and dates back to Aristotle.

A number of terms from logic are threaded into the discussion about evidence such as proposition, inference, premise, induction, deduction, abduction, and conclusion. A *proposition* is a statement or declarative sentence that may be true or false. *Inference* is a logical or conceptual process of deriving a statement from one or more other statements (Angeles, 1992, p. 145). For example, because large organizations are complex and the organization under review is large, it is reasonable to assume that the organization under review is complex. A *premise* is defined as a statement that is true or that is believed to be true; it is any statement that serves as the basis for an argument or inference (Angeles, 1992, p. 240).

A premise is composed of propositions; when taken together, they form a conclusion. For example, intensive care units within the same facility often have different lengths of stay. Yet these units are part of the same organization. One can surmise that patient acuity and practice patterns must play some part in variation of length of stay.

*Inductive reasoning* is the process of reasoning from a part to a whole, from a particular instant of something to a general statement, or from particular to universal (Angeles, 1992, p. 144). For example, if using a particular patient-turning device on one unit of a facility is effective in reducing pressure ulcers, then using the device on all other units in the facility should also be effective in reducing pressure ulcers throughout the facility. This statement may or may not be true for a variety of reasons such as variations in patient populations and acuity. *Deductive reasoning* is the process of reasoning from a general truth to a particular instant of a truth, from the general to the particular, or from the universal to the particular. For example, all men have two feet and two arms; John is a man; therefore, John has two feet and two arms. *Deduction* is a form of logical inference that proceeds from observation to a hypothesis that accounts for the reliable data (observation) and seeks to explain relevant evidence (Magnani, 2001). A *conclusion* is a statement that has been inferred from other statements. It is the logical consequence or implication of the premises of an argument (Angeles, 1992, p. 51).

## EVIDENCE

The origin of the word *evidence* comes from Middle English via Latin (*evidentia*—obvious to the eye or mind) and Old French (*evidence*—appearance from which inferences may be drawn). Evidence, as a broad and generic concept, is information presented in support of an assertion. This support may be strong or weak. The strongest type of evidence is that which provides direct proof of the truth of an assertion. At the other extreme is evidence that is merely consistent with an assertion, but does not rule out other, contradictory assertions. Further discussion of the strength of evidence is found later in this chapter.

The word *evidence* can be a noun or a verb. For purposes of this discussion, only evidence as a noun is addressed. According to Webster's Dictionary, evidence is "a condition of being evident; something that makes another thing evident; and something that tends to prove or to provide grounds for belief." Evidence is that which is accepted as conclusive (e.g., clear, obvious, acceptable, confirmed) support of a statement (Angeles, 1992, p. 97). To have evidence is to have some conceptual warrant for belief or action (Goodman, 2003, p. 2). Evidence has also been defined as:

- Facts or physical signs that help to prove something.
- The basis of belief; the substantiation or confirmation that is needed in order to believe that something is true (Pearson, Wiechula, Court, & Lockwood, 2005).
- The available facts and circumstances supporting or refuting a belief or proposition or indicating whether something is true or valid (Pearsall & Trumble, 1995).

## Evidence and Perspectives

Evidence can be viewed from a legal, empirical, or evidence-based perspective.

### Legal Perspective of Evidence

From a legal perspective, evidence is something presented in a legal proceeding; it is a statement of a witness. Further investigation of a variety of websites uncovers the following definitions: evidence is that which tends to prove or disprove something; grounds for belief; proof; something that makes plain or clear; and an indication or sign. Evidence is data presented to a court or jury in proof of the facts about something; it may include the testimony of witnesses, records, documents, or objects. Synonyms often used for evidence are information, knowledge, exhibit, testimony, and proof.

Review of subcategories of evidence from law offers insight into concepts useful for this discussion. For example, *clear and convincing evidence* is evidence demonstrating a high probability of truth of the factual matter under review. This definition suggests the need for high-level, reliable, and valid information, as well as some system of ranking of evidence. *Corroborating evidence* is evidence that is independent of and different from other evidence, but supplements and strengthens evidence already presented as proof. In evaluation, different kinds of information are collected from a variety of sources to provide a comprehensive view to assist the evaluator in making judgments. Evidence from a variety of sources provide for triangulation of information. *Cumulative evidence* adds additional evidence that is similar to evidence already presented as proof of the same factual matter. Collecting information over time elucidates trends and consistencies or inconsistencies important in evaluation. *Demonstrative evidence* is evidence in the form of objects (e.g., diagrams, models, tables) used to illustrate and clarify the factual matter presented. The evaluator is often responsible for synthesizing large amounts of information and presenting it in a concise, organized, and understandable form for other decision makers. Crunching of information through diagrams, dashboards, models, and other presentation strategies is commonly used. *Relevant evidence* is evidence that tends to prove or disprove an issue of fact that is of consequence to the work or project.

### Empirical Perspective of Evidence

When health professionals talk about evidence, they are generally thinking about empirical evidence. Empirical evidence (also known as scientific evidence) is information ascertained by *observation* and *experimentation* that serves to support, refute, or modify a scientific hypothesis or theory when collected and interpreted in accordance with the scientific method. *Merriam-Webster's Dictionary* defines the *scientific method* as "principles and procedures for the systematic pursuit of knowledge involving the recognition and formulation of a problem, the collection of data through *observation* and *experimentation*, and the formulation and testing of hypotheses" ("Scientific method," 2016a). The *Oxford English Dictionary* defines the *scientific method* as "a method or procedure that has characterized natural science since the 17th century, consisting of systematic observation, measurement, experimentation, formulation, testing, and modification of hypotheses" ("Scientific method," 2016b). Through the investigation of phenomenon, new knowledge, or connection or integration of previously known knowledge, occurs to further expand knowledge in a given area. Data integrity addresses the quality, measurement, and accuracy of data and is contingent on how well the data are collected and managed. Integrity is also related to empirical measurement of data, which may take the form of quantitative or qualitative research methodologies.

*Quantitative research* is the systematic empirical investigation of observable phenomena via statistical, mathematical, or computational techniques (Given, 2008). The focus of quantitative research is to develop and employ mathematical models, theories, and/or hypotheses pertinent to the phenomena. The measurement process is central to quantitative research because it provides the fundamental connection between empirical observation and mathematical expression of quantitative relationships (Given, 2008). Quantitative data are any data that are in numerical form, such as statistics or percentages. This means that the quantitative investigator asks a specific, narrow question and collects a sample of numerical data from observable phenomena or from study participants. The investigator analyzes the data using statistics. The findings may be generalized to some larger population. Quantitative methodologies have been the dominant approach to empirical research recognized for methodological rigor, and the randomized control trial (RCT) is the gold standard for high-quality research.

In the last three decades, the value of qualitative methodologies has been recognized in knowledge development. By comparison, *qualitative research* addresses broad questions and collects word data about phenomena or from participants. The investigator searches for themes and describes the information in themes and patterns exclusive to that set of participants so that generalizability is not an expectation. Qualitative methods are often used when there is little known about a phenomenon in order to define the dimensions of the concept for further clarification and concept development.

### Evidence-Based Practice Perspective of Evidence

In evidence-based practice, the term *evidence* is used deliberately instead of *proof*. This distinction is important because it emphasizes that evidence is not the same as proof. Evidence can be so weak that it is not convincing, and thus has little or no value, or it can be so strong that no one doubts its correctness. Therefore, it is important to be able to determine which evidence is the most authoritative. A number of levels of evidence pyramids have been developed for this purpose and specify a hierarchical order for various research designs based on their internal validity (Center for Evidence-Based Management, n.d.).

## Data, Information, Knowledge, and Understanding

The words *data, information, knowledge,* and *understanding* are often used interchangeably in practice and evaluation. According to Graves and Corcoran (1989), *datum* (singular; plural: *data*) is a single entity that has been described objectively and has not been interpreted. An example of datum is a single blood pressure or apical pulse value. *Information* is defined as data that have been interpreted, organized, or structured (American Nurses Association [ANA], 2001). An example of information is an evaluator noticing a trend in gradually rising systolic blood pressure when a 48-hour period of time is reviewed. *Knowledge* is defined as information that has been synthesized so that relationships are identified and formalized (ANA, 2001). An example of knowledge is realizing that the rising systolic blood pressure in a brain-injured patient could be a sign of increased intracranial pressure.

A review of the framework proposed by Ackoff (1989) helps differentiate data, information, and knowledge. He proposed that the content of the human mind can be classified into five categories: data, information, knowledge, understanding, and wisdom. In addition to defining data, information, and knowledge, he also included the terms *understanding* and *wisdom* (see Table 2.1). *Understanding* is described as a cognitive and analytical process of applying and appreciating relationships. *Wisdom* has many definitions that include an ethical and moral tone. Frances Hutcheson said that wisdom denotes the pursuit of the best ends by the best means (Knowles, 1999, p. 396).

**TABLE 2.1  Data, Information, Knowledge, Understanding, and Wisdom Model**

| Term | Definition/Description | Example |
|---|---|---|
| Data | Symbols<br>Exists in and of itself and has no significance beyond its existence<br>Does not have meaning by itself<br>Exists in both usable and nonusable forms | Single blood pressure, pulse, or serum glucose reading<br>Overall budget amount |
| Information | Data that are processed and have been given meaning by way of connecting it to something<br>The meaning provided may or may not be useful<br>Provides answers to "who," "what," "where," and "when" questions | Notice trend regarding decrease in satisfaction score after elimination of receptionist in clinic |
| Knowledge | Application of data and information<br>Collection of information organized to be useful<br>It is not at the level of integration<br>Provides answers to how something works<br>Answers "how" questions | Recognizing the fit of using complexity science as a framework to understanding implementation of electronic medical records in a health care organization |
| Understanding | A cognitive and analytical process of applying and appreciating relationships<br>Process by which knowledge can be synthesized into new knowledge by combining other knowledge with current knowledge to create something new | A teacher understands the relationship between using multiple methods of instruction and particular learning styles of students in mastering competencies |
| Wisdom | Evaluated understanding based on an integration and synthesis of cumulative knowledge and experience and inclusion of a moral and ethical context to provide insight and high-level understanding to complex and not easily answered questions | Ability to appreciate the ethical and moral impact of providing access to care for all members of a society |

In describing the Ackoff model, Bellinger, Castro, and Mills (2004) note that the first four categories are related to the past and address what has happened or what is known. The fifth category, wisdom, focuses on the future because it incorporates vision and design. With wisdom, the future can be created, thus extending vision and understanding of the past and present.

Rycroft-Malone et al. (2004) provide an interesting discussion about knowledge. Knowledge has been divided into *propositional* and *nonpropositional knowledge* (Eraut, 1985, 2000; see Table 2.2). The formal-explicit characteristics of propositional knowledge come from organized knowledge derived from rigorous research methods that can be generalized and disseminated through publications, presentations, and other media. By comparison, the informal-implicit characteristics of nonpropositional knowledge come from professional/discipline-specific knowledge and personal knowledge that an individual brings to a particular situation without the primary purpose of transferability (Eraut, 2000; Higgs & Titchen, 1995). Nonpropositional knowledge may become propositional knowledge when tacit knowledge accumulates and is tested using rigorous research methodologies that yield results that can then become generalizable to other populations. Although knowledge based on research with the resulting propositional knowledge has been viewed as higher level knowledge than nonpropositional knowledge, it is becoming clearer that both categories of knowledge are needed to work together in synergy to provide the most comprehensive body of evidence for understanding clinical practice.

## Empiricism and Positivism

Historically, evidence has its roots in empiricism and positivism, a philosophical view that has greatly influenced the perceptions of knowledge in nursing for decades (Billay, Myrick, Luhanga, & Yonge, 2007). *Empiricism* is a branch of philosophy that ties knowledge to experience. It states that all ideas are abstractions formed by combining and recombining what is experienced. Experience is the sole source of knowledge, and all that we know is ultimately dependent upon data from the senses. Information provided by the senses serves as the basic building block for all knowledge. *Positivism* is an outgrowth of traditional empiricism attributed to Comte, the 19th century French philosopher, and is based on the belief that the highest or only form of knowledge is the description of sensory phenomena. Comte expounded three stages of human belief; the theological, the metaphysical, and the positive. Positivism was so named because it confined

**TABLE 2.2  Comparison of Propositional Knowledge and Nonpropositional Knowledge**

| Propositional Knowledge | Nonpropositional Knowledge |
| --- | --- |
| Formal | Informal |
| Explicit | Implicit |
| Derived from research and scholarly work | Derived primarily from practice |
| Focused on generalizability | Focused on an individual; linked to experience and cognition resources of an individual |

itself to what is positively given, thus avoiding all speculation (Blackburn, 2008, p. 283). From a positivist perspective, knowledge is equated to truth that can be discovered.

From an empirical framework, all evidence comes exclusively from one's experiences. What one sees, hears, and feels through touch, smells, or tastes are interpreted; that interpretation is one's source of knowledge and the evidence for making sense of everything. Yet, an empirical approach to evidence and knowledge is dependent upon a number of interrelated factors that include: what one experiences as one lives; awareness of those experiences; how one processes and thinks about the experiences (perception); how one talks about those experiences; and how we diagram or sketch the experiences. Therefore, the sources of evidence based on empiricism are personal observations and experiences along with one's interpretation of those observations or experiences. An example of current work grounded in the empirical tradition is exemplified by the definition of evidence provided by Guyatt, Rennie, Meade, and Cook (2008), who have published extensively about evidence-based practice. They define *evidence* as an empirical observation that constitutes potential evidence whether systematically collected or not. Copi and Cohen (2009), in their classic book on logic, note that evidence ultimately refers to experience.

Many would argue that this is a narrow perspective of evidence for the 21st century and one that is prone to bias, which is discussed later in this chapter. Goldberg (2006) argues that rather than empirical evidence increasing certainty by factoring out the subjective and contextual components of everyday experience that bias understanding, empirical evidence obscures the subjective elements that inescapably enter all forms of human inquiry. From this perspective, evidence is not objective or neutral, but rather part of a social system of knowledge production. Although health professionals have been taught to value empirical knowledge above all forms of knowledge, new paradigms are challenging these beliefs and are redefining how health professionals think about the bases of health care and practice.

Another approach to evidence is to examine how we know. Carper (1978), in a seminal article, described four fundamental patterns of knowing in nursing. The first pattern of knowing is *empirical knowledge*. The basis of this pattern is positivism, "which believes that objective data, measurement, and generalizability are essential to the generation and dissemination of [nursing] knowledge" (Streubert-Speziale & Carpenter, 2003, p. 4). An example of empirical knowing is knowledge from the physical and biological sciences that helps nurses to understand laws of movement and human physiology. The second pattern of knowing is *aesthetics*. It involves the subjective experience and the creative aspect of nursing care. This concept is more difficult to define, but Fawcett, Watson, Neuman, Hinton-Walker, and Fitzpatrick, (2001, p. 6) proposed that aesthetic knowing is "the 'artful' performance of manual and technical skills." It answers the question of "how" a nursing act is performed rather than the key elements of the act. Aesthetic knowing has to do with style and delivery, which is personalized by the nurse for a particular patient. The third way of knowing is *personal knowing*, which involves the nurse as a person. The nurse is present or connects with others, a process often referred to as the therapeutic nurse–patient relationship (Fawcett et al., 2001) or intersubjectivity, the subject-to-subject relationship involving true presence (Parse, 1981, 1992). Presence refers to being totally focused and "being there" with authenticity and honesty in open, honest, and genuine communications. The fourth pattern of knowing is *ethical knowing*, which addresses the ethical and moral component of practice. It guides the nurse about how to behave in a given situation and emanates from an individual's sense of right and wrong. It requires the nurse to understand various philosophical perspectives and accepted standards of conduct and practice regarding what is good, right, and desirable (Billay et al., 2007).

Other scholars have added to Carper's work, including White (1995), who suggested that the fifth way of knowing is *sociopolitical* knowing. This form of knowing relates to how nurses address cultural differences of patients, political awareness, and policy issues and adds to the contextual component of individualized care. What is clear from this brief overview of knowing is that no single pattern of knowing should be used in isolation from the others because the practice of nursing relies on all five ways of knowing to provide quality care. Knowing is a form of the stream of evidence that guides practice including the dimension of evaluation.

## Other Perspectives of Evidence and Knowledge

Empiricism and positivism have had critics, beginning with philosophers such as Dewey and others who believed that knowledge was not something that must correspond to some antecedent truth, superimposed reality, or predefined description of the world; rather, knowledge is something emergent that is always interactive with experience and action, and, as such, requires continuous interpretation or revised description (Mantzoukas, 2007). Mantzoukas goes on to say that knowledge is inextricably linked with action, and is specific. Good action is described as that which works and is effective. Knowledge and advancement of knowledge emerge from our interpretive descriptions of the effectiveness or noneffectiveness of our experiences and actions (Gallagher, 1964). Building on the concept that knowledge emerges from actions and practice experiences, Schön (1983) proposed the concept of reflection as a means of acquiring and developing professional knowledge. Schön (1983, 1987) reasoned that research-based knowledge driven by theory resulted in linear, certain, and clear-cut solutions. By comparison, practice is nonlinear, uncertain, complex, and conflicting. Therefore, positivism-based research knowledge does not provide all of the answers to practitioners and does not guarantee best practice. The messy world of practice is often nonlinear and is better understood from the perspective of nonlinear complexity science.

Practitioners can use reflective techniques to identify and frame unique problematic situations and find workable unique solutions. By consciously and methodically analyzing the problematic situation and action taken, lessons learned can inform future practice regarding what works and what is more effective. Reflection offers a means for explicating practice, analyzing decision-making processes, and ensuring individualized and unique best practice and care. Reflection is described as a process of transforming unconscious types of knowledge and practices into conscious, explicit, and logically articulated knowledge and practices that allow for transparent and justifiable clinical decision making (Freshwater, Taylor, & Sherwood, 2008; Johns & Freshwater, 2005; Mantzoukas, 2007).

Nursing's thought leaders have built on the concept of reflection in many ways, including elucidating intuitive knowledge in nursing practice. Mitchell (1994) defines *intuition* as the instant understanding of knowledge without evidence of sensible thought. In addressing clinical intuition, Benner and Tanner (1987) write that intuition is understanding without rationale. Intuition is a process of arriving at accurate conclusions based on relatively small amounts of knowledge and/or information (Westcott, cited in Benner & Tanner, 1987). In the renowned book, *From Novice to Expert: Excellence and Power in Clinical Nursing Practice* (1984), Benner reports on research that investigated how nurses make clinical decisions based on different levels of experience. The levels of nursing practice are novice, advanced beginner, competent, proficient, and expert. Inherent in the notion of the expert nurse is intuitive knowing, which is also called intuitive knowledge. It is intuitive knowledge and judgment that separates expert judgment from that of a beginner (Benner & Tanner, 1987, p. 23). According to Benner and other nurse scholars, intuition is a source of knowledge in nursing to be valued and embraced. Some authors refer to intuition as tacit knowledge. *Tacit knowledge* is defined as "a state of a person or a relation between people that is not expressed, or one of which the subject may be unaware, but which can be inferred from their other capacities or activities" (Blackburn, 2008, p. 358). Blackburn (2008, p. 358) also defines *tacit communications* as the unexpressed recognition of the position of others that leads to strategies from common activity. It is knowledge that is so embedded and integrated into one's thinking that there may not even be conscious awareness of its presence.

Reflection provides structure and guidance to transpose unconscious and intuitive types of knowledge to conscious knowledge and allows for linkages to be developed with previous knowledge and experience, formal theories, and research knowledge to provide the best sources of evidence for professional practice and care.

## SOURCES OF EVIDENCE

To answer the question, "Where does evidence come from?" there are many ways to think about the sources of evidence. One way to classify the sources of evidence is through primary, secondary, and tertiary sources. *Primary sources* of evidence refer to information in its original form. That is, information that has not been interpreted, condensed, or evaluated. It is the original thinking, reports, discoveries, or shared new insights. Primary sources represent the first time the material has been released in physical, print, or electronic format. Examples of primary sources include journal articles of original research published in peer review journals; survey results; proceedings of meetings, conferences, or symposia; newspaper or electronic media postings; patient medical records; and data sets, such as national census descriptive statistics (University of Maryland Libraries, 2006). *Secondary sources* of evidence are accounts that are removed from the event or information and are provided after the fact. They describe, interpret, analyze, or evaluate information provided from primary sources. Examples of secondary sources are biographies, commentaries, monographs, textbooks, review articles, critiques, or opinion articles. *Tertiary sources* of evidence are works that include both primary and secondary resources in a special subject area that have been synthesized, reformatted, and condensed to a convenient and easy-to-read format. It may also include compilations of primary and secondary sources of information that recommend how to use the information. Examples of tertiary sources are clinical guidelines, manuals, handbooks, and practice protocols.

Evidence can come from external and internal sources. *External evidence* is generated through rigorous research such as RCTs and can be generalized to other settings. Melnyk and Fineout-Overholt (2015) point out that an important question to consider when applying external evidence to a project is can the same results be achieved in a different setting? In other words, does the research evidence translate and transfer to a real-world setting and project? By contrast, *internal evidence* is evidence generated through practice initiatives such as outcomes management and quality improvement projects that were conducted to improve care or outcomes in the setting in which the change was initiated.

Another way to think about the sources of evidence is based on qualitative and quantitative methods. *Qualitative methods* are used to investigate a phenomenon or area of interest through the collection of (nonnumeric) narrative materials using a variety of methods to collect the data. By comparison, *quantitative methods* collect data in a quantified (numeric) form; the focus of the investigation lends itself to precise measurement and quantification. This raises the question of value. Is evidence from one method of investigation better when conducting an evaluation? The response to that question is, it depends. It depends upon the elements of the evaluation and what evidence you are trying to collect. Some questions are answerable by qualitative methods. For example, if the evaluator wishes to determine how staff nurses feel about a seminal event in a clinical unit, then qualitative methods such as semistructured interviews are appropriate to tap into those personal responses. However, if the evaluator wishes to determine the demographic characteristics of the nursing staff employed in a cardiovascular service, then a quantitative method such as a forced-choice questionnaire is appropriate. In most evaluations, both qualitative and quantitative methods are needed to collect all of the evidence necessary to complete a comprehensive evaluation.

Still another perspective about the sources of evidence is practitioner-generated evidence called reflective knowledge, which was previously discussed in this chapter. The fundamental basis of reflection is primarily the experiences of the practitioner and the conscious effort of the practitioner to link this reflective knowledge with other types of knowledge to be applied to the current situation of interest. Understanding reflective knowledge and how it is used in practice and evaluation is complex and slowly evolving.

## CLASSIFICATION OF DATA SETS BY SIZE: BIG DATA

The remarkable rapid development of computer technology capacity that can support exabytes ($2.5 \times 10^{18}$) of data has made it possible to work with large data sets. Professional publications and national conferences capture this interest across multiple disciplines with the buzzword of *big data*. The word *big* refers to size; simple logic would suggest that if there are big data sets then there must also be small and medium size data sets. The next logical step is to define each category into some quantifiable fashion, and this is where the clarity and boundaries of definitions end. The term *big data* is a broad and evolving term that describes any voluminous amount of structured, semistructured, and unstructured data that has the potential to be mined for information. Although big data currently does not refer to any specific quantity, the term is often used when speaking about petabytes and exabytes of data (DeMauro, Greco, & Grimaldi, 2015). A common definition of big data is based on the three Vs of volume, velocity, and variety, to which have been added variability, veracity, and complexity. A recent consensual definition states that "big data represents the information assets characterized by such a high volume, velocity, and variety to require specific technology and analytical methods for its transformation into value" (De Mauro et al., 2015). The following describes the three Vs plus other characteristics addressed in the consensual definition.

### Volume

The quantity of generated data is important to the context of big data, the bigness of data, and its potential usefulness. Multiple factors have contributed to the increase in data volume, including accumulating previously collected stored data, unstructured data from social media, and increasing use of new sources of data collection and storage such as electronic medical records. A substantial decrease in the cost of data storage has supported further increases in the volume of data and has precipitated issues about the determination of relevance within large data sets and how to use analytics to create value from relevant data.

### Velocity

The term *velocity* refers to the speed of generation of data. The amount of data generated each day is unprecedented and will only increase in the future. How to organize and access these data streams for added value is challenging.

### Variety

Data come in all types of formats including structured and unstructured forms. The challenge is to manage, merge, and administer their use according to ethical and constructive practices.

### Variability

The term *variability* in this context refers to the inconsistency that can be evident in the data at times, thus hampering the process of being able to handle and manage the data effectively.

### Veracity

The quality of the data being captured can vary greatly. Statistical techniques are used to examine data before data analysis for quality. Verification of the "cleanliness" of data is critical because it directly affects the accuracy of analysis of the data set.

### Complexity

Data management can become a very complex process, especially when large volumes of data come from multiple sources. These data need to be linked, connected, and correlated in order to be able to grasp the information that is supposed to be conveyed by these data.

Magaoulas and Lorica (2009) note that the term *big data* is relative, and it depends on the capabilities of the users and their tools. What is considered big data today will become ordinary data in the not too distant future. Some organizations are overwhelmed with the volume of data they generate daily, thus requiring new data management procedures, while others are able to manage the ever increasing volume of data, at least for the foreseeable future.

Returning to the original question posed in the beginning of this section regarding the definition of small, medium, and big data sets, it is clear that the term *big data* is a relative term. A general understanding is that big data will always be more than conventional techniques and personal computers can manage. An example of a big data set is the Healthcare Effectiveness Data and Information Set (HEDIS), a dataset used by more than 90% of American health care plans to measure performance on dimensions of care and service. If the ability of a personal computer to handle analytics is a marker for size, then small and medium size data sets are manageable with a personal computer. Small and medium size data sets are also relative, and classification of data set by size is left to the reader to determine.

## QUALITY OF EVIDENCE

Quality is a notion that has to do with value to the beholder, thus suggesting a degree of subjectivity. The quality of evidence can be examined from a number of perspectives. Because evaluation is based on the accumulation and organization of evidence, examining the quality of evidence is briefly addressed in this section.

### Strength of Evidence and Evidence Hierarchies

An important distinction is made between strength of evidence systems and evidence hierarchies. Evidence hierarchies focus on the study design, with meta-analysis and systematic reviews of RCTs positioned at the highest level. By comparison, strength of evidence systems incorporates not only study design, but also other components such as presence or absence of bias, quality of the evidence, and precision of estimates (Owens et al., 2010). Yet, the domains included in the strength of evidence systems are not uniform, thus contributing to the confusion of grading evidence. See Table 2.3 for an example of levels of evidence based on a hierarchy of evidence for intervention/treatment questions. Burns, Rohrich, and Chung (2011) provide examples of hierarchies developed by several professional organizations.

Given the movement of the last 25 years to evidence-based practice, several evidence hierarchies have been developed by a number of scholars and organizations to grade scientific evidence according to the quality and strength of the empirical evidence for clinical practice. These hierarchies are specifically designed for scientific evidence, most often from publications reporting systematic reviews, RCTs, quasi-experimental designs, qualitative studies, case reports, and other forms of research. These hierarchies are further discussed in Chapter 10. Hierarchies are helpful when a review of the literature is conducted to determine the state of the science about a particular area of interest addressed through RCTs

TABLE 2.3   Rating System for the Hierarchy of Evidence for Intervention/Treatment Questions

| Level of Evidence | Description |
|---|---|
| Level I | Evidence from a systematic review of all relevant randomized controlled trials (RCTs), or evidence-based clinical practice guidelines based on systematic reviews of RCTs (includes meta-analysis) |
| Level II | Evidence obtained from at least one well-designed RCT |
| Level III | Evidence obtained from well-designed controlled trials without randomization, quasi-experimental |
| Level IV | Evidence from well-designed case-control and cohort studies |
| Level V | Evidence from systematic reviews of descriptive and qualitative studies |
| Level VI | Evidence from a single descriptive or qualitative study |
| Level VII | Evidence from the opinion of authorities and/or reports of expert committees |

*Source:* Melnyk & Fineout-Overholt (2015).
Level I evidence is the highest level of evidence.

or to understand the constructs of interest. Not all questions lend themselves to be investigated through RCTs. When considering evidence for evaluation, several questions confront the evaluator such as: What is the strength of the evidence? What is the value of the evidence? How confident are you about the validity of the evidence? Can you trust the evidence?

Strength has to do with the capacity to exert influence. In the case of evaluation, it is the strength of the evidence that informs the evaluator about the focus of interest. Strong evidence is compelling while weak evidence contributes little or nothing to the evaluation process. Primary evidence is viewed as stronger than secondary evidence. The value of evidence requires judgment by the evaluator and is subject to bias, and often depends upon the purpose for which the evidence is to be used. Purpose helps the evaluator decide what kind of evidence is needed, in what form, and in what amount.

Value of evidence also depends upon the context and environment for which it will be used. Some evidence will be critical based on the context of an evaluation, while other information may be helpful but not critical. Evidence is used to inform decision making and judgment so that the evaluator must determine if the evidence collected is appropriate, useful, credible, accurate, and trustworthy. It may take some investigation to verify that these characteristics of evidence are present. The legitimacy of evidence is always linked to purpose. The evaluator makes a judgment on a continuous series of questions throughout the evaluation process. The evaluator's goal is to access the best available evidence possible.

The evaluator is challenged to search and find the best evidence important to the project. This requires comprehensive knowledge about collecting targeted data through a variety of sources, such as electronic databases, other repositories of information, and expert consultation. In the pursuit of the "best evidence" to evaluate anything—a program, practice change, or published guidelines—evaluation is a high-level, complex process that involves an understanding of the nature of evidence and how it is collected, used, and evaluated as a basis for decision making. In evaluation, evidence can be considered clues or pieces of a puzzle that contribute to creating an accurate picture of the focus of evaluation. It is a process to search for truth as a basis for evaluation.

## Evaluation and Finding of Credible Evidence

What should the evaluator do if the desired evidence is not available? There are times when the evaluator does not have access to the evidence that he or she would like to collect. This may be due to evidence not being recorded, the unavailability of an informant, or a limitation of access due to the confidential nature of some information or other reasons. In such a situation, the evaluator must decide how critical the information is to the evaluation process. Often, some evidence is nice to have but is not critical; in other instances, certain evidence may be critical to the evaluation. The evaluator must determine if there is other available evidence that can substitute or be a proxy for the desired evidence. It may be possible to infer from other pieces of evidence about the area of interest. If the evaluator determines that missing evidence is indeed very important in the evaluation process and is unattainable, then this information should be listed as a limitation of the evaluation.

## Bias and Validity of Evidence

In examining the quality of evidence in any evaluation, bias and validity, which influence evidence and its usefulness in the evaluation process, must be considered.

### Bias

#### Evaluator/Observer Bias

For the purposes of this chapter, *bias* is defined as any influence that produces a distortion in the result of an evaluation. It can affect the quality of evidence in both qualitative and quantitative components of an evaluation (Polit & Beck, 2012, p. 720). Bias can be further divided into bias related to the evaluator or observer and bias related to evidence and process. *Evaluator bias* can occur in a number of forms. If the evaluator interviews people in the course of the evaluation process, interviewer bias is possible. The ideal interviewer is a neutral agent through which evaluation-focused questions are passed and recorded. However, this seemingly simple notion is difficult to achieve. The respondents and interviewer interact on a human level that includes complex verbal and nonverbal communications and interactions. These interactions can affect the interviewee's responses to questions. This means the quality of the information or evidence provided is inaccurate or incomplete, thus having a negative effect on the evaluation outcome. Evaluator bias may be communicated verbally or nonverbally, and the bias may be subtle. The basis of the bias may be personal preference for the outcome of the evaluation, allegiances to stakeholders who will be affected by the evaluation outcome, or a desire to validate previously articulated beliefs or experience.

A second potential source of evaluator bias is *observer bias*; that is, the evaluator collects evidence for an evaluation by observation. Observation is often an excellent alternative to self-reporting methods with subjects. Observation is useful to record characteristics and conditions of individuals, groups, and environments; verbal and nonverbal communications; activities and behaviors; and performance characteristics. Polit and Beck (2012, p. 189) address factors that interfere with objective observations with the following:

- Observer prejudices, attitudes, and values may result in faulty inferences.
- Personal commitment may distort observations in a preferred direction.
- Anticipation of what is to be observed may affect what is observed.
- Premature decisions before adequate information is collected may result in errors of classification or conclusions.

Although observational biases cannot be removed completely, they can be minimized through the careful training of the observer and attention to bias in the study design. Structured observations help to control bias and to systematically record observations so that comparable evidence is collected for all subjects.

### Participant Bias

As with evaluator bias, there is potential bias from the participants in an evaluation. In any evaluation, evidence is often collected from people either directly or indirectly involved in the evaluation process. Participants may be a source of evidence through input from interviews or from information provided though questionnaires, documents, reports, or other sources of evidence. Bias can be introduced in a number of ways such as *nonresponse bias*, *selection bias*, and *attrition bias*. Individuals decide if they wish to participate in an evaluation. It is important for the evaluator to determine if there are any group differences between the responders and nonresponders, such as demographic, socioeconomic, or other differences that could be a source of bias. This form of bias is called *nonresponse bias*. Another form of bias is *selection bias*. The evaluator must have a representative sample to collect evidence so that there is no segment of evidence excluded from the evaluation that could distort the findings. *Attrition bias* refers to participants who remove themselves from continuation in the process. The evaluator should determine if there are any group differences between those that continue to participate and those who withdraw. The reasons for withdrawal may provide important insight about the evaluation or the evaluation process.

Participants who are directly interviewed by the evaluator may demonstrate social desirability response bias and extreme response bias. *Social desirability response bias* is noted when participants mask their true responses consistently and provide responses that are reflective of prevailing social values or professional expectations (Polit & Beck, 2012, p. 313). Another form of social desirability bias occurs when the respondent knows or has a personal relationship with the evaluator. The respondent may not wish to offend the evaluator or may not wish the responses to seem critical or unappreciative of the evaluator's efforts, so the respondent may answer in a way that he or she believes will please, or at least not offend, the evaluator. *Extreme response bias* is demonstrated by participants who distort their opinions and respond so that everything is reported as very positive or very negative. In designing an evaluation, the evaluator should take into consideration all possible sources of bias and attempt to find ways to control or minimize their influence.

### Validity

Validity is divided into internal and external validity. *Internal validity* concerns the validity of inferences that there truly is an empirical relationship or correlation between the presumed cause and the effect (Polit & Beck, 2012, p. 235). The independent variable, rather than something else, causes the outcome. The justification is based on the extent to which a study minimizes systematic error (or bias). *External validity* is the extent to which the results of a study can be confidently generalized to other situations and to other people. There are a number of threats to internal validity; these include temporal ambiguity, selection, history, maturation, mortality/attrition, and testing/instrumentation. These concepts are well described in a number of research texts and are not addressed in this chapter.

Evaluation can be a form of research, especially when it is conducted with the rigor of a scientific investigation. Many concepts addressed in research texts are applicable to evaluation. From the perspective of research design, Shadish, Cook, and Campbell (2002, p. 34) define *validity* as, "the approximate truth of an inference." Polit and Beck (2012) note that validity is not an absolute value; rather, it is a matter of degree. Moving from a perspective of validity in research to evidence, validity of evidence is the degree to which the evidence is justified, supported, and founded on truth. Therefore, the validity of evidence is critical when considering design, conduct, and analysis in evaluation.

#### Construct Validity

A special form of validity, called *construct validity*, is an important consideration in evaluation. A *construct* is an abstract (nonobservable) entity, the existence of which is postulated and explained by use of observable phenomena (Angeles, 1992, p. 55). *Construct validity* involves the validity of inferences. It is the extent to which an instrument is said to measure a theoretical construct or trait (LoBiondo-Wood & Haber, 2014, p. 576). The concept of construct validity can also be applied to evaluation. Constructs link the methods used in the evaluation to the higher order concept of interest and to the ways the resulting evidence is translated into knowledge to make decisions related to that concept. A construct in an evaluation must be defined and operationalized before the evaluator can determine the key characteristics of interest and the best way to measure those characteristics. For example, if the focus of the evaluation is to examine interprofessional collaboration on a unit, the evaluator must first describe and operationalize the concept of interprofessional collaboration. What are the key characteristics to examine? A review of the literature might reveal that interprofessional collaboration is based on mutual respect, transparency, open and honest communications, and a common goal. The evaluator would then focus on ways to collect evidence about these attributes from the team that is being evaluated. As there are a variety of methods of eliciting the evidence related to a construct, the evaluator would have to decide what methods would provide the best evidence to address the question. The evaluator may use more than one method to collect evidence, which is often necessary to provide information about different aspects of a construct.

Threats to construct validity, defined as erroneous inferences from the particular evaluation study to the higher level abstract concept, must be considered. Threats can occur if there is a mismatch between the higher level concept of interest (e.g., interprofessional collaboration) and how the evaluator has operationalized the concept for purpose of the evaluation. It can also occur if irrelevant evidence is collected and included in the evaluation process. Although the evidence may be accurate, it is irrelevant to the focus of the evaluation. Other forms of threats to construct validity include evaluator bias and participant bias, both of which were discussed earlier in this chapter. In thinking about validity, it is never a determination of either present or not present consideration; validity is always a determination of the degree of validity.

## Contextual and Environmental Dimensions of Evidence

In conducting any evaluation, the context and local environment in which the evaluation takes place is important. Stetler (2003) described this evidence source as "internal evidence," which she says comes primarily from: local systematically collected information including data about local performance, planning, quality, and outcomes; knowledge about the culture of the organization and the individuals in it; and local and national policy. The focus of the evaluation, regardless if an organization, a group, or an individual is being evaluated, has to be appreciated within the context of the environment in which it operates. There may be special contextual and environmental characteristics unique to the focus of the evaluation that must be taken into consideration. For example, if an evaluator is assisting an organization to determine its readiness to apply for the Magnet Recognition Program offered by the American Nurses Credentialing Center (ANCC), the mission, size, and community in which the organization is located should be considered. A 75-bed, acute care facility located in a rural setting may not have the infrastructure to meet the research expectations of the Magnet criteria. Such a facility may be better positioned to apply for the Pathway to Excellence Program, which is also administered by ANCC, with criteria that focuses on use of evidence-based practice rather than generation of new knowledge.

## DNPS AND EVALUATION

The interest in evidence by health professionals is related to their need to substantiate the worth of a wide variety of activities and interventions (Pearson, Wiechula, Court, & Lockwood, 2007). Basing all beliefs and practices strictly on evidence allegedly separates science from other activities (Husserl, 1982; Kuhn, 1996). The type of evidence sought by the evaluator varies according to the focus of the evaluation, which might be a clinical question, or a question about the nature of an intervention, activity, or focus of interest. The previous discussion provided a background for the evaluation in a generic sense to assist DNPs in thinking about evidence. In this final section, the evaluation process focuses on the role of DNPs in evaluation.

## Role of the DNP in Evaluation

DNPs often assume responsibility and accountability for evaluation. Evaluation of care for individual patients and populations is an integral part of care. However, DNPs may be asked to evaluate any number of practices, interventions, products, programs, and policies either as an individual evaluator or as part of a team of evaluators. Additionally, evaluation in a digital age offers new dimensions to sources of evidence as well as the collection, storage, and organization of evidence. The following provides examples of common types of evaluations that DNPs may conduct.

### Practice

For DNPs, the word *evidence* is usually synonymous with evidence-based practice. Clinical practice and the practices or processes involved in providing care are exceedingly complex. For example, the DNP may be asked to examine the hand-off practices by nurses and physicians on a unit or service line. In thinking about this request, the DNP considers the many forms of hand-offs in health care. There are nurse-to-nurse hand-offs between shifts, at mealtime, and during transfer to another unit. Physician-to-physician hand-offs occur when a patient is transferred to another unit or another hospital. In a model where physicians are employed by a health care facility to work shifts, such as a hospitalist or resident, there is physician-to-physician hand-off between shifts. The DNP evaluating hand-off practices would most likely begin with focusing on the overall evaluation and then conducting a review of the literature to understand the state of the science related to hand-offs. In the process of review, the DNP would identify key variables to address and might also find instruments useful for collecting and measuring variables of interest. The literature is often a good guide for developing a protocol for the evaluation.

Another example of practice evaluation is one that examines the effectiveness of interprofessional teams for their impact on core measures and patient or organizational outcomes. Although it is generally believed that high performance, interprofessional teams have better patient and provider outcomes, teasing out the contributions that each team member contributes to outcomes may be difficult to determine. This is an example of a complex evaluation focus that might be conducted by a team that includes an expert consult to guide the process. Sources of evidence might include review of the literature, observation, semistructured interviews, questionnaires, and mining of patient outcome data related to practice processes, cost analyses, and core measures data.

### Interventions

Although providers like to think that their practice is evidence-based, it is clear that more than half of what is done in practice has no scientific basis. DNPs understand the processes of care and how to examine processes of care with such tools as process mapping and review of the literature for best practices. For example, the nursing practice of turning a patient every 2 hours has no scientific basis. The focus of the evaluation could be to examine the practices of turning patients and the incidence of pressure ulcers in a facility. This information could be of value to a nursing practice committee charged with reviewing patient turning protocols in a long-term care facility. Sources of evidence are similar to practice inquiry and might include review of the literature, observation, semistructured interviews, questionnaires, mining of patient outcome data related to team performance, cost analyses, and core measures data.

## Products

Health care facilities must make decisions on all products, from beds to dressings to educational materials. The decision may be about including new products in a facility or replacing a newer product with an established product. The DNP is often asked to evaluate a new product and compare it with current products. The evaluation is not only based on cost, but also achievement of stated outcomes, user friendliness, time required by the care provider to use the product, and acceptability by the patient. Because products and equipment are a big part of the operating budget, decisions on product evaluation have ramifications for the cost of health care. Helpful sources of evidence might include the literature on comparative effectiveness with other similar products, interviews with current users to determine how it is used, ease of use, reliability, cost, maintenance requirements, contribution to patient care, and return on investment.

## Programs

Another type of evaluation that DNPs might conduct is that of program evaluation. The program could be a clinical program such as a community-outreach stroke prevention program, an established comprehensive heart failure program within a hospital or system, or an orientation program for newly hired registered nurses on a specialty unit such as an orthopedic service. All programs should first be effective. It is important to understand the purpose of the evaluation. Is the purpose of the evaluation for feasibility, impact on a community, or cost? The purpose will determine what evidence will need to be examined. The findings of a program evaluation may lead to a quality improvement project. In the current cost-conscious environment of quality and safety, much emphasis is being placed on comparative effectiveness evaluation to guide decision making. Sources of evidence to evaluate a program might include: the literature; descriptions of characteristics of effective high-performance programs for purposes of focused data collection and comparison; interviews with a broad range of stakeholders including providers, administrators, and recipients about effectiveness and meeting of recipients' needs; patient/client outcome data; cost analysis; analysis on return on investment; projected changes in the program for the future including need for additional resources and cost; and observations of program processes.

## Policies

Policies and procedures that guide practice and care must be evaluated and updated on a regular basis to stay current and in compliance with regulatory bodies and professional standards. The DNP is often responsible for evaluating and updating policies and procedures as an individual evaluator or as part of a committee or other group advising decision makers. For example, a policy that requires 10 units of continuing education for all nursing staff may be scheduled for review in light of changes made by the state board of nursing for relicensure. The number of continuing education units may need to be increased because of new mandatory continuing education required by the state nurse practice act. The evaluation process might include current policy, mandatory changes, financial impact on the health care facility to support the continuing education requirements, and methods of communicating the change to staff. Sources of evidence to evaluate policies include a review of the literature, interviews with stakeholders affected by the policy or policies, policy analysis with local and national compliance imperatives, potential consequences of policy change or lack of change, cost implications of policy decisions, and the social environmental impact of the policy. Much of the evidence can be collected from internal sources including people and databases, and then applied to the local and national imperatives and standards required by the organization.

## Common Sources of Evidence Used by DNPs

Common sources of evidence used by DNPs when conducting an evaluation are included in Table 2.4.

In planning any evaluation, regardless if it appears simple or complex, careful attention must be paid to models and design. Models for evaluation provide a

**TABLE 2.4  Common Sources of Evidence for DNPs**

| Source | Examples |
|---|---|
| Print and electronic sources including data mining from internal and external databases | Journals, websites, electronic databases, books, survey data, dashboards, minutes of meetings, patient medical records, internally developed databases |
| Guidelines, protocols, and authoritative publications of professional organizations and state and national reports | American Heart Association clinical practice guidelines and Institute of Medicine reports |
| Forums and consensus standards for performance, which are considered the gold standard for evidence | National Quality Forum |
| Observations | Physical examination, participatory interactions (attending meetings, demonstrations) |
| Interviews | Individuals, groups |
| Surveys/instruments | Conducted electronically (e.g., SurveyMonkey) or in paper format; reported as aggregate data |
| Experiments/comparisons | Use of comparison groups or products |
| Personal experiences | Composite of clinical, professional, and personal experiences gained in a variety of ways<br>Practice knowledge (what is learned in practice) |
| Reflections | Linking knowledge learned from patient care or other experiences with other forms of knowledge to provide best practice<br>Seeing similarities in a new patient situation with previously accumulated knowledge from other cases |

framework for the evaluation. Design includes thinking prospectively of all possible factors that could undermine the quality of the evaluation including bias and validity. Although evaluation is generally considered at the end of many processes, it should be integrated early into the planning stage of any new projects. The steps to conducting an evaluation are discussed in Chapter 1.

## SUMMARY

Evaluation is based on the collection, organization, and critical review of evidence to make decisions about value. Evidence comes from many sources and is found in many forms. The evaluator must not only understand the overall process of evaluation, but also must be able to identify and collect the necessary evidence. The quality of the evidence must be constantly considered including bias and validity of evidence that will lead to the best possible evidence that can be trusted for evaluation and decision making.

## REFERENCES

Ackoff, R. L. (1989). From data to wisdom. *Journal of Applied System Analysis, 16*(1), 3–9.

American Nurses Association. (2001). *Scope and standards of nursing informatics practice.* Washington, DC: American Nurses Publishing.

Angeles, P. A. (1992). *The HarperCollins dictionary of philosophy* (2nd ed., p. 85). New York, NY: HarperCollins Publishers.

Bellinger, G., Castro, D., & Mills, A. (2004). *Data information, knowledge, and wisdom.* Retrieved from http://www.systems-thinking.org/dikw/dikw.htm

Benner, P. (1984). *From novice to expert: Excellence and power in clinical nursing practice.* London, UK: Addison-Wesley.

Benner, P., & Tanner, C. (1987). Clinical judgment: How expert nurses use intuition. *American Journal of Nursing, 87*(1), 23–31.

Billay, D., Myrick, F., Luhanga, F., & Yonge, O. (2007). A pragmatic view of intuitive knowledge in nursing practice. *Nursing Forum, 42*(3), 147–155.

Blackburn, S. (2008). *Oxford dictionary of philosophy.* New York, NY: Oxford University Press.

Burns, P. B., Rohrich, R. J., & Chung, K. C. (2011). The levels of evidence and their role in evidence-based medicine. *Plastic Reconstructive Surgery, 128*(1), 305–310. doi:10.1097/PRS/0b013e318219c17

Carper, B. (1978). Fundamental patterns of knowing in nursing. *Advances in Nursing Science, 1*(1), 12–23.

Center for Evidence-Based Management. (n.d.). *What are the levels of evidence?* Retrieved from http://www.cebma.org/frequently-asked-questions/what-are-the-levels-of-evidence/

Copi, I. M., & Cohen, C. (2009). *Introduction to logic* (13th ed.). Upper Saddle River, NJ: Pearson Prentice Hall.

De Mauro, A., Greco, M., & Grimaldi, M. (2015). What is big data? A consensual definition and a review of key research topics. *AIP Conference Proceedings, 1644*(1), 97–104.

Dictionary.com. (2010). *Unabridged; based on the Random House Dictionary, Random House, Inc.* Retrieved from http://www.bing.com/search?q=dictionary.com&src=IE-SearchBox&FORM=IESR02&pc=EUPP_UE04

Eraut, M. (1985). Knowledge creation and knowledge use in professional contexts. *Studies in Higher Education, 10*(2), 117–133.

Eraut, M. (2000). Non-formal learning and tacit knowledge in professional work. *British Journal of Educational Psychology, 70,* 113–136.

Fawcett, J., Watson, J., Neuman, B., Hinton-Walker, P., & Fitzpatrick, J. J. (2001). On nursing theories and evidence. *Journal of Nursing Scholarship, 33*(2), 115–119.

Freshwater, D., Taylor, B. J., & Sherwood, G. (Eds.). (2008). *International textbook of reflective practice in nursing.* Oxford, UK: John Wiley & Sons.

Gallagher, T. K. (1964). *The philosophy of knowledge.* New York, NY: Sheed and Ward.

Given, L. M. (2008). *The Sage encyclopedia of qualitative research methods.* Los Angeles, CA: Sage Publications.

Goldberg, M. J. (2006). On evidence and evidence-based medicine: Lessons from the philosophy of science. *Social Science and Medicine, 62*(11), 2621–2632.

Goodman, K. W. (2003). *Ethics and evidence-based medicine: Fallibility and responsibility in clinical science.* Cambridge, UK: Cambridge University Press.

Graves, J. R., & Corcoran, S. (1989). The study of nursing informatics. *IMAGE: Journal of Nursing Scholarship, 21*(4), 227–231.

Guyatt, G., Rennie, D., Meade, M. O., & Cook, D. (2008). *Users' guide to the medical literature* (2nd ed.). New York, NY: McGraw-Hill.

Higgs, J., & Titchen, A. (1995). The nature, generation and verification of knowledge. *Physiotherapy, 81*(9), 521–530.

Husserl, E. (1982). *Ideas pertaining to a pure phenomenology and a phenomenological philosophy: First book: General introduction to a pure phenomenology* (F. Kersten, Trans.). The Hague, Netherlands: Nijoff.

Johns, C., & Freshwater, D. (2005). *Transforming nursing through reflective practice* (2nd ed.). Oxford, UK: Blackwell Publishing.

Knowles, E. (Ed.). (1999). *The Oxford dictionary of quotations* (5th ed., p. 396). Oxford, UK: Oxford University Press.

Kuhn, T. (1996). *The structure of scientific revolutions* (3rd ed.). Chicago, IL: University of Chicago Press.

LoBiondo-Wood, G., & Haber, J. (2014). *Nursing research: Methods and critical appraisal for evidence-based practice* (8th ed.). St Louis, MO: Elsevier Mosby.

Magaoulas, R., & Lorica, B. (2009). *Introduction to big data.* Released 2.0. Sebastopol, CA: O'Reilly Media.

Magnani, L. (2001). *Abduction, reason, and science: Processes of discovery and explanation.* New York, NY: Kluwer Academic Plenum Publishers.

Mantzoukas, S. (2007). A review of evidence-based practice, nursing research, and reflection: Leveling the hierarchy. *Journal of Clinical Nursing, 17*(2), 214–223.

Melnyk, B., & Fineout-Overholt, E. (2015). *Evidence-based practice in nursing and healthcare* (3rd ed.). Philadelphia, PA: Lippincott Williams & Wilkins.

Mitchell, G. J. (1994). Intuitive knowing: Exposing a myth in theory development. *Nursing Science Quarterly, 7*(1), 2–3.

Owens, D. K., Lohr, K. N., Atkins, D., Treadwell, J. R., Reston, J. T., Bass, E. B., . . . Helfand, M. (2010). AHRQ series paper 5: Grading the strength of a body of evidence when comparing medical interventions–Agency for Healthcare Research and Quality and the Effective Health-Care Program. *Journal of Clinical Epidemiology, 63*(5), 513–523.

Parse, R. R. (1981). *Man-living-health: A theory of nursing*. New York, NY: John Wiley & Sons.

Parse, R. R. (1992). Human becoming: Parse's theory of nursing. *Nursing Science Quarterly, 5*(1), 35–42.

Pearsall, J., & Trumble, B. (Eds.). (1995). *The Oxford encyclopedia dictionary* (2nd ed.). New York, NY: Oxford University Press.

Pearson, A., Wiechula, R., Court, A., & Lockwood, C. (2005). The JBI model of evidence-based healthcare. *International Journal of Evidence-Based Healthcare, 3*, 207–215.

Pearson, A., Wiechula, R., Court, A., & Lockwood, C. (2007). A re-consideration of what constitutes "evidence" in the health care professions. *Nursing Science Quarterly, 20*(1), 85–88.

Polit, D. F., & Beck, C. T. (2012). *Nursing research: Generating and assessing evidence for nursing practice* (9th ed.). Philadelphia, PA: Wolters Kluwer/Lippincott Williams & Wilkins.

Rycroft-Malone, J., Seers, K., Titchen, A., Harvey, G., Kitson, A., & McCormack, B. (2004, July). What counts as evidence in evidence-based practice? *Journal of Advanced Nursing, 47*(1), 81–90.

Schön, D. (1983). *The reflective practitioner*. London, UK: Temple Smith.

Schön, D. (1987). *Educating the reflective practitioner*. San Francisco, CA: Jossey-Bass.

Scientific method. (2016a) Retrieved from *Merriam-Webster dictionary online*. Retrieved from http://www.merriam-webster.com/dictionary/scientific%20method

Scientific method. (2016b). *Oxford dictionary online*. Retrieved from http://www.oxforddictionaries.com/us/definition/american_english/scientific-method

Shadish, W. R., Cook, T. D., & Campbell, D. T. (2002). *Experimental and quasi-experimental designs for generalized causal inference*. Boston, MA: Houghton Mifflin.

Stetler, C. (2003). The role of the organization in translating research into evidence-based practice. *Outcomes Management for Nursing Practice, 7*(3), 97–103.

Streubert-Speziale, H. J., & Carpenter, D. R. (2003). *Qualitative research in nursing: Advancing the humanistic imperative* (2nd ed.). Philadelphia, PA: Lippincott.

University of Maryland Libraries. (2006). *Primary, secondary, and tertiary sources*. Retrieved from http://www.lib.imd.edu/guides/promary-sources.html

White, J. (1995). Patterns of knowing: Review, critique, and update. *Advances in Nursing Science, 17*(4), 73–86.

# CHAPTER THREE

# CONCEPTUAL MODELS FOR EVALUATION IN ADVANCED NURSING PRACTICE

Christine A. Brosnan

> *Do not go where the path may lead, go instead where there is no path*
> *and leave a trail.*
> —*Ralph Waldo Emerson*

## EVALUATION: AN ESSENTIAL STEP IN NURSING

Nurses in undergraduate and graduate programs are taught to assess patient needs, diagnose patient problems, plan for the care of patients, implement that plan of care, and then evaluate the results of the care provided (Potter & Perry, 2009). Following the mandate of *The Essentials of Doctoral Education for Advanced Nursing Practice* (American Association of Colleges of Nursing, 2006), graduate education programs have expanded curriculum content related to evaluation. As a result of this upgraded training, practitioners should be able to engage more fully in quality improvement and other evaluation activities. Early evaluations focused primarily on comparing the value of advanced practice nursing to medical care (Kleinpell, 2009). Today, as health professionals and patients become more comfortable with the advanced practice role, the scope and depth of evaluations are increasing.

While nursing is an essential component of the health care delivery system, other providers also directly impact health status and outcomes. Medicine, respiratory therapy, physical therapy, and pharmacy are some examples of disciplines to include in a comprehensive evaluation of patient care. The definition of *patient/client* and the focus of an evaluation have also expanded in advanced practice. As noted in Chapter 1, *patient* may now be defined as an individual, a group, a community, or a population affected by the health care activity being evaluated. The evaluation may not focus solely on direct patient care. The DNP nurse may be asked to participate in the evaluation of technologies, programs, guidelines/protocols, information systems, health education programs, and policies. Depending upon knowledge, experience, and skill set, the nurse may be a leader or a member of an interdisciplinary evaluation team.

## OVERVIEW

The conceptual foundation that supports the expanded scope of evaluation is interdisciplinary and continues to evolve. This chapter describes five approaches to evaluating the quality of health care, two methods for facilitating change based on evaluation, and three tool kits for care improvement.

The first evaluative approach, Donabedian's conceptual model, introduced in the first chapter, is discussed here in more depth. Not only is his model directly applied in health care evaluation, but his concepts have also been adapted for use in the development of alternative evaluation models.

The second approach, the effectiveness–efficiency–equity conceptual frame-work developed by Aday, Begley, Lairson, and Balkrishnan (2004), is briefly mentioned in this chapter and is described more completely in Chapter 13. It has applications across a variety of settings and types of perspectives. It is particularly relevant to the evaluation of policies affecting populations.

Logic models, the third approach, provide a blueprint to guide the evaluation process and illustrate how the components of the evaluation process relate to each other. Logic models are quite popular, particularly among funding agencies.

The fourth approach, monitoring and evaluating health systems strengthening, is a conceptual framework developed by the World Health Organization (WHO) and other international organizations (Boerma et al., 2009). The framework is especially useful for the evaluation of very large health care systems, such as those at the national level.

Finally, the Triple Aim framework was briefly described in Chapter 1 and will be reviewed more fully in this chapter (Berwick, Nolon, & Whittington, 2008). It has gained widespread acceptance because it is a comprehensive approach to evaluate the effectiveness and efficiency of care provided to both individuals and populations.

This chapter also discusses two approaches that facilitate health care change. While neither approach includes all the components of a comprehensive evaluation, each has been successful in improving performance. The first approach, the Iowa Model of Evidence-Based Practice to Promote Quality Care, has evolved over the years (Titler, Steelman, Budreau, Buckwalter, & Goode, 2001). It started as a method to find valid and reliable scientific information that providers could integrate and apply in patient care. It is now a multifaceted model used to guide the practitioner through a comprehensive change process. The second approach is the Promoting Action on Research Implementation in Health Services Framework (PARIHS). This conceptual framework has gained recognition because it offers a thorough and effective structure to direct the implementation of the change process in an interdisciplinary setting (Botti et al., 2014).

Finally, the following tools will be briefly reviewed: plan-do-study-act (PDSA), root cause analysis (RCA), and program evaluation and review technique (PERT). Each has a distinct purpose and they all have gained widespread acceptance in quality improvement activities.

## APPROACHES TO EVALUATION

### Donabedian's Conceptual Model: S-P-O Model

Donabedian's contribution to developing a systematic and objective method of ensuring the quality of health care evolved over four decades beginning in 1966 when he first introduced his model for evaluating quality. He observed that quality means different things to different people: "The definition of quality may be almost anything anyone wishes it to be, although it is, ordinarily, a reflection of values and goals current in the medical care system and in the larger society of which it is a part" (Donabedian, 1966, p. 167). He suggested that one could evaluate quality using three approaches individually or in combination. One could focus on the structure of care, on the process of care, or on the outcome of care. Donabedian identified basic problems in successfully conducting systematic and objective evaluations regardless of approach. These include: (a) a lack of valid and reliable measures, (b) the limitations of data sources and standards of measurement, (c) inadequate measurement scales, and (d) difficulty in establishing the link among each of the three approaches (structure, process, and outcome [S-P-O]). Donabedian spent the rest of his professional career (and his life) examining these concerns and their relevance to improving the health of patients.

### Health and Health Care

At the most basic level, health focuses on biophysical status (Donabedian, 1987). Practitioners assess the baseline health status of a patient, diagnose the condition, develop a plan of care, and intervene with evidence-based treatment. Outcome evaluation focuses primarily on the positive or negative changes in health status that result from the treatment provided. For example, in evaluating the outcome of individual care, a practitioner might measure the change in temperature and laboratory values after an acutely ill pediatric patient who has been diagnosed with H3N2 influenza is treated appropriately with medication and IV fluids. In evaluating a program, a practitioner may measure the change in the number of cases of H3N2 diagnosed in a community as a result of a vaccine program. In evaluating population health, a practitioner may measure the change in the number of deaths caused by H3N2 in a city among individuals who did receive the vaccine and those who did not.

An expanded description of health includes a sense of well-being that can be associated with quality of life (Donabedian, 1987, 2003). Determining the effect of an intervention or program on quality of life is challenging. For instance, a pacemaker inserted in the chest of a patient with dementia may improve the patient's health status but may not improve the patient's sense of well-being. Individuals differ and that makes it difficult to define and measure quality of life. Consider two patients who must have a below-the-knee amputation as a result of diabetes mellitus complications. One patient may have strong family and social supports, adapt to the disability, and rate the resultant quality of life as good. The other patient may have fewer resources and judge quality of life as poor. Health service researchers have spent decades developing measures that attempt to quantify and standardize the term. Quality of life is discussed in greater detail in Chapter 5.

Evaluation functions at the macro, meso, and micro levels. Periodically, it is important to examine the totality of care provided by a nation (macro level) or regional health system (meso level) to meet the health care needs of a population. Care provided to individual patients and groups of patients at the micro level should be monitored more frequently. If health care at the micro level is found to be less than optimum, practitioners can make appropriate changes that will theoretically impact care at the macro and meso levels. Quality improvement at all three levels provides the most comprehensive analysis (Donabedian, 1987).

DNPs frequently participate in monitoring activities and Donabedian's framework provides a method for deciding what indicators to monitor (Donabedian, 2003). Some indicators are externally imposed, such as those required by regulatory organizations and agencies in order to maintain accreditation or to establish a unique status. The Joint Commission, Centers for Medicare and Medicaid Services, and the American Nurses Credentialing Center Magnet Recognition Program are examples of external influences on monitoring health care.

Other quality improvement indicators arise from local institutional concerns. These may focus on specific internal indicators selected either as a result of administrative planning or because an adverse event presents an opportunity for further examination. As an example of administrative planning, the director of nursing of a medical clinic establishes an interdisciplinary quality improvement committee to identify problem areas and concerns. The committee requests chart audits and surveys to detect untoward trends that merit further study. The committee reports to the director that during the past year, the number of patients with diabetes mellitus returning for periodic eye examinations has decreased. The committee recommends that all patients receive letters reminding them about their next scheduled follow-up visit and a brief statement about the importance of eye examinations. The committee further suggests that the number of patients returning for follow-up be reanalyzed in 1 year.

An adverse event or a sudden rise in complaints may trigger monitoring activities. As an example, the director of quality improvement notices a 50% increase in the number of patient complaints related to the timeliness of receiving pain medication. The director asks the quality improvement committee to examine the problem and report the findings. Chart audits, staffing records, and interviews reveal a problem of nighttime understaffing. The chairperson of the quality improvement committee forwards the report to the director of nursing for feedback and recommendations.

It is not feasible to evaluate all indicators at the same time; therefore, priorities must be established. There is no hard and fast rule in setting priorities, but problems that pose a direct risk to patient health should be a primary concern. Practitioners also need to consider the extent of the problem and the feasibility of fixing the problem (Donabedian, 2003).

### Defining the Pathways to Quality: Structure, Process, and Outcome

At the most fundamental level, quality is an assessment of the "technical performance of individual health care practitioners" (Donabedian, 1987, p. 75). An expanded description provides contextual components of the interaction between patient and practitioner. Contextual components include: patient adherence to practitioner recommendations, the barriers and facilitators to obtaining health, and the hospital or clinic environment.

Donabedian's model lays out three approaches or pathways to evaluating health care: structure, process, and outcome. *Structure* refers to the administrative support provided for quality care and the environment in which health care occurs. Adequacy of supplies and equipment, number and proficiency of health care personnel, the hospital environment, and barriers and facilitators to access are structural components (Donabedian, 1987, 2003). Tarlov et al. (1989) also included patient characteristics like age, comorbidity, risk, and beliefs under the category of structure (see Table 3.1).

**TABLE 3.1   The Medical Outcomes Study's conceptual framework**

| Structure of Care | Process of Care | Outcomes |
|---|---|---|
| Systems characteristics<br>Organization<br>Specialty mix<br>Financial incentives<br>Work load<br>Access/convenience | Technical style<br>Visits<br>Medications<br>Referrals<br>Test ordering<br>Hospitalizations<br>Expenditures<br>Continuity of care<br>Coordination | Clinical end points<br>Symptoms and signs<br>Laboratory values<br>Death |
| Provider characteristics<br>Age<br>Gender<br>Specialty training<br>Economic incentives<br>Beliefs/attitudes<br>Preferences<br>Job satisfaction | Interpersonal style<br>Interpersonal manner<br>Patient participation<br>Counseling<br>Communication level | Functional status<br>Physical<br>Mental<br>Social<br>Role |
| Patient characteristics<br>Age<br>Gender<br>Diagnosis/condition<br>Severity<br>Comorbid conditions<br>Health habits<br>Beliefs/attitudes<br>Preferences | | General well-being<br>Health perceptions<br>Energy/fatigue<br>Pain<br>Life satisfaction |
| | | Satisfaction with care<br>Access<br>Convenience<br>Financial coverage<br>Quality<br>General |

Adapted from Tarlove et al. (1989). Copyright 1989 by the *Journal of the American Medical Association*. Used with permission.

*Process* comprises practitioner–patient interactions and the practitioners' technical proficiency in their therapeutic relationships with patients. Process indicators offer a direct approach to evaluating health care quality because health care that meets best practice standards in a specific time and place is quality care. Inherent in the selection of process criteria is the assumption that a strong link exists between how providers interact with patients and the outcomes of care (Donabedian, 1966, 1978, 2003). The type and number of diagnostic tests ordered, differential diagnoses listed, interpretation of test results, treatment prescribed, and type of patient education are all process characteristics (Donabedian, 2003; Tarlov et al., 1989). Process indicators reflect current standards of practice and, as a result, evolve over time (Larson & Muller, 2002).

*Outcomes* refer to a measurable change in patient health status that results from health care delivered (Donabedian, 1988, 2003). Measuring outcomes does not provide as direct a path as process in evaluating quality, but outcomes are "the ultimate validators of the effectiveness and quality of medical care" (Donabedian, 1966, p. 169). An advantage of outcomes is that they are recognizable to both practitioners and patients. Practitioners can measure the effect of a treatment and patients can report if a treatment made them feel better or worse. Another advantage is that desired outcomes may be standardized across settings. A 10% reduction of nosocomial infections in a hospital is a beneficial outcome that can be compared to other hospitals regardless of geographic location.

Outcomes may be generic or specific to a disease (Donabedian, 2003). Generic outcomes such as mortality and life expectancy are generally influenced by more than disease and reflect the culture and values of family and society. Disease-specific outcomes provide a better link to the quality of health care provided. For example, a practitioner determines that mortality among a group of patients with atherosclerosis is higher than among patients without atherosclerosis (a generic outcome). Unless investigated further, the practitioner cannot conclude that the higher mortality is a direct result of atherosclerosis because it could have been caused by other factors common to the age group at risk for atherosclerosis, such as cancer, accidents, pneumonia, and so on. On the other hand, an evaluator might audit clinic records to determine the range of high-density lipoprotein (HDL) and low-density lipoprotein (LDL) cholesterol values in patients with atherosclerosis and hyperlipidemia (a disease-specific end point). Determining that 90% of patients have cholesterol values within a normal range after 1 year of treatment provides evidence that intervention has been effective in lowering cholesterol.

When we focus on only one path to quality, we assume that there is a strong correlation among structure–process–outcome (Donabedian, 1987; Larson & Muller, 2002). If we evaluate only outcome, we may assume that the change in health status was a result of the structure and/or process of care. For example, a practitioner presumes that a decrease in blood pressure in a hypertensive patient indicates that the treatment prescribed was correct. However, in actuality, the patient stopped taking the prescribed medication because of the unpleasant side effects associated with it. The patient's blood pressure decreased after the patient resigned from a stressful job. In this case, the practitioner wrongly assumed that there was a link between the medication (process) and improved health status (outcome).

Establishing links among the approaches to quality can be challenging, although a valid and reliable link must be demonstrated if the evaluation is to be trusted (Donabedian, 1978). Over time, evaluators have found a stronger correlation between process and outcome indicators than between structure and process or between structure and outcome indicators. This may be due to a lack of research in establishing the effect of structure on quality. It does not mean that structural indicators should be ignored; rather, each approach should be viewed as providing unique and complementary information. Taken together, they provide the most comprehensive evaluation of quality care (Donabedian, 1978, 2003).

### Criteria and Standards

Criteria, standards, and norms are key components in Donabedian's framework, yet their definition and application often lack clarity and consistency across evaluations (Donabedian, 1981, 1982). Donabedian addressed this problem by comparing and contrasting the terms. He described *criterion* as "an attribute of structure, process, or outcome that is used to draw an inference about quality" (Donabedian, 2003, p. 60). He defined a *standard* as a "specified quantitative measure of magnitude or frequency that specifies what is good or less so" (Donabedian, 2003, p. 60). Acting together, criteria and standards are the means by which evaluators actualize the conceptual model of S-P-O.

For example, a structural criterion for providing quality care in a nursing home (NH) might be the number of registered nurses who staff the facility; the associated standard might be that the facility will not have less than one registered nurse on each shift (Table 3.2). A process criterion might be the number and percent of patients assessed for decubitus ulcers; the associated standard might be that 100% of patients will be assessed daily for pressure ulcers. An outcome criterion might be the number of patients with pressure ulcers; the associated standard might be that no patient will develop a pressure ulcer.

**TABLE 3.2  Examples of Criteria and Standards**

| Approach | Criterion | Standard |
|---|---|---|
| Structure | RNs staffing a nursing home<br>Protocol for screening patients with diabetes mellitus | No less than one RN on each shift<br>Protocol will include measuring HbA1c and blood pressure at each clinic visit |
| Process | Patients assessed for pressure ulcers<br>Patients tested for HbA1c and high blood pressure | 100% of patients will be assessed daily for pressure ulcers<br>100% of patients will have HbA1c and blood pressure measured |
| Outcomes | Patients diagnosed with pressure ulcers<br>Level of HbA1c and blood pressure | No patient will develop a pressure ulcer<br>80% of patients will have HbA1c < 7 and blood pressure < 140/80 |

## Role of Patient/Consumer

Patients play a vital role in evaluating the quality of health care. As one-half of the practitioner–patient dyad, they are well qualified to provide certain input about their care. For example, patients are certainly qualified to rate the amenities of care that form the contextual and environmental experience (structure). Was the room clean and odor free? Was the food tasty and delivered promptly? Was parking available and affordable?

Patients also provide a unique perspective in rating the technical proficiency and interpersonal skills of their practitioners (process). Did the practitioner explain the problem and interventions clearly? Did the practitioner appear caring? Did the practitioner spend time answering questions? Was the staff pleasant and respectful? Although they may not understand the intricacies of technology, patients do know if a procedure made them feel better or worse (an outcome). Did treatment improve their ability to perform activities of daily living? Did treatment enable them to return to work (Donabedian, 1980, 1992, 2003)?

Evaluators must bear in mind that, for a variety of reasons, patients are not always the best judges of quality. The amenities that please one patient may cause distress in another. For example, one patient's hospital experience may be improved by having a roommate while another patient prefers to be alone. Some patients focus on interpersonal relationships while others are more concerned with technical performance. Expectations of successful outcome may or may not be realistic. Regardless of limitations, patient input is an essential component in determining quality of care (Donabedian, 1987, 1992, 2003; Larson & Muller, 2002).

### Application of the S-P-O Conceptual Model

From a practical perspective, the most important attribute of the S-P-O model is how robust it has proven to be over time. The concepts are so universally accepted that practitioners may assume that the categories of S-P-O have always been part of quality evaluation. In fact, the model has evolved and adapted as practitioners increasingly apply it in innovative and novel ways. Three studies that illustrate how Donabedian's model adapts to a variety of settings and clinical specialties are presented in Table 3.3 and discussed in the following text.

Kilbourne, Fullerton, Dausey, Pincus, and Hermann (2010) were concerned that patients with major mental health disorders frequently receive less than optimal care when they are diagnosed with accompanying substance abuse and medical problems. Using Donabedian's model, they sought to develop a method to identify S-P-O measures with the goal of improving quality of care. They identified structural measures including the availability of medical care practitioners, practitioners with substance abuse knowledge, readiness of hospital beds for patients with dual diagnoses, and patient compliance with evidence-based treatment protocols. Process measures focused on screening and treatment for substance abuse and diagnosis of problems related to diabetes mellitus and hypertension, comorbidities common in this patient population. Process measures were linked to outcomes that included patient satisfaction, morbidity, and mortality data. The authors noted that it was not difficult to obtain data about structural measures because there was no need to rely on patient records, but it was difficult to establish the link between structure and process and between structure and outcome. They determined that the comprehensiveness of the S-P-O

**TABLE 3.3   Examples of Evaluative Studies Using Structure–Process–Outcome**

| Study | Structure | Process | Outcome | Findings/ Conclusions |
|---|---|---|---|---|
| **Kilbourne et al. (2010)** | | | | |
| Developed a framework to measure quality of care in patients with mental disorders and comorbidities | Number of general practitioners available<br>Percent of mental health practitioners with knowledge of substance abuse<br>Number of dual-diagnosis beds available<br>Compliance to evidence-based care | Percent of patients receiving recommended screening for lipids and hypertension<br>Percent of patients who had ocular and foot assessments<br>Percent of patients with substance use screening<br>Percent of patients receiving substance use care | Percent with acceptable screening results<br>Patient satisfaction<br>Mortality<br>Addiction severity index changes<br>Percent going back to work | Authors plan to use the framework and evaluate results |
| **Shield et al. (2014)** | | | | |
| Developed a model to represent the effect of medical staff on the quality of care in nursing homes | Type of staffing-open versus closed<br>Number of staff<br>Staff attendance | Communication<br>Coordination<br>Presence at staff meetings | Emergency visits<br>Readmission<br>Pain control | Donabedian's model clarified variable interactions and advanced research |
| **Holt et al. (2014)** | | | | |
| Integrative review assessed the characteristics of NMHCs | Holistic care<br>Facilities<br>Faculty providers<br>Grants<br>Vulnerable population | Health education programs<br>Screening programs<br>Chronic disease care<br>Midwifery care<br>Referral care | Patient satisfaction<br>Increased detection of disease<br>Increased vaccines<br>Better birth outcomes | Donabedian's model proved valuable in evaluating quality of care and in developing an evidence-based description of NMHCs |

NMHC, nurse-managed health center.

Model was an advantage in successfully evaluating care provided to this patient population. They resolved to apply and assess the validity of Donabedian's model in future studies.

Shield et al. (2014) evaluated the structure of care and its link to process and outcome in a series of interrelated studies focused on the effectiveness of medical staff in NHs. Physicians, nurse practitioners (NPs), and physician assistants were categorized as medical staff. Using data from studies and surveys that they had conducted, the authors adapted Donabedian's model to interpret interactions in the clinical setting of a NH. Based on the results, the authors concluded that regulating the frequency and length of attendance by the medical staff (e.g., in a closed staff model) increases medical presence in the NH. Medical presence was associated with better communication and coordination of care. They also noted that geriatric NPs were perceived to provide higher quality care than physician assistants or other types of NPs. The authors concluded that this study enabled them to more clearly define links among the variables in their model, to ascertain which interactions increased quality of care, and to determine future research topics.

Holt, Zabler, and Baisch (2014) applied Donabedian's model to guide an integrative review of the literature that examined the characteristics of nurse-managed health centers (NMHCs) within the context of health care quality. Their review yielded 59 articles that were included in the study. The authors then used qualitative analysis to categorize the articles under the classifications of structure, process, and outcome. As a result of the review, the authors were able to develop an evidence-based description of NMHCs that will facilitate the continuing examination of this model of care and its comparison with other health care models.

Although these examples represent disparate uses of Donabedian's S-P-O Model, all have in common a precise identification of the aspects of structure, process, or outcome as they relate to the study. In each case, the model facilitates an objective and systematic assessment of health care quality and a direction for future evaluations.

## Conceptual Framework: Effectiveness–Efficiency–Equity

Aday collaborated with economists, physicians, and other health service researchers in developing an integrated and comprehensive framework that evaluates health policies based on three principal criteria: effectiveness, efficiency, and equity (Aday & Andersen, 1974; Aday et al., 1999, 2004). Aday's framework is eclectic, integrating some of Donabedian's concepts with constructs from epidemiology, sociology, ethics, economics, and the behavioral sciences. The framework addresses the interactive nature of policy and health care quality by providing practitioners with methodologies to measure the impact of policy and the skills to influence policy changes. Depending upon the goal, evaluation may be at the micro, meso, or macro level.

In the effectiveness–efficiency–equity framework, health care policies are viewed from the perspective of the practitioner/researcher who seeks to understand the intricacies and variety of policies at the local, state, and federal levels (Aday et al., 2004). The practitioner examines the positive and negative ways that policy affects the health status of individuals, communities, and populations; compares and contrasts the impact of alternate health care programs; and offers recommendations to administrators and lawmakers who ultimately make health care policy decisions (Aday & Andersen, 1984; Phillips, Mayer, & Aday, 2000; Quill, Aday, Hacker, & Reagan, 1999).

Aday and colleagues adapted Donabedian's S-P-O Model to categorize the components of their framework and to provide an approach for evaluation. The system for delivering health care, the population projected to need health care, and the setting in which the population lives comprise the structure of care. The attained access to health care and the health risks of the patients seeking care comprise the process of care. The health status of individuals and populations comprise the outcome of care. Effectiveness, efficiency, and equity in health care are the criteria on which these outcomes are evaluated.

The authors defined *effectiveness* as "the degree to which improvements in health now attainable, are, in fact, attained" (Aday et al., 2004, p. 57). In analyzing effectiveness, the practitioner includes not only improvements resulting from the health services provided, but also improvements associated with the familial, cultural, and environmental settings. Effectiveness can further be evaluated at the micro (clinical) and macro (population) levels. Clinical effectiveness relates primarily to changes in the health status of individuals through the health care provided. Population effectiveness relates to changes in the overall health status of populations achieved through health care and environmental factors (Aday et al., 2004).

*Efficiency* refers to both the production and allocation of health care services. Aday et al. (2004, p. 121) refer to production efficiency as "producing a given level of output at a minimum cost." They refer to allocative efficiency as the "attainment of the 'right,' or most valued, mix of outputs" (Aday et al., 2004, p. 121). Efficiency can be viewed from a macro or micro perspective (Aday et al., 2004). The DNP nurse will not normally be involved in evaluating efficiency at the macro level, but may be called upon to collaborate with other health professionals in conducting micro level evaluations. For example, the practitioner may be asked to determine the best combination of supplies, equipment, and human resources (the inputs) needed to efficiently produce a health care service (Aday et al., 2004). A practitioner may also be part of a team conducting a cost-effectiveness, cost-benefit, or cost-utility analysis of a technology, service, or program. These evaluation methodologies are commonly used and will be described in Chapter 5.

*Equity* refers to "maximizing the fairness in the distribution of health care (procedural equity) and minimizing the disparities in health across groups (substantive equity)" (Aday et al., 2004, p. 189). Indicators of procedural equity include equality of input into policy decisions, types of facilities and providers available, payment sources, number of services provided, and patient satisfaction. Indicators of disparity in health groups include inequalities with regard to clinical indicators and to population rates of morbidity and mortality. A DNP may be called on to collect information about one or more of these indicators in order to determine the equity of current health policies in an agency, community, or population. In evaluating equity, the practitioner examines factors that facilitate and factors that hinder the fair and just distribution of health care across all demographic and clinical groups (Aday et al., 1999, 2004).

The effectiveness–efficiency–equity framework is discussed more extensively in Chapter 13 because of its relevance to health policy.

## Logic Models

Logic models also have components similar to the S-P-O Model. However, logic models provide a more detailed blueprint of how to plan, implement, and measure performance. Emphasis is placed on first defining end points and then deciding on the activities and inputs needed to achieve them. Each component of a logic model is connected to and is a consequence of a prior component. The approach is iterative because activities may be modified if end points are not attained. Logic models are frequently used by health professionals from nonprofit organizations who are concerned with evaluating mission-motivated rather than profit-motivated end points (Chen, 2005; Fitzpatrick, Sanders, & Worthen, 2004). They may be applied at the macro, meso, or micro level.

Logic models are concerned with the inputs (also called resources), activities, and end points of a program. End points may be referred to as outputs, outcomes, or impact. Figure 3.1 presents an example of a logic model used by the Centers for Disease Control and Prevention (CDC) Division for Heart Disease and Stroke Prevention (2011). Inputs refer to structural components such as organizational framework, administrative guidelines and protocols, number of health care providers, health care environment, and financial resources. Program activities are the processes that take place as a program is implemented. These may include health care interventions, educational activities, or technological services.

Logic models use distinct end points defined by scope and time (Fitzpatrick et al., 2004). Although the number of end points may vary, there are generally three types of end points described in a logic model. The first end point is output. Outputs are immediate consequences of activities; for example, the number and types of patients receiving a particular health care intervention, the quantity of health education pamphlets delivered to patients, or the total number of hours of screening provided to a community group outcomes provide evaluators with a specific timeline to measure program performance. They may be short term, mid-term, or long term depending upon the project. Outcomes focus on improvements in health status including cognitive, behavioral, and attitudinal change. In some logic models, the term *impact* is used to represent a long-term end point such as a change in policy or population health. There are a number of guidelines available online that facilitate the creation of logic models including those developed by the W. K. Kellogg Foundation (2004) and the CDC Division for Heart Disease and Stroke Prevention.

### Application of Logic Models

Logic models have been used extensively in a variety of health care programs including a statewide heart disease and stroke prevention program (Sitaker, Jernigan, Ladd, & Patanian, 2008), a teenage pregnancy prevention program (Hulton, 2007), the creation of a DNP orthopedic clinical specialty (Instone &

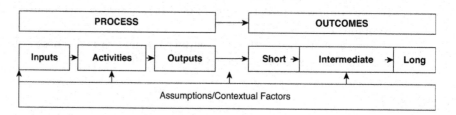

**Figure 3.1**  Layout of a general logic model.
*Source:* Centers for Disease Control and Prevention (2011). Reprinted with permission.

Palmer, 2013), and the collaboration of a School of Nursing and a Veteran Affairs (VA) Medical Center to develop a VA Nursing Academy (Harper, Selleck, Eagerton, & Froelich, 2015). Two examples along with selected variables are provided in the following text and in Table 3.4.

Harper, Selleck, Eagerton, & Froelich described the collaboration between the Birmingham VA Medical Center and the University of Alabama at Birmingham School of Nursing (SON) to form the Birmingham VA Nursing Academy. Formation of the Academy was part of a 5-year grant funded by the Veterans Administration. The objectives of this alliance of academia and service included the recruitment of graduates from the SON to work at the VA Medical Center, the integration of veteran-related content into the curriculum at the SON, and improvement in the quality of care delivered to veterans. The authors applied the logic model to provide organization and direction for both institutions as they continue their partnership.

**TABLE 3.4  Examples of Studies That Applied the Logic Model**

| Study | Inputs | Activities | Outputs | Outcomes |
|---|---|---|---|---|
| **Harper et al. (2015)** | | | | |
| Examined a joint effort to establish the VA Nursing Academy | Shared objectives Combined Advisory Council VA nurses SON faculty | Create programs for: veteran-specific simulation, shared staff between the VA, and the SON Formative evaluation | Veteran focused lectures to students Faculty working at the VA VA staff teaching at SON Summative evaluation plan | Over 2,000 BSN students participated in VA-specific educational programs Increased support for veteran students Increased quality of care for veterans |
| **Instone and Palmer (2013)** | | | | |
| Developed a plan to include orthopedic content into a DNP program | Orthopedic certification DNP programs Experienced faculty | Administrative approval Local resources Program personnel Potential students | Didactic orthopedic course Clinical practice | Graduation rates Certification exam pass rates Faculty and student satisfaction Orthopedic nursing employment Increased number of low-income clients receiving care from DNPs |

Instone and Palmer (2013) observed that because of an aging population and an insufficient supply of orthopedic surgeons, an unmet need exists for practitioners with the education and experience to provide quality care to patients with orthopedic problems. NPs trained in this specialty at the master's level currently provide care to this population; however, the emergence of the DNP presents an opportunity to expand the number and expertise of orthopedic providers. The authors asserted that a realistic solution is to place orthopedic content and practice into the DNP program as a specialty area. They applied the logic model to provide a blueprint for action. In order to be eligible to take the orthopedic nursing certification examination, students must accrue at least 2,500 hours of clinical training. Some or all of this training may fit into the clinical concentration of the DNP educational program. They concluded that increasing the number of DNPs trained as orthopedic specialists allows nurses to collaborate with physicians in a partnership to improve the quality of care for all patients with orthopedic problems, particularly those from vulnerable populations who have historically lacked access to care.

## Conceptual Framework: Monitoring and Evaluation of Health Systems Strengthening

National leaders have long recognized the need to measure the health status of citizens and the benefit of comparing standard health outcomes in one nation to those of other nations. The framework for monitoring and evaluation of health systems strengthening was developed in response to this need through the collaborative efforts of several international organizations including the WHO, the World Bank, the Global Alliance for Vaccines and Immunisation (GAVI), and the Global Fund (Boerma et al., 2009). This macro level framework shares components with the basic logic model described previously. It also provides guidelines for standardizing terms, indicators, and methods with the goal of improving the quality and comprehensiveness of health care evaluation within and among individual countries. Although it is recommended for use at the national level, the framework is also suitable for use at a regional or state level.

The Monitoring and Evaluation (M&E) Framework (Figure 3.2) consists of four main indicator domains: inputs and processes, outputs, outcomes, and impact. The *inputs and processes* domain contains governance, health financing, infrastructure, workforce, and supplies. The *outputs* domain contains services readiness and access, as well as intervention quality, safety, and efficiency. The *outcomes* domain contains coverage of interventions and risk behaviors and factors. The *impact* domain contains improved health outcomes and equity, social and financial risk protection, and responsiveness.

An important component of the M&E Framework is the use of valid and reliable core indicators across the domains. The authors recommended that evaluators not only develop indicators relevant to their own target population, but also avail themselves of internationally accepted indicators when appropriate. As in every evaluation, sources for data collection should be relevant and feasible. Such sources include but are not limited to surveys, clinical trials, large national databases, registries, and hospital records. Once obtained, data are analyzed using a variety

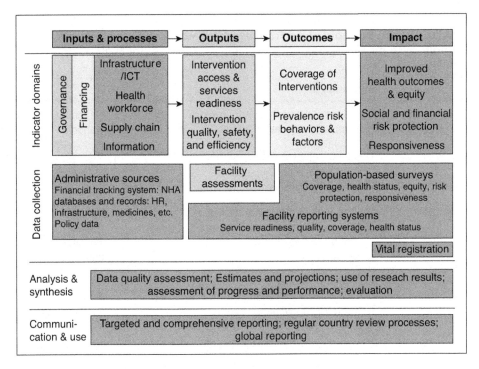

**Figure 3.2** Monitoring and evaluation of health systems reform/strengthening.
*Source:* Boerma et al. (2009). Reprinted with permission.

of statistical tests. Results are first reported to the decision makers who requested the information, and then disseminated to a wider audience in the form of papers and publications. The ultimate benefit of many nations using the same framework, definitions, indicators, and methods, and then sharing their results, is an increase in the validity of the findings and a better chance that health care programs will be effective, efficient, and equitable.

## Application of the Monitoring and Evaluation of Health Systems Strengthening Framework

As an example, a DNP might be a member of an evaluation team that is asked to examine the quality of newborn care in a southwestern region of the United States (Table 3.5). One of the initial decisions the team makes is to choose indicators and sources to evaluate the four domains (inputs and processes, outputs, outcomes, and impact). Under the domain of inputs and processes, indicators might include hospital expenditures (health financing), number of registered nurses (workforce), neonatal intensive care units (infrastructure), and average cost for ventilators and incubators (supplies). National health databases, registries, surveys, and assessments of clinical and hospital facilities are good sources for these data.

Under the output domain, indicators might include utilization of registered nurses (service readiness), location of facilities (access), and neonatal case fatality

**TABLE 3.5  An Example of the Framework for Monitoring and Evaluation of Health Systems Strengthening: Indicators and Sources for Evaluating Quality of Newborn Care**

| Domain | Indicators | Sources |
|---|---|---|
| Inputs and process | 1. Expenditures for hospital newborn facilities<br>2. Number of registered nurses/10,000 population<br>3. Number of neonatal intensive care units per 10,000 population<br>4. Average cost for ventilators and incubators | 1. National health databases<br>2. National nurse registries<br>3. Hospital surveys<br>4. Hospital surveys and facility assessment |
| Outputs | 1. Utilization of registered nurses<br>2. Geographic location of newborn facilities in relation to population<br>3. Neonatal case fatality | 1. Survey<br>2. Survey<br>3. Hospital records and national databases |
| Outcomes | 1. Neonatal aftercare home coverage<br>2. Immunization coverage<br>3. Newborn screening for hearing coverage<br>4. Breastfeeding for 6 months | 1. Survey<br>2. Medical records<br>3. National registries<br>4. Medical records |
| Impact | 1. Child mortality (under 5 years)<br>2. Hearing disabilities diagnosed in children under 5 years | 1. Vital statistics<br>2. Survey and medical records |

(quality and safety). Surveys, registries, hospital records, and national databases are generally used as sources for these types of indicators. Under the outcomes domain, indicators might include use of aftercare home coverage, immunization coverage, and newborn screening for hearing coverage (coverage of interventions) and breastfeeding for 6 months (risk factors and behaviors). Data could be collected through surveys and medical record review. Impact indicators include child mortality and hearing disabilities diagnosed. Information related to these impact indicators might be obtained from vital statistics, surveys, and health records.

## The Triple Aim Framework

In 2007, a group of researchers organized by the Institute for Health Improvement (IHI) developed the Triple Aim framework, an ambitious attempt to guide the work of organizations and other entities seeking to improve the quality of health care (Institute for Healthcare Improvement, 2015a; Lewis, 2014; Whittington, Nolan, Lewis, & Torres, 2015). The first aim of the framework is to improve the health experiences of individuals. In defining health experience, the architects of the Triple Aim referred to the six dimensions of quality described by the Institute of Medicine. These dimensions are safety, effectiveness, patient-centeredness, timeliness, efficiency, and equity (Institute of Medicine, 2001).

The second aim is to advance population health. In many instances, this can be accomplished through public health activities, such as providing nutrition education and increasing the number of individuals who are immunized. These interventions may not involve expensive high-tech procedures but can have a large impact on the health of communities.

The third aim is to decrease the per person cost of health care. The United States' low position among developed countries ranked on the basis of health care indicators is incongruent with the cost of health care, which surpasses the spending of all the other developed countries. There are many reasons for this paradox including excessive administrative costs, the extensive use of expensive high-tech interventions, greater charges for health products and services in the United States compared with other countries, and the prevalent perception among health care providers that they must practice "defensive medicine" (Reinhardt, 2008).

Berwick et al. (2008) stressed that the position of "integrator" is essential to the success of the Triple Aim framework. The integrator is a recognized group responsible for coordinating all health care activities of the organization as well as implementing the components of the Triple Aim strategy. These components include: encouraging individuals and families to become more involved in their own health care, changing the way in which primary care is delivered, controlling the delivery of resources to populations, educating the population about the cost of health care, and providing a link between the organization and the larger health care system. The authors cited Kaiser Permanente as an example of an integrator.

### An Organized Approach to Improving Quality

IHI uses the phrase "science of improvement" to describe the steps in a process designed to move organizations and communities toward achieving their objectives. To be successful, organizations should have (a) well-defined goals, (b) an appropriate rubric for measuring success, (c) an explanation of how the concepts they develop will result in desired change, (d) a plan that directs activities, (e) a commitment to implementing the plan on a small scale to determine its impact, (f) a method to represent systems interactions, and (g) the ability to learn through experimentation (Institute for Healthcare Improvement, 2015b).

One key to successful implementation of this model of improvement is the use of valid and reliable measures. IHI urged organizations to combine process and outcome measures as well as balancing measures. The latter are used to be sure that one activity does not offset the desired effect of another activity.

The IHI also developed metrics, referred to as "whole system measures," which are linked to each of the aims and may be added to the existing metrics of an organization. Thus, progress toward achieving the three aims can be compared across organizations and populations. For example, patient experience is measured through surveys and indicators linked to the Institute of Medicine's six dimensions of quality. Population health is quantified using functional health status, risk status, disease burden, and mortality. Per capita cost is calculated using patient cost and hospital utilization rates (Nelson, Lloyd, & Nolan, 2007).

### Application of the Triple Aim Framework

The Triple Aim has become widely accepted as a guide to evaluating performance quality. In 2007, the IHI invited national and international participation to evaluate the performance of the framework (Whittington et al., 2015). A total of 141 entities took part including hospitals, insurance companies, and public health agencies. Some of these organizations were quite successful in applying the framework; others were less successful. The investigators observed that organizations had difficulty achieving all three aims and that the greatest challenge was decreasing health cost. This was largely due to the reluctance of organizations to eliminate sources of revenue. The investigators concluded that the following principles increased the chances of success: a solid foundation, services appropriate for the population, and a long-term educational program about Triple Aim strategies.

In 2010, Dr. Donald Berwick, Administrator for Medicare and Medicaid Services (CMS), recommended using the framework to improve the quality of health care for Medicare and Medicaid enrollees (Fleming, 2010). His recommendation along with passage of the Affordable Care Act encouraged organizations to apply the framework in a variety of health care settings. Ouslander and Maslow (2012) discussed the importance of developing valid measures that are aligned with the Triple Aim for patients in long-term care. Potter et al. (2013) used the framework to create a research protocol to support quality care for patients with inborn errors of metabolism. Christopher (2014) discussed the relevance of Triple Aim to the Visiting Nurse Services of New York.

One article has particular relevance to DNPs. Hoyle and Johnson (2015) discussed the impact of health care reform on the nursing profession, and the related requests from organizations like the Institute of Medicine (2010) and American Association of Colleges of Nursing (2006) for educational initiatives to develop increased leadership abilities among advanced practice nurses. These recommendations provided the impetus for faculty at the University of Washington, School of Nursing, to offer DNP students the education and experience to increase their proficiency in quality improvement activities. The authors described a DNP–Family Nurse Practitioner curriculum that is aligned with the goals of the Triple Aim. Students were introduced to quality improvement strategies, tools, and processes that they then applied in the clinical setting. Ongoing evaluation was conducted using a clinical evaluation instrument, along with peer, faculty, and agency feedback.

In another example of the flexibility of the Triple Aim framework, Prior, McManus, White, and Davidson (2014) observed that children with chronic diseases frequently have a difficult time transitioning from pediatric to adult clinical settings. The authors utilized the Triple Aim framework to conduct a systematic literature review designed to examine measures associated with the transition process. There were 33 studies included in the final review. Of these, the most studies focused on diabetes mellitus (12). Other conditions included were transplants, sickle cell disease, cystic fibrosis, and HIV. Health care measures were classified using the Triple Aim. The authors concluded that studies examining transition care often employ methodologies and tools that are inconsistent, and whose validity and reliability have not been established. They recommended that experts in the field work together to create measures that are applicable across a wide variety of chronic disease states. Selected measures associated with this study are provided in Table 3.6.

**TABLE 3.6  An Example of the Triple Aim Framework With Selected Measures**

| Study | Patient Measures | Population Measures | Cost Measures |
|---|---|---|---|
| **Prior et al. (2014)** | | | |
| Conducted a literature review to determine the classification of transition measures | Positive care experience Challenges to care | Compliance disease-specific measures Self-care abilities | Health care use Cost of care |

## APPROACHES TO CHANGE

### The Iowa Model of Evidence-Based Practice to Promote Quality Care

The Iowa Model is a comprehensive paradigm that has gained wide popularity in guiding the change process in health care settings (Titler et al., 2001). The first step in the process is to detect "triggers," which are described as clinical questions or problems that require further investigation. Triggers may be found through a number of sources including clinical experience, current literature, guidelines, and patient feedback (Dang et al., 2015).

The next step is to determine the importance of the problem to the organization's administrators because their commitment to the change process is essential for its success. Once their approval is obtained, the DNP creates a team with the ability to solve the problem. Depending on the issue, the team may be composed of representatives from several disciplines who have expertise in the relevant clinical area.

The team is responsible for deciding on the methodology of the review of research literature, inclusion and exclusion criteria, and analysis of the results and conclusions drawn. If there is insufficient evidence in the literature, the team may decide to conduct a research study on the topic. If this is not practical, another option is to use other kinds of validation for the proposed solution, which may come from expert panels, case reports, and science or theoretical principles. One or more pilot tests that verify the conclusions are conducted before extensive changes are put in place. If pilot testing is successful, the team then plans a strategy to implement change. During the entire process, the team carefully examines the benefits and risks of the new treatment or procedure; they are then ready to adjust the plan if it is not successful. If a decision is made, based on the evidence, to implement a change in clinical practice, the team works with staff to promote a smooth transition. After the new practice is in place, evaluation based on structure, process, and outcome indicators continues to provide further evidence of the impact of the change on quality of care (Dang et al., 2015; Titler et al., 2001).

The following example is a novel application of the model. Pittman, Beeson, Kitterman, Lancaster, and Shelly (2015) were concerned about the increased incidence of hospital-acquired pressure ulcers related to the use of medical devices, which can comprise 50% of reported cases. The authors set up a task force of nurses from different areas of the hospital where patients were at risk for developing ulcers. They reached consensus that the incidence of pressure ulcers from medical devices was indeed a cause of concern at their hospital. They established that it was also a priority of hospital administrators. The task force developed a methodology for reviewing the literature and obtained pertinent data. They also accessed findings from clinical conferences, government publications, and clinical experts. They incorporated their findings into a position statement that will direct future education, research, and clinical practice at their facility. One immediate impact of the position statement was a 33% decrease in pressure ulcers over a 1-year period.

### Promoting Action on Research Implementation in Health Services

The PARIHS framework creates a path for DNPs to integrate research into practice. It incorporates three major elements and accompanying subelements that give direction in determining the success or failure of an intervention. The major elements are evidence, context, and facilitation. Evidence is drawn from studies, literature, clinical wisdom, patient feedback, and local indications. Context comprises the cultural background of the clinical setting, the type of leadership provided, and the scope and depth of evaluation activities. Facilitation refers to how well health professionals collaborate with each other to transition research into positive patient outcomes (Dang et al., 2015; Kitson et al., 2008).

In an example that also addressed the problem of pressure ulcers, Sving, Högman, Mamhidir, and Gunningberg (2014) described a quasi-experimental study on the integration of current evidence into clinical practice on preventing pressure ulcers. The PARIHS framework provided the structure that enabled investigators to evaluate the positive or negative impact of the evidence, context, and facilitation indicators on the success of the change process. The study was conducted by an interdisciplinary team in a Swedish general hospital and involved a sample of approximately 506 patients and 275 nurses. The team concluded that performance goals were not being met because of insufficient expertise, time, and resources. An intervention that incorporated a pressure ulcer prevention training program was provided to nurses. The program included periodic evaluations to assess cognitive learning.

The authors found that the intervention was significantly linked to an increase in nurses' knowledge about pressure ulcers and in activities directed toward preventing them. However, there was no significant change in the prevalence of pressure ulcers among patients. The authors determined that the PARIHS framework was helpful in determining the enablers and barriers to the change process.

## TOOLS

There are a number of tools commonly used in quality improvement that are helpful in ensuring that the change process flows smoothly. Three of these tools are briefly discussed in the following text and examples are presented in Table 3.7.

### PDSA: Plan-Do-Study-Act

PDSA is a circular process composed of four phases and is frequently used alongside the Triple Aim framework (Minnesota Department of Health, 2014; Whittington et al., 2015). The first step in the "Plan" phase is creating a team whose members have the skills to solve the problem at hand. The team is responsible for determining the goals of the project, delineating the problem based on available evidence, examining the causes of the problem, and creating options for its resolution. In the "Do" phase, the team tests a plan, and in the "Study" phase, the team decides if the plan has improved outcomes. If the plan is successful, it becomes part of the standard practice in the "Act" phase. If not successful, the team returns to the first phase.

### Root Cause Analysis

RCA is a process of identifying the basic mechanism responsible for an adverse event or a latent adverse event (one that may occur in the future). As the cause in question has already taken place, the process is retrospective. The RCA approaches

**TABLE 3.7  Examples of Tools Used in Quality Improvement**

| Tool | Example |
|---|---|
| Plan-do-study-act (PDSA) | Graudins et al. (2015) tested an audit tool to establish the frequency of missed medication doses and their effect on patient safety. The tool was first assessed through pilot testing. The PDSA enabled the researchers to gather input from hospital personnel to decide if further changes to the audit tool were indicated. |
| Root cause analysis (RCA) | Tschannen et al. (2015) described a senior level course that teaches quality improvement skills to undergraduate nurses. In addition to classroom content, senior students organized RCA projects in the clinical setting. Teams of four to five students collaborated with hospital unit personnel to conduct analysis of identified problems including the following areas: communication, restraints, falls, and pressure ulcers. Evaluative comments by hospital staff noted that the RCAs improved staff performance and patient outcomes. |
| Program evaluation and review technique (PERT) | Girija and Bhat (2013) conducted an exploratory study focused on the efficiency of the emergency department (ED) of a teaching hospital. The sample included 100 randomly observed patients admitted to the ED over a 60-day period. Using the PERT process, activities of hospital personnel and the time to complete activities were defined and analyzed. Results indicated that a visit could be expected to last 84.89 minutes. |

problems in a logical and objective manner with the intent to focus on the entire system and to refrain from placing blame on individuals (Agency for Healthcare Research and Quality, 2014).

## Program Evaluation and Review Technique

PERT is a tool used to increase the efficiency of an intervention or program by decreasing the time and cost entailed. This is accomplished through assessing the activities involved and determining the most expeditious way to proceed. PERT is most successful with large, multifaceted, and complicated projects (Improhealth Collaborative, 2015).

## SUMMARY

This chapter explored approaches to comprehensively evaluate health care and to improve performance. Each of the approaches described has proven to be beneficial and each provides the DNP with a structure to systematically and objectively examine interventions, programs, policies, and technologies that affect individuals, groups, and populations.

As a member of an evaluation team, the DNP will select the model that best fits the purpose of the evaluation. Once the model is chosen, the team must address the challenges inherent in conducting evaluations. Methodological challenges involve selecting valid and reliable measures, establishing associations between the components of the model, and determining the most relevant data sources, data collection methods, and types of analyses. After the results of the evaluation are determined, the team must decide on an appropriate way to disseminate their findings. Team members should also be ready to report the strengths and weaknesses of the evaluation itself.

## REFERENCES

Aday, L. A., & Andersen, R. (1974). A framework for the study of access to medical care. *Health Services Research, 9*(3), 208–220.

Aday, L. A., & Andersen, R. (1984). The national profile of access to medical care: Where do we stand? *AJPH, 74*(12), 1331–1339.

Aday, L. A., Begley, C. E., Lairson, D. R., & Balkrishnan, R. (2004). *Evaluating the healthcare system* (3rd ed.). Chicago, IL: Health Administration Press.

Aday, L. A., Begley, C. E., Lairson, D. R., Slater, C. H., Richard, A. J., & Menloya, I. D. (1999). A framework for assessing the effectiveness, efficiency, and equity of behavioral healthcare. *American Journal of Managed Care, 5*, SP25–SP44.

Agency for Healthcare Research and Quality. (2014, August). *Root cause analysis.* Retrieved from http://www.psnet.ahrq.gov/primer.aspx?primerID=10

American Association of Colleges of Nursing. (2006). *The essentials of doctoral education for advanced nursing practice.* Washington, DC: Author.

Berwick, D. M., Nolon, T. W., & Whittington, J. (2008). The Triple Aim: Care, health, and cost. *Health Affairs, 27*(3), 759–769.

Boerma, T., Abou-Zahr, C., Bos, E., Hansen, P., Addai, E., & Low-Beer, D. (2009, November). *Monitoring and evaluation of health systems strengthening.* Geneva, Switzerland: World Health Organization. Retrieved from http://www.who.int/healthinfo/HSS_MandE_framework_Nov_2009.pdf

Botti, M., Kent, B., Bucknall, T., Duke, M., Johnstone, M.-J., Considine, J., . . . Cohen, E. (2014). Development of a management algorithm for post-operative pain (MAPP) after total knee and total hip replacement: Study rationale and design. *Implementation Science, 9*(10), 1–11. doi:10.1186/s13012-014-0110-3

Centers for Disease Control and Prevention Division for Heart Disease and Stroke Prevention. (2011). *State heart disease and stroke prevention program. Evaluation guide: Developing and using a logic model.* Retrieved from http://www.cdc.gov/DHDSP/index.htm

Chen, H. T. (2005). *Practical program evaluation.* Thousand Oaks, CA: Sage Publications, Inc.

Christopher, M. A. (2014). The role of nursing and population health in achieving the Triple Aim. *Home Healthcare Nurse, 32*(8), 505–506.

Dang, D., Melnyk, B. M., Fineout-Overholt, E., Ciliska, D., DiCenso, A., Cullen, L., .. Dang, D. (2015). Models to guide implementation and sustainability of evidence-based practice. In B. M. Melnyk & E. Fineout-Overholt (Eds.), *Evidence-based practice in nursing & healthcare* (pp. 274–315). Philadelphia, PA: Wolters Kluwer.

Donabedian, A. (1966). Evaluating the quality of medical care. *Milbank Memorial Fund Quarterly, 44*(Suppl. 3), 166–206.

Donabedian, A. (1978). The quality of medical care. *Science, 200*(4344), 856–864.

Donabedian, A. (1980). *Explorations in quality assessment and monitoring: Vol. I. The definitions of quality and approaches to its assessment.* Ann Arbor, MI: Health Administration Press.

Donabedian, A. (1981). Criteria, norms and standards of quality: What do they mean? *AJPH, 71*(4), 409–412.

Donabedian, A. (1982). *Explorations in quality assessment and monitoring: Vol. II. The criteria and standards of quality*. Ann Arbor, MI: Health Administration Press.

Donabedian, A. (1987). Commentary on some studies of the quality of care. *Health Care Financing Review/Annual Supplement*, 75–85.

Donabedian, A. (1988). Quality assessment and assurance: Unity of purpose, diversity of means. *Inquiry, 25*, 173–192.

Donabedian, A. (1992). The Lichfield lecture. Quality assurance in health care: Consumers' role. *Quality Health Care, 1*, 247–251.

Donabedian, A. (2003). *An introduction to quality assurance in health care*. New York, NY: Oxford University Press.

Fitzpatrick, J. A., Sanders, J. R., & Worthen, B. R. (2004). *Program evaluation: Alternative approaches and practical guidelines* (3rd ed.). Boston, MA: Pearson Education.

Fleming, C. (2010, September 14). *Berwick brings the "Triple Aim" to CMS*. Retrieved from http://healthaffairs.org/blog/2010/09/14/berwick-brings-the-triple-aim-to-cms/

Girija, V. R., & Bhat, M. S. (2013). Process flow analysis in the emergency department of a tertiary care hospital using program evaluation and review technique (PERT). *Journal of Health Management, 15*(3), 353–359.

Graudins, L. V., Ingram, C., Smith, B. T., Ewing, W. J., & Vandevreede, M. (2015). Multicentre study to develop a medication safety package for decreasing inpatient harm from omission of time-critical medications. *International Journal for Quality in Health Care, 27*(1), 67–74.

Harper, D. C., Selleck, C. S., Eagerton, G., & Froelich, K. (2015). Partnership to improve quality care for veterans: The VA Nursing Academy. *Journal of Professional Nursing, 31*(1), 57–63.

Holt, J., Zabler, B., & Baisch, M. J. (2014). Evidence-based characteristics of nurse-managed health centers for quality and outcomes. *Nursing Outlook, 62*(6), 428–439.

Hoyle, C., & Johnson, G. (2015). Building skills in organizational and systems change. *Nurse Practitioner, 40*(4), 15–23.

Hulton, L. J. (2007). An evaluation of a school-based teenage pregnancy prevention program using a logic model framework. *The Journal of School Nursing, 23*(2), 104–110.

Improhealth Collaborative. (2015). *Program evaluation and review techniques (PERT)*. Retrieved from http://www.improhealth.org.fileadmin/Documents/Improvement_Tools/PERT.pdf

Institute for Healthcare Improvement. (2015a). *Initiatives*. Retrieved from http://www.ihi.org/Engage/Initiatives/TripleAim/pages/default.aspx

Institute for Healthcare Improvement. (2015b). *Science of improvement*. Retrieved from http://www.ihi.org/about/Pages/ScienceofImprovement.aspx

Institute of Medicine. (2001). *Crossing the quality chasm: A new health system for the 21st century*. Washington, DC: National Academies Press.

Institute of Medicine. (2010). *The future of nursing: Leading change, advancing health*. Washington, DC: National Academies Press.

Instone, S. L., & Palmer, D. M. (2013). Bringing the Institute of Medicine's report to life: Developing a doctor of nursing practice orthopedic residency. *Journal of Nursing Education, 52*(2), 116–119.

Kilbourne, A. M., Fullerton, C., Dausey, D., Pincus, H. A., & Hermann, R. C. (2010). A framework for measuring quality and promoting accountability across silos: The case of mental disorders and co-occurring conditions. *Quality and Safety in Health Care, 19*, 113–116.

Kitson, A. L., Rycroft-Malone, J., Harvey, G., McCormack, B., Seers, K., & Titchen, A. (2008). Evaluating the successful implementation of evidence into practice using the PARIHS framework: Theoretical and practical challenges. *Implementation Science, 3*(1) 1–12. doi:10.1186/1748-5908-3-1

Kleinpell, R. M. (2009). *Outcome assessment in advanced practice nursing.* New York, NY: Springer Publishing Company.

Larson, J. S., & Muller, A. (2002). Managing the quality of health care. *Journal of Health and Human Services Administration, Winter,* 261–280.

Lewis, N. (2014, October 21). *Re: A primer on defining the Triple Aim* [Web log message]. Retrieved from http://www.ihi.org/resources/Pages/Publications/PrimerDefiningTripleAim.aspx

Minnesota Department of Health. (2014, March). *PDSA: Plan-do-study-act.* Retrieved from www .health.state.mn.us/qi

Nelson, M. L. A., Lloyd, R. C., & Nolan, T. W. (2007). *Whole system measures, IHI innovation series white paper.* Cambridge, MA: Massachusetts Institute for healthcare improvement. Retrieved from http://www.ihi.org/resources/Pages/IHIWhitePapers/WholeSystemMeasuresWhitePaper.aspx

Ouslander, J. G., & Maslow, K. (2012). Geriatrics and the Triple Aim: Defining preventable hospitalizations in the long-term care population. *JAGS, 60*(12), 2313–2318.

Phillips, K. A., Mayer, M. L., & Aday, L. A. (2000). Barriers to care among racial/ethnic groups under managed care. *Health Affairs, 19*(4), 65–75.

Pittman, J., Beeson, T., Kitterman, J., Lancaster, S., & Shelly, A. (2015). Medical device-related hospital acquired pressure ulcers. Development of an evidence-based position statement. *Journal of Wound, Ostomy and Continence Nurses, 42*(2), 151–154.

Potter, B. K., Chakraborty, P., Kronick, J. B., Wilson, K., Coyle, D., Feigenbaum, A., & Syrowatka, A. (2013). Achieving the "Triple Aim" for inborn errors of metabolism: A review of challenges to outcomes research and presentation of a new practice-based evidence framework. *Genetics in Medicine, 15*(6), 415–422.

Potter, P. A., & Perry, A. G. (2009). *Fundamentals of nursing.* St. Louis, MO: Mosby Elsevier.

Prior, M., McManus, M., White, P., & Davidson, L. (2014). Measuring the "Triple Aim" in transition care: A systematic review. *Pediatrics, 134*(6), e1649–1661.

Quill, B. E., Aday, L. A., Hacker, C. S., & Reagan, J. K. (1999). Policy incongruence and public health professionals' dissonance: The case of immigrants and welfare policy. *Journal of Immigrant Health, 1*(1), 9–18.

Reinhardt, U. E. (2008, November 14). *Why does U.S. health care cost so much? (Part I).* Retrieved from http://www.blogs.nytimes.com/2008/11/14/why-does-us-health-care-cost-so-much-part-1/?

Shield, R., Rosenthal, M., Wetle, T., Tyler, D., Clark, M., & Intrator, O. (2014). Medical staff involvement in nursing homes: Development of a conceptual model and research agenda. *Journal of Applied Gerontology, 33*(1), 75–96.

Sitaker, M., Jernigan, J., Ladd, S., & Patanian, M. (2008). Adapting logic models over time: The Washington State Health Disease and Stroke Prevention Program experience. *Preventing Chronic Disease, 5*(2), 1–8.

Sving, E., Högman, M., Mamhidir, A.-G., & Gunningberg, L. (2014). Getting evidence-based pressure ulcer prevention into practice: A multi-faceted unit-tailored intervention in a hospital setting. *International Wound Journal,* 1–10. doi:10.1111/iwj.12337

Tarlov, A. R., Ware, J. E., Greenfield, S., Nelson, E. C., Perrin, E., & Zubkoff, M. (1989). The medical outcomes study. *JAMA, 262*(7), 925–930.

Titler, M. G., Steelman, V. J., Budreau, G., Buckwalter, K. C., & Goode, C. J. (2001). The Iowa model of evidence-based practice to promote quality care. *Critical Care Nursing Clinics of North America, 13*(4), 497–509.

Tschannen, D., Aebersold, M., Kocan, M. J., Lundy, F., & Potempa, K. (2015). Improving patient care through student leadership in team quality improvement projects. *Journal of Nursing Care Quality*, *30*(2), 181–186.

W. K. Kellogg Foundation. (2004). *Logic model development guide.* Retrieved from http://www .wkkf.org/resource-directory/resource/2006/02/wk-kellogg-foundation-logic-model-development- guide

Whittington, J. W., Nolan, K., Lewis, N., & Torres, T. (2015). Pursuing the Triple Aim: The first 7 years. *Milbank Quarterly*, *93*(2), 263–300.

# CHAPTER FOUR

# EVALUATION AND OUTCOMES

Christine A. Brosnan and Patrick G. Brosnan

> *True genius resides in the capacity for evaluation of uncertain,*
> *hazardous, and conflicting information.*
> —*Winston Churchill*

The previous chapters reviewed the major issues driving health care evaluation in the United States and the context in which doctor of nursing practice (DNP) graduates and other health professionals seek to improve the quality of that care. The chapters discussed acquisition and use of evidence, and the various approaches to quality improvement. Chapter 4 builds on that content to explore the association between evaluation and outcomes in greater depth. This chapter describes recent changes in and challenges to quality measurement, the development of patient-centered outcomes, and sources for valid and reliable measures. The role of comparative effectiveness research (CER) in establishing effective treatment in a real-world context is reviewed and examples provided.

## EXPLORING QUALITY IMPROVEMENT

During the past 50 years, health service researchers, health care professionals, consumers, and stakeholders have continued to search for the elusive path to quality improvement. Researchers became increasingly interested in identifying clinical trials in which health-related variables could be compared across studies through either qualitative synthesis or statistical testing of aggregated data. Literature synthesis and meta-analysis studies now provide an evidence base for practice and for developing health care guidelines (Chassin & Loeb, 2011).

Utilization review committees and professional standards review organizations, which grew out of the Medicare legislation of 1965, came to be viewed as conduits for improving quality in participating hospitals (Chassin & Loeb, 2011). In 1994, the Clinton administration proposed legislation known as the Health Security Act (Mariner, 1994). Although the bill was not approved by Congress, the Health Security Act provided an impetus for an expanded discussion of more comprehensive quality improvement activities. These activities included the development of quality measures, the creation of computer centers to store data collected from hospitals and other clinical facilities, and the formation of health care standards (Sadeghi, Barzi, Mikhail, & Shabot, 2013).

The Joint Commission (TJC), originally called The Joint Commission on Accreditation of Health Care Organizations, encouraged the use of evidence-based performance metrics and the application of Donabedian's structure-process-outcome indicators in evaluating hospital quality (Chassin & Loeb, 2011). In 1999, the Agency for Health Care Policy and Research was renamed the Agency for Healthcare Research and Quality (AHRQ) and was charged with gathering and disseminating evidence on best health care practices. The National Quality Forum, a not-for-profit-organization formed in the same year, was tasked with supporting the application and dissemination of quality metrics (Sadeghi et al., 2013). In 2001, the report *Crossing the Quality Chasm* recommended redesigning the health care system to place quality improvement in the forefront (Institute of Medicine [IOM], 2001). The Affordable Care Act of 2010 contained major initiatives designed to improve health outcomes, along with incentives to help accomplish the goal.

Today, there are numerous governmental and nonprofit entities striving to construct the most direct path to quality improvement. Governmental entities such as AHRQ, Centers for Medicare & Medicaid Services (CMS), and the National Quality Measures Clearinghouse (NQMC) contain sections devoted to reviewing and disseminating valid and reliable metrics. Nonprofit organizations including the IOM, TJC, the National Committee for Quality Assurance, and the Institute for Health Improvement offer guidance to providers, patients, and health care facilities who seek to measure quality care (Sadeghi et al., 2013).

## DEVELOPING PATIENT-CENTERED OUTCOMES

In 1966, Donabedian stated that outcomes were "the ultimate validators of the effectiveness and quality of medical care" (Donabedian, 1966, p. 169). Practically, however, outcome measures are more difficult to develop and collect than process measures. Outcome is more patient centered than process, and thus harder to identify and link with a specific treatment or intervention (Chin, 2014). Changes in health status often occur because of complex interactions and cannot always be attributed to a linear association of one provider to one patient. Donabedian discussed the concept of *attribution* and the possibility of weighting all factors that contribute to a change in health status. Thus, under certain circumstances, the contributions of physicians, nurses, therapists, pharmacists, families, and patients might be identified, measured, and analyzed to determine their impact on outcomes (Donabedian, 2003).

Process includes provider interactions, which are often easier to identify and describe than outcomes. They are also more apt to align with health care guidelines, which tend to focus on what a caregiver does. Process measures may be obtained by documenting the number of procedures billed, the amount of immunizations provided, or the number of patients screened for hypertension. Porter (2010) asserted that the majority of measures currently collected are process measures; and that, while they may reflect current quality standards, they do not necessarily correlate with patient health status. Over time, experts in the field have reached the general consensus that more needs to be done to develop and use valid and reliable patient-centered outcome measures (Cassel et al., 2014; Lee, 2010; Porter, 2010).

An outcome refers to a change in patient health status that results from health care delivered (Donabedian, 1988, 2003). In the earlier example, an outcome measure might refer to disability or death among those patients who were billed for a specific procedure, who received immunizations, or who were screened for hypertension. Donabedian's guidelines for developing outcomes (Donabedian, 2003) are listed in Exhibit 4.1. While appearing straightforward, the guidelines are complex and require a serious commitment of resources. For example, the fourth guideline admonishes the evaluator to monitor outcomes not only for how great a difference an intervention made, but also for how long the change in health status was maintained. And the sixth guideline recommends collecting data for the amount of time it takes for the change to become apparent. The guidelines also include the need to make judgments. The fifth guideline suggests that some individuals will want to trade quantity of life for quality of life and that the individual's desires must be considered. Finally, the cost of the intervention must be considered because dollars spent on evaluating one health care intervention will not be available to spend on another alternative. This is known as an *opportunity cost* and will be discussed in the next chapter.

Donabedian (2003) listed four types of outcomes: (a) alteration in health status; (b) alteration in patient knowledge; (c) alteration in patient or family activities; and (d) patient and family satisfaction. He classified outcomes as clinical, physiological-biochemical, physical, psychological, social, integrative, and evaluative.

---

**EXHIBIT 4.1**

**Guidelines for the Development of Outcomes as an Indicator of Quality**

1. The outcome selected should be relevant to the objective of care; it stands for what the clinician is aiming for.
2. The outcome must be achievable by good care. This means that the methods for this are available and under the control of the health care system.
3. The outcome, whether good or bad, must be attributable first to health care, and then, to the contribution of the practitioner or other person whose performance is being assessed.
4. The duration of the outcome as well as its magnitude should be taken into account.
5. As a corollary, the trade-off between levels and duration of alterative outcomes may be considered. For example, a shorter life at a higher level of function may have to be weighed against a longer life with greater disability.
6. As another corollary, information on the relevant outcome must be available, which is not an easy matter, especially when obtaining the information requires follow-up over long periods.
7. It is necessary to track not only the consequences of taking action but also the consequences of not taking action in order to obtain a complete picture of performance.
8. Finally, the outcome cannot stand alone. The means used to achieve the outcome also have to be considered, unless it is assumed that resources are unlimited, which almost always is far from true.

*Source:* Donabedian (2003). Used with permission.

There are a variety of perspectives through which to view outcomes. Aday, Begley, Lairson, and Balkrishnan (2004) categorized outcomes from a population perspective and a clinical perspective. They further divided clinical outcomes into system, institution, and patient subcategories. An example of a population outcome is the incidence of measles in a city between January 1st and December 31st. In a system or health care facility, the outcome might be the diagnosis of the disease on the first visit. For an individual patient, the outcome may be recovery without sequellae.

Regardless of the perspective, if an intervention involves more than one person, the only way to aggregate and analyze outcomes is to measure them. The following section presents measures that are frequently used in health care evaluation.

## CREATING MEANINGFUL OUTCOME MEASURES

### Measuring Health Care Outcomes

Evaluators quantify health care outcomes using counts, means, or medians. For example, they may calculate the number of adverse events, the mean systolic and diastolic blood pressure, or the median length of hospital stay. They also use proportions and percentages. Proportions are calculated by counting the number of persons with the outcome of interest and dividing that number by the number of all persons treated during a specified period of time (Romano, Hussey, & Ritley, 2010). For example, 600 out of 1,000 patients (60%) surveyed during 2015 at a city hospital said they were satisfied with the care they received during their hospital stay. Other outcomes associated with percentages include symptoms, pressure ulcers, falls, and readmission within 30 days.

Rates, proportions, and ratios are used as measures of disease frequency and are often used to evaluate health outcomes, particularly in large health care facilities, communities, and populations. A description of commonly used frequencies is provided in Table 4.1. Two major types of frequency are prevalence and incidence. Prevalence refers to the proportion or percent of the total number of individuals in a population who are known to have an existing condition at a particular point in time (Greenberg, 2015; Hennekens & Buring, 1987). Prevalence is useful in determining if a chronic condition such as diabetes or cardiovascular disease is becoming more common and in estimating the total number of patients who need treatment.

Cumulative incidence refers to new events in a population at risk during a certain time interval. The population at risk is defined as all members of that population who are susceptible to the outcome of interest. For instance, a member of the population that is a prevalent case is not at risk of becoming an incident (i.e., new) case. Incidence rates are essential to studies of causes of disease because they are used to make inferences about risk or probability of disease (Greenberg, 2015; Hennekens & Buring, 1987).

Morbidity and mortality are particular types of incidence. Morbidity refers to the appearance of diagnosable disease and mortality refers to death. All-cause mortality, cause-specific mortality, and case fatality provide different kinds of information. All-cause mortality includes everyone who died in

**TABLE 4.1   Selected Measures Used in Evaluating Treatment Outcomes**

| Measure | Description |
| --- | --- |
| Cumulative incidence | $$\frac{\text{Number of new occurrences in a population}}{\text{All individuals at risk in the population}}$$ |
| Prevalence | $$\frac{\text{Number of persons who have an existing condition}}{\text{Entire population}}$$ |
| All-cause mortality | $$\frac{\text{Number of persons who died from all causes}}{\text{All persons in the population}}$$ |
| Cause-specific mortality | $$\frac{\text{Number of persons who died from a specific disorder}}{\text{All persons in the population}}$$ |
| Case fatality rate | $$\frac{\text{Number of persons who died from a specific disorder}}{\text{Number of persons with the disorder}}$$ |
| Relative risk | $$\frac{\text{Incidence among persons exposed}}{\text{Incidence among persons not exposed}}$$ |
| Relative risk reduction | 1 *minus* the relative risk |
| Absolute risk reduction | Incidence of outcome in the treated population *minus* the incidence of outcome in the untreated population |
| Number needed to treat | $$\frac{1}{\text{Absolute risk reduction}}$$ |
| Number needed to screen | $$\frac{\text{Number Needed to Treat}}{\text{Disease prevalence}}$$ |

*Sources:* Hennekens and Buring (1987); Kendrach, Covington, McCarthy, and Harris (1997); Rembold (1998).

a specific place during a specific time period divided by the total population. In cause-specific mortality, the numerator includes only those individuals dying from a particular disorder in the total population. In case fatality, the numerator includes the individuals who died from a certain disorder and the denominator includes only those who have the disorder. When calculating the frequency of less common diseases, rates are often multiplied by 1,000, 10,000, or 100,000 so that they may be expressed as a whole number (Greenberg, 2015; Hennekens & Buring, 1987).

Measures of association compare rates in populations to estimate the probable amount of benefit or harm caused by an agent of interest. In *relative risk* (RR), the incidence of a studied event in an exposed population is divided by the incidence in an unexposed population. The exposure may refer to an environmental factor, disorder, diagnostic test, or treatment. A result less than one indicates lower risk (for harm or benefit) and a result greater than one indicates more risk (for harm or benefit) to the exposed population. A value of one indicates that the exposure had little or no effect. The result may be expressed as a percent (Greenberg, 2015; Hennekens & Buring, 1987). For example, compared with a population of adults who were not exposed, a population exposed to a carcinogen over a 5-year period had an RR of 1.07 or a 7% greater risk of developing cancer than those never exposed to the carcinogen. In discussing a benefit of treatment, epidemiologists sometimes refer to *relative risk reduction* (RRR), which is 1-relative risk (Kendrach, Covington, McCarthy, & Harris, 1997). For instance, if 93 of 1,000 patients treated for hypertension go on to have strokes, and 100 of 1,000 untreated patients have strokes, the RR of stroke is 0.93 and the RRR is 1 minus 0.93, which is 7%. This is the percentage of baseline risk that is reduced with treatment.

Absolute risk reduction (ARR) is obtained by subtracting the incidence of an outcome among untreated persons from the incidence among treated persons. ARR, which is generally expressed as a percentage, is a meaningful way to compare the results of randomized controlled trials (RCTs) because it estimates the actual benefit of the experimental treatment to a population. Its magnitude depends on the baseline risk that occurs in the absence of the experimental treatment (Greenberg, 2015; Kendrach et al., 1997). RRR compares only the numerators of risk but ARR compares the denominators as well. RRR would be the same 7% if stroke decreased from 100 to 93 per 1,000 or from 100 to 93 per 100,000, but ARR would fall from 0.07% to 0.00007%.

A measure frequently used along with the ARR is the *number needed to treat (NNT)*. The NNT offers health care providers and decision makers an estimate of the total sum of individuals who must receive an intervention before obtaining a beneficial (or preventing a harmful) result. The NNT (Greenberg, 2015) is the inverse of the ARR (1 divided by ARR).

### Determining the Effectiveness of Treatment

For example, a researcher studying disease X conducts an RCT of an intervention, and finds that subjects given treatment A are less likely to have an unwanted outcome than those given no treatment. This desired result may be expressed as an RR, the incidence of the unwanted outcome among the treated patients divided by the incidence of the unwanted outcome among untreated patients. In this study, 1 out of 1,000 patients treated with medication A have the targeted unwanted outcome during the study period and 5 of 1,000 untreated patients have the unwanted outcome during the same period. The RR for the unwanted outcome is 20% (0.001/0.005) and the RRR is 80% (1 minus 20%). The researcher correctly proclaims that treatment A reduced the risk of disease X by 80%. However, before adopting the treatment a decision maker with finite resources must consider the impact of treatment for other diseases in the same population.

For example, assume that disease Y has the same unwanted outcomes but is more prevalent than disease X. In a similar study of disease Y, 100 of 1,000 patients treated with medication B have the targeted unwanted outcome during the study period, and 500 of 1,000 untreated patients have the unwanted outcome during the same period. The RR for the unwanted outcome is 20% (0.1 for persons on treatment B divided by 0.5 for persons not receiving treatment). The RRR is 80% (1 minus 20%). Both results seem equally positive, and may be reported so, but to a society considering programs based on effectiveness and cost, the impact is different because of the higher prevalence of the unwanted result in the population with disease Y. The risk changed from 0.005 to 0.001 in the study of disease X and 0.5 to 0.1 in the study of disease Y. The ARR for treatment of disease X is 0.004 and the ARR of disease Y is 0.4.

In the first example (disease X), only 4 patients are helped by treatment, but in the second scenario (disease Y) 400 patients benefited because the risk of the unwanted outcome in the 1,000 untreated subjects with diseases X and Y is different. Assuming that the unwanted outcomes of the diseases are similar, a decision maker with limited resources who had to choose between these competing interventions would probably elect to implement the treatment for disease Y because the impact on the population will be greater.

Another way to interpret the data is by using the NNT, which is the inverse of the ARR. In disease Y, the ARR is 0.4 and the NNT is 2.5 (1 divided by 0.4). This means that only 2.5 patients need to receive treatment B before one unwanted outcome is prevented. Practically, if 1,000 patients are treated, 400 patients will avoid the unwanted outcome. Applying the NNT with disease X (with an ARR of 0.004 and an NNT of 1/0.004 or 250), 1,000 patients need to receive treatment A in order for four patients to avoid an unwanted outcome. Thus, 250 patients need treatment to save one patient, and after 1,000 treatments only four patients benefit. A decision maker may consider not only the impact of the interventions but also the cost. If the cost of treatment is $10,000 for both disease X and disease Y, a patient with disease Y can be saved from the unwanted outcome for $25,000 but society would need to spend $2,500,000 to prevent an unwanted outcome with disease X. The price of the proposed intervention multiplied by the NNT determines the cost of the benefit but, of course, high NNT may be tolerable for inexpensive interventions.

These calculations depend on evidence-based data, usually from one or more RCTs about a disorder with a known prevalence, treated in a specified manner to avoid a specific unwanted outcome. Calculating the NNT is only useful if the source studies are well conducted and comparable (Greenberg, 2015).

## Measuring Screening Outcomes

Screening involves testing individuals who seem healthy now, to find out if they may have a disorder that has not yet been diagnosed but can be cured or helped with treatment before symptoms develop. According to Wilson and Jungner (1968), screening can be universal (all individuals are screened) or focused (only individuals at high risk are screened). Screening is not diagnostic. There will be, depending on the screening test, a few or many persons with positive results who are later found not to have the disorder. And, depending on the test, there will be a few or many persons with negative results who are later diagnosed with the disorder when they manifest symptoms. There are specific measures that apply to all screening tests that can be used to evaluate validity and reliability. Knowing how these measures work together will help the DNP evaluate and compare screening programs.

Every screening test has four possible outcomes. A positive test result is a *true positive (TP)* if, after diagnostic follow-up, an individual is found to have the disorder. A positive test result is a *false positive (FP)* if, after diagnostic follow-up, an individual is found not to have the disorder. A negative test result is *true negative (TN)* if an individual does not go on to develop the disorder. A negative test is *false negative (FN)* if, despite the negative result, an individual develops symptoms and is found to have the disorder (Greenberg, 2015; Guyatt, Sackett, & Haynes, 2006; Hennekens & Buring, 1987).

### Determining the Effectiveness of Screening

Let us assume that there is a chronic condition called beta disorder that children develop early in life. Beta disorder occurs in an estimated 1/5,000 young children and causes seizures. There is no easy way to establish if some children are at higher risk for the disorder than others. A screening test becomes available that measures the amount of beta micrograms in the blood. If there are 75 or more micrograms, the test is positive. If there are less than 75 mcg per deciliter, the test is negative. A positive screen can be confirmed and the disorder diagnosed with additional blood tests and with magnetic resonance imaging (MRI). The diagnosed disorder is treatable with daily injections.

A universal screening program becomes available and all parents are encouraged to have their children tested before 12 months of age. As Table 4.2 indicates, out of 1,000,000 children screened, 10,196 children tested positive for the disorder, including 198 children who after follow-up with further blood tests and an MRI were diagnosed with beta disorder (TP) and 9,998 children who after further diagnostic tests were found to be healthy (FP). There were 989,804 children who tested negative for the disorder, including 989,802 children who never developed the disorder (TN) and 2 children who later developed symptoms and were subsequently diagnosed with beta disorder (FN).

*Sensitivity* is the chance that a child with the disorder has a positive test. It is calculated by counting the number of children who had TP tests and dividing it by the number of children tested who went on to be diagnosed with the disorder. The sensitivity of the beta screening test was 99%. *Specificity* is the chance that a child without the disorder had a negative test. It is calculated by counting the number of children who had TN tests and dividing it by the number of children tested who did not have the disorder. The specificity of the beta test was 99%. *Positive predictive*

### TABLE 4.2 Results of a Screening Program to Identify Children With Beta Disorder

| Screening Test | Beta Disorder Present | Beta Disorder Absent | Total |
|---|---|---|---|
| Positive | 198 | 9,998 | 10,196 |
| Negative | 2 | 989,802 | 989,804 |
| **Total** | **200** | **999,800** | **1,000,000** |

| Screening Measures | | | Results |
|---|---|---|---|
| Sensitivity = TP/TP + FN = 198/198 + 2 | | | 99% |
| Specificity = TN/TN + FP = 989,802/989,802 + 9,998 | | | 99% |
| Positive predictive value = TP/TP + FP = 198/198 + 9,998 | | | 1.9% |
| Negative predictive value = TN/TN + FN = 989,802/989,802 + 2 | | | 99.9% |

*value* is the chance that a child with a positive test has the disorder. It is calculated by counting the number of children who had a TP test and dividing it by the number of all children with positive tests. The positive predictive value of the beta test was 1.9%. *Negative predictive value* is the chance that a child with a negative test did not have the disorder. It is calculated by counting the number of children who had a TN test and dividing it by the number of all children with negative tests. The negative predictive value of the beta test was 99.9% (Greenberg, 2015; Guyatt et al., 2006; Hennekens & Buring, 1987).

Both sensitivity and specificity should be as close to 100% as possible, although they tend to have an inverse association. The beta screening test had a high sensitivity (99%) and specificity (99%) and negative predictive value (99.9%). However, the test had a low positive predictive value of 1.9%, which means that the chance of a positive test accurately predicting the presence of the disorder was extremely small. As a consequence, the concerned parents of the 9,998 children with FP screening results may spend time and money taking their perfectly healthy children for follow-up blood tests and MRIs that were not needed. Positive predictive values tend to be small when the prevalence of the screened-for disorder in a population is low (Greenberg, 2015; Hennekens & Buring, 1987).

Recently, there has been interest in applying the concept of NNT to screening for more common adult disorders whose risks lie dormant in the population (Rembold, 1998). This introduces another layer of complexity but can yield useful public health information if done correctly. Number needed to screen (NNS) is the NNT derived from an RCT of treatment in the targeted disease divided by the prevalence of undiagnosed target cases in the population. To apply NNS, an evaluator needs a reliable estimate of the prevalence of undetected target disease in the general population as defined by the same diagnostic criteria that were used to include subjects in the reference RCT. Using the number of positive screens in the asymptomatic population is not recommended, because screens typically find many mild cases that may not have the same outcome risk that subjects in the RCT had.

Let us use disease Y, discussed in the prior section, as an example. With an ARR of 0.4 and an NNT of 2.5, treating the disease is beneficial, but there is a problem. Very few affected people know they have the disease in time for treatment to help. Assume that a blood test is developed that can identify 100% of the affected individuals (not likely, but for simplicity) at a cost of $10 per screen. A study of 1,000 randomly chosen subjects finds 21 individuals who would have qualified for the study, and that only one of these knew he had the problem. The researchers assume that screening 1,000 individuals will identify 20 new individuals (2%) who might benefit from treatment. In this example, 2% of the population has undiagnosed treatable disease Y during a specific time period. Based on the NNT of 2.5 from the treatment RCT and the 2% prevalence of undiagnosed cases, the NNS is 125 (2.5 divided by 0.02). This is the number of people from the general population who must be screened and, if positive, treated to save one person from the targeted bad outcome.

Determining the effectiveness of a screening test is complex, involving issues intrinsic to the test and to the natural history of the target disease. The results of a screening test are not definitive but must be confirmed by further study. No screen has only TPs and TNs; and even if a test has a 99% sensitivity and specificity there remains much work to be done in clearing FPs and FNs. Screening is not meant to diagnose a disorder but only to identify individuals who *may* have it. Buried in the statistics of sensitivity and specificity are technical aspects of the applied test, principally expressed as validity and reliability.

Discussions of validity and reliability are about how confident we can be acting on the test data. Validity refers to the accuracy of the test method in detecting its target indicator. In the earlier pediatric screening example, this would be the test's accuracy in finding a beta level of 75 mg/dL as assessed by repeated measurement of known standards, and not by its ability to diagnose the target disease. Reliability is the ability of a specific test to reproduce the same result every time within one and repeated assays, which is of course influenced by test method and operator skill. For a test to be reliable, everyone involved must conduct the screen using the same methods. When those conducting the tests vary in their amount of training, experience, and expertise, it is hard to know how confident to be about the results. Vision screening conducted in a school setting is one example. When testing is done by volunteers, school nurses, or optometrists, each using slightly different methods, reliability may be questionable (Powell & Hatt, 2009).

Besides understanding the test methods, one must know the natural history of the target disease. In addition to identifying the treatable disease, many screening tests also pick up previously unseen mild forms of the disorder which may not need treatment, or abnormalities that will never progress to disease status. Deciding whether treatment might be beneficial or harmful can be difficult for the provider and anxiety producing for the patient in cases where the natural history is insufficiently understood (Welch, 2015). Screening may help to answer our questions about the natural history of the disease but such screening may come under the purview of research.

Another important consideration related to an understanding of the target disease is the availability of treatment. The DNP should be able to assure individuals that treatment is available for those with a positive screen and diagnosis. If treatment is unavailable, the ethical issues of screening become more complex. Screening may be done for genetic counselling to the patient's benefit or for research, and the DNP should be clear about the primary purpose of the screening test.

Further, consider whether treatment initiated at an asymptomatic stage of the disease process leads to better outcomes than treatment initiated after the disease becomes clinically apparent. Finally, if physical symptoms of a condition can be easily identified and treatment started without a screening test, then screening makes no difference (Wilson & Jungner, 1968). Every intervention has risk and screening is no exception.

## A MAZE OF MEASURES

During the last 10 years, the U.S. health care system has made great progress in creating quality measures (Scott & Jha, 2014). In fact, thousands of measures have been described. Meyer et al. (2012) concluded that this proliferation of quality measures is a costly endeavor and threatens to dilute their influence on health care. Cassel et al. (2014) observed that while over 500 measures were used by state and regional entities, 80% of them were applied in only one program. They recommended that health care evaluators collaborate in developing a limited set of metrics that are balanced and targeted to provide information critical to quality improvement.

One way to control the growing maze of measures is to organize them into coherent and manageable domains. Fortunately, the quality domains described by the IOM in *Crossing the Quality Chasm* (2001) appear to meet this need. Safe, timely, effective, efficient, equitable, and patient-centered health care has become the sine qua non of quality improvement. The IOM domains are widely accepted by health care facilities, providers, governmental agencies, and consumers as theoretically sound and practical (Greenberg, 2015; Sadeghi et al., 2013). They have been incorporated into the Triple Aim framework (Institute for Healthcare Improvement, 2015) and serve as a framework for research studies. Used in conjunction with Donabedian's approaches of structure–process–outcome, they can facilitate a comprehensive and comprehensible evaluation of health care (Greenberg, 2015).

## SOURCES OF MEASURES

There are numerous online resources that provide valid and reliable quality measures that may be used in a variety of settings. Perhaps the most inclusive resource is the NQMC (www.qualitymeasures.ahrq.gov). The NQMC is an enterprise supported by AHRQ and the U.S. Department of Health and Human Services. It provides a website with information including tutorials on such topics as establishing the validity of quality measures and deciding which outcome metrics are appropriate for specific health care settings (Sadeghi et al., 2013).

In describing the essential characteristics of quality measures, the NQMC recommended that they (a) respond to a situation that needs improvement, cover a variety of demographic groups, and be significant to stakeholders, providers, public health officials, and patients; (b) have a foundation in clinical evidence; (c) be valid, reliable, understandable, and permit case-mix adjustment; and (d) have available data sources and clear, precise methodologies. Data sources for measures include electronic health records, surveys, imaging and laboratory data, organizational protocols, provider attributes, public health, and registry information (Greenberg, 2015; NQMC, 2015a).

Risk adjustment is a critical consideration in outcome measurement. Individuals receiving health care vary by age, gender, socioeconomic status, race/ethnicity, education, and so on, and these demographic variables impact how patients respond to health care. Comorbidities must be taken into account as they make treatment more complex and sometimes less effective. In cases with a wide variety of risks, large sample sizes are needed to calculate meaningful outcome measures (Aday et al., 2004; NQMC, 2015a; Porter, 2010).

In addition to providing information, the NQMC contains an extensive database of quality measures. The database is an outgrowth of prior AHRQ programs that offered consumers, providers, hospitals, and agencies a central location for accessing valid and reliable quality metrics. The Computerized Needs-Oriented Quality Measurement Evaluation System (CONQUEST) and the Expansion of Quality of Care Measures (C-SPAN) are two of the measure sets found on the NQMC site.

The NQMC has two main groups of measures: those related to health care delivery and those related to population health. A structure–process–outcome

**EXHIBIT 4.2**

**Example of Measures From the National Quality Measures Clearinghouse**

Primary Measure Domain

| Institute of Medicine | Structure | Process | Outcome |
|---|---|---|---|
| Effectiveness domain | "Percent of clinicians who have education and training regarding palliative care concepts." (McCusker et al., 2013) | "Percent of adult patients with a serious illness who have a symptom assessment documented in the medical record." (McCusker et al., 2013) | "Percent of 4-hour intervals (on Day Zero and Day One) of ICU admission for which the documented pain score was less than or equal to 3." (VHA, Inc., 2006) |

Adapted from NQMC (2015b).

approach is used in both groups of measures and the description of quality is derived from the IOM. Efficiency is incorporated as an aspect of quality measurement because in any realistic appraisal the use of resources must be considered. Measures included in the database must meet a rigorous screening process to ensure that they are current, evidence-based, valid, and reliable (NQMC, 2015a).

The site contains thousands of measures listed under a number of categories including topic, organization, domain, and endorsement by the National Quality Forum. One of the most useful tools on the site is a matrix that allows users to select among numerous domains those in which they are most interested. An example using the domains "Institute of Medicine" and "Primary Measure" is presented in Exhibit 4.2. Primary measures represent the main focus of an intervention as opposed to secondary measures, which represent a subordinate focus. The structure–process–outcome measures in the exhibit relate to palliative care for adults (NQMC, 2015b).

## COMPARATIVE EFFECTIVENESS RESEARCH

RCTs may establish that an intervention is efficacious under ideal conditions, but most health care is not provided under ideal conditions. An objective of CER is to evaluate alternative interventions in order to determine the most effective means available to improve health outcomes in actual health care settings (IOM, 2009). The aim is to disseminate the evidence-based findings to practitioners, patients, consumers, stakeholders, and policy makers who will then use the knowledge to make informed decisions about health care. The methodology of CER includes clinical trials, observational studies, secondary data analysis, meta-analysis, literature synthesis, and computer modeling (Kaiser Family Foundation, 2009; Titler & Pressler, 2011).

A good example of CER is a study by Voss et al. (2011) in which the authors applied the findings of a prior RCT (Coleman, Parry, Chalmers, & Min, 2006) to their own clinical setting. The RCT had established the efficacy of care transition interventions among a sample of Medicare patients who had been admitted to a health care facility with diagnoses of cardiac or respiratory disorders. The intervention included a transition coach who visited patients at the hospital and at home, and followed up with telephone calls. The setting was an integrated hospital system. The outcome was 30-day readmission.

Voss et al. sought to determine the effectiveness of the same intervention by applying it in nonintegrated hospital settings using a quasi-experimental prospective cohort design. The study group consisted of 257 fee-for-service Medicare patients who were compared with internal controls ($n = 736$) and external controls ($n = 14,514$). Results indicated that 12.8% of patients who received the transition intervention were readmitted within 30 days compared with 18.6% in the internal and 20% in the external control group. The authors concluded that these significant findings provided good evidence that care transition interventions were effective in a real-world health care setting.

In another interesting example, Xian et al. (2015) studied the link between warfarin treatment and outcomes among elderly patients who experienced ischemic stroke and atrial fibrillation. Based on the results of RCTs, clinical guidelines support the use of warfarin, but questions remained regarding its benefit in older populations and those at increased risk for hemorrhage. The researchers used an observational design and registry data. During the entire study process, they consulted groups of patients about outcomes that were most important to them. The study was sponsored by the Patient-Centered Outcomes Research Institute (PCORI).

The study population included 12,552 persons discharged to the community from 1,487 hospitals during a 3-year period. The mean age of the 11,039 persons (88% of the study population) in the warfarin treatment group was 80.1, compared with 83.1 in the group with no anticoagulation treatment. Results indicated that warfarin significantly increased both the amount of patient time at home and time without a major cardiovascular event. There was also a significant decrease in all-cause mortality. These findings were apparent even among the most elderly patients, females, and those who had experienced devastating strokes. Providers sometimes hesitate in prescribing warfarin to these groups, thinking that the medication places them at higher risk. However, this study demonstrated in an actual community setting that warfarin was effective for these patients.

PCORI, established in 2010, continues to support CER by increasing the number and quality of patient-centered comparison studies, disseminating results, encouraging implementation of findings in a timely manner, and persuading other entities to support research that is shown to be beneficial in a real-world setting. Through September 2013, PCORI committed more than $300 million in funding to studies that addressed national priorities including the assessment of prevention, diagnosis, and treatment alternatives for health problems ($116 million), the improvement of health care systems ($77 million), the communication and dissemination of health care research ($42 million), addressing disparities in access and treatment ($52 million), and increasing the rate of patient outcome and methodological research ($28 million). In September 2014, the PCORI Board of Governors approved the recommended FY2015 budget of $463 million to support new research studies and to sustain current programs. PCORI administrators anticipate that $1.5 billion in funding will be provided to researchers between 2014 and 2017 (Gabriel & Normand, 2012; Newhouse, Barksdale, & Miller, 2015; PCORI, 2014; Selby & Lipstein, 2014).

## CHALLENGES TO QUALITY MEASUREMENT

Developing health care quality measures is a work in progress. The Affordable Care Act and PCORI provide enormous incentives to develop and use valid and reliable measures to improve health status, but there is a long way to go before their recommendations are realized. Some of the biggest challenges are discussed here.

First, as noted earlier, evaluators can lose their way amid the maze of measurements and methods. There are thousands of quality measures; some are valid, reliable, evidence based, and transparent, and some are not. Some measures evaluate quality improvement on the margins instead of measuring the total effect on health status (Cassel et al., 2014). Some measures overlap. At times, evaluators seem to miss the big picture of quality as a change in patient health status while focusing on the individual pixels of care (Sadeghi et al., 2013).

The sheer number of measures used internally by health care entities, and mandated by external regulatory agencies, insurance companies, and other payers, has increased the cost of quality improvement activities. It is estimated that some systems spend 1% of net patient revenue on these activities. Administrators and policy makers have called for the development of a critical but limited cluster of quality measures for submission to external agencies. This would allow health entities to spend a larger portion of their quality improvement budget on applying measures most specific to their current needs for quality improvement (Cassel et al., 2014; Meyer et al., 2012).

Second, the difficulty in linking structure–process–outcome still exists, and as measures proliferate the problem will only worsen. One cannot simply assume that a compliant administration policy or provider performance produces a good patient outcome unless the association is identified, described, and measured. If a linkage of structure–process–outcome is established and the outcome is positive, the cause of the success can clearly be recognized. Conversely, if the outcome is not positive, one can trace back to process and structure to identify the problem (Donabedian, 2003).

A third challenge is the difficulty in attributing outcomes to particular activities or persons. Outcomes are not physician outcomes or nursing outcomes; they are patient outcomes. Today, health care is delivered by a system that includes administrators, health care professionals, ancillary health personnel, families, and patients (Sadeghi et al., 2013). Weighting the contribution of each of these entities is difficult. There have been attempts to use algorithms or modeling to weight each contribution to a patient outcome (Titler, Shever, Kanak, Picone, & Qin, 2011), but even if weighting could be apportioned, the attribution might still vary among individual providers, facilities, and geographic locations. So far, national guidelines for delineating attribution are not available (Romano et al., 2010).

The challenges are great but DNPs along with policy makers, patients, and other health professionals are making good strides toward quality improvement.

And, as long as the focus remains on the destination, outcomes will continue to improve. As noted in *Crossing the Quality Chasm*, "Perfect care may be a long way off, but much better care is within our grasp" (IOM, 2001, p. 20).

## REFERENCES

Aday, L. A., Begley, C. E., Lairson, D. R., & Balkrishnan, R. (2004). *Evaluating the healthcare system* (3rd ed.). Chicago, IL: Health Administration Press.

Cassel, C. K., Conway, P. H., Delbanco, S. F., Jha, A. K., Saunders, R. S., & Lee, T. H. (2014). Getting more performance from performance measurement. *New England Journal of Medicine, 371*(23), 2145–2147.

Chassin, M. R., & Loeb, J. M. (2011). The ongoing quality improvement journey: Next stop, high reliability. *Health Affairs, 30*(4), 559–568.

Chin, M. H. (2014). How to achieve health equity. *New England Journal of Medicine, 371*(24), 2331–2332.

Coleman, E. A., Parry, C., Chalmers, S., & Minn, S. J. (2006). The care transitions intervention: Results of a randomized controlled trial. *Archives of Internal Medicine, 166*(17), 1822–1828.

Donabedian, A. (1966). Evaluating the quality of medical care. *Milbank Memorial Fund Quarterly, 44*(Suppl. 3), 166–206.

Donabedian, A. (1988). The quality of care. How can it be assessed? *JAMA, 260*(12), 1743–1749.

Donabedian, A. (2003). *An introduction to quality assurance in health care.* Oxford, UK: Oxford University Press.

Gabriel, S. E., & Normand, S. -L. T. (2012). Getting the methods right—the foundation of patient-centered outcomes research. *New England Journal of Medicine, 367*(9), 787–790.

Greenberg, R. S. (2015). *Medical epidemiology, population health and effective health care* (5th ed.). New York, NY: McGraw Hill Education.

Guyatt, G. H., Sackett, D. L., & Haynes, R. B. (2006). Evaluating diagnostic tests. In R. B. Haynes, D. L. Sackett, G. H. Guyatt, & P. Tugwell (Eds.), *Clinical epidemiology* (3rd ed., pp. 273–322). Philadelphia, PA: Lippincott Williams & Wilkins.

Hennekens, C. H., & Buring, J. E. (1987). *Epidemiology in medicine.* Boston, MA: Little, Brown and Company.

Institute for Healthcare Improvement. (2015). *Initiatives.* Retrieved from http://www.ihi.org/Engage/Initiatives/TripleAim/pages/default.aspx

Institute of Medicine. (2001). *Crossing the quality chasm: A new health system for the 21st century.* Washington, DC: National Academies Press.

Institute of Medicine. (2009). *Initital national priorities for comparative effectiveness research.* Washington, DC: National Academies Press.

Kaiser Family Foundation. (2009, October). Explaining health reform: What is comparative effectiveness research? *Focus on Health Reform.* Retrieved from https://kaiserfamilyfoundation.files.wordpress.com/2013/01/7946.pdf

Kendrach, M. G., Covington, T. R., McCarthy, M. W., & Harris, M. C. (1997). Calculating risks and number-needed-to-treat: A method of data interpretation. *Journal of Managed Care Pharmacy, 3*(2), 179–183.

Lee, T. H. (2010). Putting the value framework to work. *New England Journal of Medicine, 363*(26), 2481–2483.

Mariner, W. R. (1994). Patients' rights to care under Clinton's Health Security Act: The structure of reform. *American Journal of Public Health, 84*(8), 1330–1335.

McCusker, M., Ceronsky, L., Crone, C., Epstein, H., Greene, B., Halvorson, J., ... Setterlund L. (2013). *Palliative care for adults.* Bloomington, MN: Institute for Clinical Systems Improvement (ICSI).

Meyer, G. S., Nelson, E. C., Pryor, D. B., James, B., Swensen S. J., Kaplan, G. S., . . . Hunt, G. C. (2012). More quality measures versus measuring what matters: A call for balance and parsimony. *BMJ Quality & Safety, 21,* 964–968. doi:10.1136/bmjqs-2012-001081

National Quality Measures Clearinghouse. (2015a). *Tutorials on quality measures.* Retrieved from http://www.qualitymeasures.ahrq.gov/tutorial/

National Quality Measures Clearinghouse. (2015b). *Matrix.* Retrieved from http://www .qualitymeasures.ahrq.gov/matrix.aspx

Newhouse, R., Barksdale, D. J., & Miller, J. A. (2015). The Patient-Centered Outcomes Research Institute, research done differently. *Nursing Research, 64*(1), 72–77.

PCORI. (2014, September 16). *PCORI Board approves 2015 budget and release of draft proposal on peer review for public comment.* Retrieved from http://www.pcori.org/news-release/pcori-board-approves-2015-budget-and-release-draft-proposal-peer-review-public-comment

Porter, M. E. (2010). What is value in health care? *New England Journal of Medicine, 363*(26), 2477–2481.

Powell, C., & Hatt, S. R. (2009). Vision screening for amblyopia in childhood (review). *The Cochrane Collaboration.* Retrieved from http://www.conchranelibrary.com DOI:10.1002/14651858. CD005020.pub3

Rembold, C. M. (1998). Number needed to screen: Development of a statistic for disease screening. *BMJ, 317,* 307–312.

Romano, P., Hussey, P., & Ritley, D. (2010). *Selecting quality and resource use measures: A decision guide for community quality collaboratives* (AHRQ Publication No. 09(10)-0073). Retrieved from http:// www.ahrq.gov/professionals/quality-patient-safety/quality-resources/tools/perfmeasguide/ index.html

Sadeghi, S., Barzi, A., Mikhail, O., & Shabot, M. M. (2013). *Improving quality and strategy.* Burlington, MA: Jones & Bartlett Learning.

Scott, K. W., & Jha, A. K. (2014). Putting quality on the global health agenda. *New England Journal of Medicine, 371*(1), 3–5.

Selby, J. V., & Lipstein, S. H. (2014). PCORI at 3 years—Progress, lessons, and plans. *New England Journal of Medicine, 370*(7), 592–595.

Titler, M. G., & Pressler, S. J. (2011). Advancing effectiveness science: An opportunity for nursing. *Research and Theory for Nursing Practice: An International Journal, 25*(2), 75–79.

Titler, M. G., Shever, L. L., Kanak, M. F., Picone, D. M., & Qin, R. (2011). Factors associated with falls during hospitalization in an older adult population. *Research and Theory for Nursing Practice, 25*(2), 127–148.

VHA Inc. (2016). *TICU care and communication bundle: Care and communication quality measures.* Irving, TX: Author.

Voss, R., Gardner, R., Baier, R., Butterfield, K., Lehrman, S., & Gravenstein, S. (2011). The care transitions intervention, translating from efficacy to effectiveness. *Archives of Internal Medicine, 171*(14), 1232–1237.

Welch, G. (2015). *Less medicine, more health.* Boston, MA: Beacon Press.

Wilson, J. M., & Jungner, G. (1968). *Principles and practice of screening for disease, Public Health Papers 34.* Geneva, Switzerland: World Health Organization.

Xian, Y., Wu, J., O'Brien, E. C., Fonarow, G. C., Olson, D. W., Schwamm, L. H., . . . Hernandez, A. F. (2015). Real world effectiveness of warfarin among ischemic stroke patients with atrial fibrillation: observational analysis from Patient-Centered Research into Outcomes Stroke Patients Prefer and Effectiveness Research (PROSPER) study. *BMJ, 351,* 1–8. doi:101136/bmj.h3786

# CHAPTER FIVE

# ECONOMIC EVALUATION

Christine A. Brosnan and J. Michael Swint

> *There can be economy only when there is efficiency.*
> —*Benjamin Disraeli*

Doctors of nursing practice (DNPs) are being encouraged to assume greater responsibility in determining the economic efficiency of health care interventions, programs, and delivery systems. The American Association of Colleges of Nursing's (AACN, 2006) *The Essentials of Doctoral Education for Advanced Nursing Practice* directed the DNP to "evaluate the cost effectiveness of care and use principles of economics and finance to redesign effective and realistic care delivery strategies . . . [and] design, direct, and evaluate quality improvement methodologies to promote safe, timely, effective, efficient, equitable, and patient-centered care."

This chapter discusses the increasing importance of economic evaluation, also known as efficiency evaluation, in the provision of health care (Drummond, Sculpher, Torrance, O'Brien, & Stoddart, 2005). The chapter explores the application of economic principles in comparing health care cost and outcomes at the macroeconomic and microeconomic levels. The chapter also reviews the essential concepts and assumptions that support the economic evaluation of health care interventions and programs. The implications of *utility theory* and its impact on health care decisions are discussed. Approaches to valuing health status, including *quality adjusted life years* (QALYs), are explained.

Key terms that provide the basis for different types of economic evaluation are provided in Table 5.1. The chapter reviews the importance of establishing a *perspective* when planning an economic evaluation and discusses the need to *discount* costs and outcomes that occur in the future. The chapter explains the distinction between *costs* and *charges*, and discusses why the addition of a *sensitivity analysis* is generally recommended after the results of an efficiency analysis are determined.

This chapter familiarizes the DNP with frequently used methods of evaluating health care outcomes along with examples of their application. The implications of the Affordable Care Act (ACA) on health care financing and comparative effectiveness research (CER) are described. The role of the DNP in applying and participating in economic evaluations is discussed. The chapter presents a guide for critiquing economic evaluations.

**TABLE 5.1 Definition of Economic Terms**

| Term | Definition |
|---|---|
| Charge | The amount of money an institution bills for an item or service (Finkler, 1982). |
| Cost | The amount of resources used to produce an item or service (Finkler, 1982). |
| Cost-benefit analysis | A comparison evaluation of two or more interventions in which costs and end points are calculated in dollars (Drummond, Sculpher, Torrance, O'Brien, & Stoddart, 2005; Torrance, Siegel, & Luce, 1996). |
| Cost-effectiveness analysis | A comparison evaluation of two or more interventions in which costs are calculated in dollars and end points are calculated in health-related units (Drummond et al., 2005; Garber, Weinstein, Torrance, & Kamlet, 1996). |
| Cost-utility analysis | A comparison evaluation of two or more interventions in which costs are calculated in dollars and end points are calculated in quality of life units (Drummond et al., 2005; Torrance et al., 1996). |
| Direct cost | The money paid for health care (Luce, Manning, Siegel, & Lipscomb, 1996). |
| Discounting | The calculation of the current value of future costs that is applied to the results of the cost analysis (Muennig, 2008). |
| Incremental cost | The extra cost and outcome produced by the intervention of interest vs. an alternative intervention or no intervention at all (Drummond et al., 2005). |
| Opportunity cost | Represents the value of benefits lost when investment in one intervention precludes investment in another alternative that might be more helpful (Russell, Gold, et al., 1996; Russell, Siegel, et al., 1996). |
| Sensitivity analysis | A comparison of a range of costs and end points applied to the results of a study because methods used in the economic analysis were not exact (Manning, Fryback, & Weinstein, 1996; Weinstein, Siegel, Gold, Kamlet, & Russell, 1996). |
| Perspective | A point of view that reflects the scope of economic responsibility and benefits; it establishes the extent of cost and end point data that must be collected (Russell, Gold, et al., 1996a; Russell, Siegel, et al., 1996). |
| Quality adjusted life year | An end point that combines the probability of quantity of life and quality of life years (Drummond et al., 2005). |
| Utility | The preference that individuals have for a specific end point(s) (Drummond et al., 2005). |

## VALUING HEALTH STATUS

There are basic items that we all value and for which we are generally willing to pay. These items include shelter, food, clothing, and health care. How much each person is willing to pay depends not only upon the resources available, but also on the value that is attached to a specific item. One person may spend 10% of the family budget on clothing, leaving 90% available for other necessities. Another person may feel compelled to spend 30% on clothing, leaving 70% available for necessities. People recognize that their budgets are limited and so they must prioritize their needs, determine their expenses, and adjust their allocations. There is always the risk that those spending 30% on clothing will wind up looking worse than those spending 10%, but that is the chance that they are willing to take. Economists refer to the preference that people have for a particular end point or end points as their *utility* (Drummond et al., 2005).

Individuals also value health status and are willing to pay for staying healthy and, if they are sick, to pay for effective treatment. However, the path to obtaining preferred health outcomes is not as straightforward as it is for other preferences. Treatment A may be much more costly than Treatment B and the effectiveness of each may not be clear. Even if Treatment A has been shown to be more effective than Treatment B, some individuals may not be able to afford it. Traditionally, society has acknowledged the benefits of a healthy population and has tried to provide essential health care services for those who did not have the means to pay for them, although significant inequities in the availability of health care services exist in the United States.

Over time it has become clear that the amount of money available to spend on health care is finite, and that spiraling costs pose a threat to society. Hiatt (1975) discussed this problem in the context of a "medical commons," the term *commons* referring to a public area used for grazing cattle (Hardin, 1968). In this example, each farmer wanted to use as much of the commons as possible to feed his herd. Over time farmers kept placing additional cattle onto the commons. The herds grew fat and the farmers prospered, but the unrestricted use eventually resulted in overgrazing and the ultimate destruction of the commons.

Hiatt observed that we inhabit a medical commons in which all individuals want to purchase as much health care as they feel they need. But meeting every individual's perceived need may cost more than society can spend. An unchecked expansion of health spending may eventually mean that society will not be able to provide for other basic items such as education, law enforcement, and defense. Underfunding of these essential items may, in turn, lead to a paradoxical diminishing of our common society's health and welfare (Muennig & Glied, 2010). Some limitation of societal support may be needed, and those purchases with the highest cost and least benefit would be logical targets for elimination. In the last few decades, there have been national initiatives to examine costs associated with health care spending compared with the associated benefits accrued.

## A MACROECONOMIC PERSPECTIVE ON COST AND OUTCOME

As part of its mission, the World Health Organization (WHO) collects health data from over 190 countries and uses standard indicators to compare health care costs and outcomes across nations (2016a). Costs are expressed as the amount and percent of the gross domestic product (GDP) spent on health care. GDP refers to the final market value of all goods and services produced in a country in a given period of time (World Bank, 2011). National leaders analyze GDP over time and compare their own country's GDP to other countries in order to monitor a country's economic well-being. Health status is measured using standard indicators of mortality and morbidity obtained from national registries. The most recent results, which can be found on the WHO website (2016b), provide a rough estimate of the benefits achieved for the amount of resources spent.

A comparison of cost and health status for selected countries is presented in Table 5.2. The cost of health care is expressed in: (a) total international dollars spent for each person and (b) total percent of GDP spent on health care. Purchasing-power parity (PPP) states that the exchange rate between one currency and another is in equilibrium when their domestic purchasing powers at that rate of exchange are equivalent (World Bank, 2011). In other words, it shows how much of a country's currency is needed in that country to buy what $1 would buy in the United States. Health status is expressed by: (a) probability of dying under 5 years of age per 1,000 live births and (b) healthy life expectancy at birth for males and females. In 2013, the United States spent more on health care than each of the other countries listed. With $9,146 in per capita health care spending, the United States was about 2.5 times higher than Japan, Italy, and the United Kingdom, and about twice as high in expenditures as Canada and France. The percent of GDP spent on health care in the United States (17.1%) represented a higher percentage on health spending than the other countries.

Despite this effort, U.S. health outcomes did not appear to reflect the generous health expenditures. In 2013, the United States had the highest child mortality (6.9/1,000) among the countries listed except for Mexico, whose expenditures were $1,061 per capita. Compared with the United States, life expectancy for males and females was higher in Canada, France, Italy, Japan, Switzerland, and the United Kingdom.

These estimates point to the possibility that decision makers in the United States may not always choose the most efficient treatment options. Muennig and Glied (2010) proposed three possible reasons for the discrepancy: (a) spending on expensive health care interventions may be forcing budgetary constraints in effective public health programs; (b) the increased cost of health care results in an increase in insurance premiums that in turn causes a loss of insurance for those who can no longer afford it; and (c) risks associated with unnecessary interventions may result in an increase in adverse events, causing an escalation of morbidity or mortality. While most economically advanced countries have virtually universal coverage, until recently, the United States has been an outlier in this regard. Of course, we must also recognize that the health of the population is significantly affected by the many social determinants of health; for example, an incidence of smoking that remains too high and the obesity epidemic and resultant increase in the incidence of type 2 diabetes mellitus. In addition, we must address the challenge of allocating scarce resources between prevention and cure.

## CONCEPTS AND ASSUMPTIONS

The conceptual basis for economic analysis can be found in social welfare theories, particularly those theories dealing with how utilities are allocated in a society (Weinstein & Stason, 1977). As discussed, we assume that good health care is a desired utility, but the resources available for providing health care are limited. How do we as individuals and groups decide what allocation of health resources will most benefit society?

**TABLE 5.2  Cost and Health Status Indicators for Selected Countries**

| Variable | Year | Country | | | | | | | |
|---|---|---|---|---|---|---|---|---|---|
| | | United States | Canada | Mexico | Japan | Italy | France | United Kingdom | Switzerland |
| **Cost** | | | | | | | | | |
| Per capita, total health expenditures, US$ purchasing-power parity[a] | 2004 | 6,401 | 3,236 | 689 | 2,348 | 2,367 | 3,077 | 2,536 | 3,947 |
| | 2008 | 7,825 | 4,030 | 892 | 2,882 | 3,027 | 3,736 | 3,204 | 4,969 |
| | 2013 | 9,146 | 4,759 | 1,061 | 3,741 | 3,126 | 4,334 | 3,311 | 6,187 |
| Total expenditure on health as a percent of GDP[a] | 2004 | 15.2 | 9.6 | 6.0 | 8.0 | 8.5 | 10.9 | 7.9 | 11.0 |
| | 2008 | 16.1 | 10.0 | 5.8 | 8.6 | 8.9 | 10.9 | 8.8 | 10.3 |
| | 2013 | 17.1 | 10.9 | 6.2 | 10.3 | 9.1 | 11.7 | 9.1 | 11.5 |
| **Effect** | | | | | | | | | |
| Child mortality/ 1,000 <5 years[b] | 2004 | 8.1 | 6.1 | 20.4 | 3.9 | 4.5 | 4.7 | 6.1 | 5.2 |
| | 2008 | 7.7 | 5.8 | 17.9 | 3.4 | 4.1 | 4.3 | 5.6 | 4.7 |
| | 2013 | 6.9 | 5.2 | 14.5 | 2.9 | 3.7 | 4.4 | 4.6 | 4.2 |
| Life expectancy (male/female)[c] | 2004 | 75/80 | 78/82 | 72/77 | 79/86 | 78/84 | 77/84 | 77/81 | 79/84 |
| | 2008 | 75/80 | 78/83 | 73/78 | 79/86 | 79/84 | 78/84 | 78/82 | 80/85 |
| | 2013 | 76/81 | 80/84 | 73/78 | 80/87 | 80/85 | 79/85 | 79/83 | 81/85 |

[a] Cost data available from WHO. Retrieved from www.apps.who.int/gho/data/node.country.country-ITA?lang=en

[b] Child mortality data retrieved from www.childmortality.org/childmortality@unicef.org, September 9, 2015. Estimates generated by the UN Interagency Group for Child Mortality Estimation (IGME) in 2015.

[c] Life expectancy data from WHO. Retrieved from www.apps.who.int/gho/data/view.main.680

Decisions about funding one health care program over another are made every day. At times, decisions are based more on the political environment or popular backing and less on the proven benefit of an intervention. Politics and societal support are important considerations, but decision makers should also consider the most effective use of scarce resources. Health economic evaluations collect, analyze, and synthesize objective information about the cost and outcome of health interventions. An intervention may be a treatment, program, or technology (Muennig, 2008). The evaluator compares two or more alternatives, although in some cases the alternative may be the status quo. Evaluations that do not meet the criteria of comparing both cost and outcomes of two or more interventions are called partial evaluations.

*Willingness-to-pay* (WTP) is one approach economists use when assessing which interventions provide the most benefit to society. In this approach, decisions about allocating health care are influenced by the value of the intervention and what society is prepared to pay. WTP seeks to inform decisions by making objective information about the perceived value and benefit of a treatment or service available to those responsible for making health care choices (Drummond et al., 2005).

It seems obvious that determining the efficiency of an unsuccessful intervention is nonsensical, but it is worth stating again that an intervention must be effective to be cost effective. "If something is not worth doing, it is not worth doing well!" (Drummond et al., 2005, p. 31). Unnecessary or harmful health care not only wastes money and places patients at risk, but it also deprives patients of receiving effective health care because of limited resources.

*Opportunity cost* represents the benefits foregone when using resources for one health care intervention instead of an alternative intervention (Russell, Siegel, et al., 1996). For instance, in considering effective but mutually exclusive interventions (due to budget limitations), the opportunity costs of investing in tuberculosis control instead of investing in diabetes control are the benefits of improved diabetes control that are foregone.

A related concern is that an economic analysis may be viewed as a way to find out how much money a hospital or clinic can make from an intervention. For example, a hospital administrator asks how long a new piece of equipment will take to pay for itself before making a profit. While it is important that hospitals make a profit (as in "no margin, no mission"), the primary focus of an economic analysis is to determine the most efficient way to improve a *patient's health status*, not a *hospital's financial health status* (Porter, 2010).

Establishing the effectiveness of interventions has always presented a challenge to practitioners and researchers (Brook & Lohr, 1985; Buerhaus, 1998; Williamson, 1978). One challenge has been the compatibility of research design and economic analysis. Traditionally, evaluators have relied on randomized controlled trials (RCTs), prospective trials, cohort studies, modeling, and meta-analyses to compare the benefits among alternate interventions (Torrance et al., 1996). Each of these research designs has strengths and limitations. The gold standard of cost-effectiveness studies has been an economic analysis alongside an RCT (Drummond et al., 2005). However, experts caution that the economic results might not be practical because the findings obtained under the ideal conditions of an RCT (the efficacy of an intervention) do not represent the findings obtained under real-world conditions (the effectiveness of an intervention). They also suggest that in many cases the results of an RCT are not generalizable (Adams, McCall, Gray, Orza, & Chalmers, 1992; Drummond et al., 2005; Sloan & Hsieh, 2012).

Muennig (2008) recommended applying the standards as described in the levels of evidence when evaluating the quality of studies (the levels of evidence will be discussed in Chapter 10). Recently, CER has become more popular because in these types of studies researchers attempt to evaluate health care interventions in actual health care settings. Regardless of flaws, using a systematic and objective method to establish the change in health status is preferable to intuition, guess-work, or no method at all.

## A GENERAL DESCRIPTION OF ECONOMIC EVALUATION

There are three types of comparative economic evaluations discussed in this chapter: cost-effectiveness analysis (CEA), cost-utility analysis (CUA), and cost-benefit analysis (CBA). They each represent a full analysis in that the evaluator is describing, measuring, and valuing the costs and outcomes of two or more alternative interventions (Drummond et al., 2005).

Typically, the results of an economic analysis have been presented as a ratio with cost in the numerator and outcome in the denominator. We will discuss some recent modifications to this. A practitioner will not only want to know the cost and outcome of an intervention, but also the *incremental cost effectiveness ratio* (ICER), which represents the incremental cost and incremental outcome of an intervention when compared with one or more interventions. In this context, incremental findings refer to the alteration in cost and outcome produced by the intervention of interest versus the alternative (Drummond et al., 2005). The findings can be represented in the following ratio adapted from Muennig (2008):

$$\frac{\text{Cost of intervention A} - \text{Cost of intervention B}}{\text{Outcome of intervention A} - \text{Outcome of intervention B}}$$

A *CEA* is a comparative evaluation of two or more interventions in which costs are calculated in dollars (or the local currency) and end points are calculated in health-related units. The health-related units may focus on outcomes such as lives saved or years of living saved, or they may focus on clinical indicators achieved, such as a decrease in blood pressure or cholesterol (Drummond et al., 2005; Garber et al., 1996). The results are given in a ratio with costs in the numerator and health-related units in the denominator (Table 5.1). A *CUA* is a comparative evaluation of two or more interventions in which costs are calculated in dollars (or the local currency) and end points are calculated in quality of life units (Drummond et al., 2005; Torrance et al., 1996). Whereas a CEA looks at objective health-related outcomes, in a CUA affected and unaffected individuals are asked how they value the outcomes that were or might be achieved. It is an attempt to incorporate the values of the patient (or potential patient) in the decision-making calculus. Because the denominator is a change in health status, many economists refer to CUA as a type of CEA rather than a different type of analysis (Muennig, 2008; Sloan & Hsieh, 2012). A *CBA* is a comparative evaluation of two or more interventions in which the costs and end points are calculated in dollars (or the local currency). The results are given in a ratio or as dollars saved or lost (Drummond et al., 2005;

Torrance et al., 1996). CUAs and CBAs allow the comparison of investments across alternative interventions (e.g., tuberculosis vs. diabetes), whereas a CEA does not. These three types of analyses are similar comparative evaluations in that all measure costs the same way, but they measure and value outcomes differently. Each method provides a unique type of information that may be useful in helping to answer different questions. Occasionally, alternative interventions are evaluated using all three methods simultaneously.

Sometimes it is impractical or not feasible to conduct a full economic evaluation, and an analyst will choose to conduct a partial evaluation. There are two types of partial evaluations. In the first type, an evaluator describes the cost and/or outcomes of an intervention without a comparison (a cost description, an outcome description, or a cost-outcome description). In the second type, an evaluator compares only the costs of two or more alternatives or only the outcomes of two or more alternatives (Drummond et al., 2005).

Before conducting an economic evaluation, an analyst must first decide on the *perspective* of the analysis. Perspective reflects the scope of economic responsibility for costs and outcomes, and it establishes the extent of cost and end point information that must be collected (Russell, Gold, et al., 1996; Russell, Siegel, et al., 1996). For example, a practitioner who conducted an annual diabetes mellitus screening program for a local health clinic may want to determine the cost and outcomes of the intervention from the perspective of the clinic. Cost information would be limited to clinic expenses and outcomes would be limited to the consequences of the program for the clinic population. On the other hand, a practitioner who conducted a state screening program for lead poisoning in children would take a broader, state-level perspective. The collection of cost information would expand to include societal costs at the state level, which might consist of the cost of blood collection, testing the blood, following up abnormal blood tests, diagnosis, and treatment. Outcomes would expand to include the benefits and risks (if any) of the state screening program on the population of the state. If the perspective of an analysis is not specified, economists use the societal perspective as the default perspective.

Once the perspective of an analysis has been established, the evaluator can begin to collect *cost* data. The evaluator must first decide what costs should be described, measured, and valued. The *ingredients approach* is one method used to make this determination, in which the cost categories of personnel, supplies and equipment, and overhead comprise the components of the cost analysis (Drummond et al., 2005). *Cost* represents the amount of resources used to produce an item or service and is usually lower than the amount presented as the charge for an item or unit of service. It is preferable to apply cost whenever possible as it more closely reflects actual resource usage. *Charge* represents the amount of money a patient is billed for an item or service. In a sense, it is the asking price and may be only roughly related to the actual resources used for the item or unit of service. Hospital and clinic bills may contain expenditures not intrinsic to the cost of the intervention that were added to increase profits or to offset expenditures in another area (Finkler, 1982). However, Medicare payments are based on the estimated cost of an item or health service unit. As a consequence, Medicare reimbursement is a good data source for establishing the value of health care interventions (Muennig, 2008).

All direct costs are generally included in a cost analysis. *Direct costs* may be described as the expenditures paid for health care. *Indirect costs* include productivity losses a patient and family may experience as a result of treatment, including days away from work and time traveled to and from a clinic or hospital (Luce et al., 1996; Muennig, 2008; Sloan & Hsieh, 2012). They may also include other costs, such as the cost to the patient for hiring a caretaker after discharge. Indirect costs may be particularly important to collect when the evaluation takes a societal perspective. Describing, measuring, and valuing indirect costs can be difficult and problematic. If an evaluator decides that the inclusion of indirect costs is not feasible, the exclusion should be noted in the evaluation report.

The cost and consequences of an intervention should be adjusted on the basis of timing differences. The adjustment is made when the cost or consequences of an intervention occur in different time periods. This adjustment process is called *discounting*. It involves calculating the current value of future costs and outcomes, and applying the rate to the results of the analysis. The rationale for discounting is in part the perception that money spent today is worth more to individuals than money spent one or more years from now. Currently, suggested discount rates for the United States range from 3% to 5%. It is not uncommon to discount cost at one rate (e.g., 3%) for the base case and to provide lower and higher rates (e.g., 1% and 5%) for alternative estimations. By varying the rates, an evaluator hopes to offer a range of probable cost approximations (Lipscomb, Weinstein, & Torrance, 1996; Weinstein et al., 1996). In addition to an adjustment for timing, a cost analysis should indicate the country and year of the currency being used (e.g., 2016 U.S. dollars).

There is no perfect economic evaluation. The results of evaluations are frequently approximations because cost and outcome data are uncertain or limited. The result of an analysis that is likely to be the most accurate estimate is referred to as a base case (Russell, Siegel, et al., 1996). Economists then use *sensitivity analysis* to adjust for the imprecision inherent in the process. In a sensitivity analysis, the analyst varies significant parameters (e.g., the discount rate) and cost and outcome information to determine how these changes impact the findings of an economic evaluation (Manning et al., 1996; Muennig, 2008; Weinstein et al., 1996). A sensitivity analysis may indicate that the findings of the evaluation are robust or that one or more components need further investigation.

Economists recommend that, whenever feasible, timing adjustments and sensitivity analyses should be applied to outcomes of care as well as to costs, recalling that costs are opportunity costs or foregone health outcomes (Drummond et al., 2005). When an economic evaluation is completed, the results of the study along with limitations, implications, and recommendations are submitted in a report to decision makers. Economists have developed guidelines for conducting economic evaluations (Exhibit 5.1) that DNPs can use to determine the quality of the studies and the feasibility of applying the results to their practice.

Efficiency should not be the only determining factor in deciding among alternative interventions; rather, it is one of many factors in the evaluation process. Other factors include agency policies, legislative mandates, ethical concerns, and input from the general public and support groups (Brosnan & Swint, 2001).

---

**EXHIBIT 5.1**

**A Guide for Evaluating Economic Studies**

1. Was a well-defined question posed in answerable form?
2. Was a comprehensive description of the competing alternatives given? In other words, can you tell who did what to whom, where, and how often?
3. Was the effectiveness of the programs or services established?
4. Were all the important and relevant costs and consequences for each alternative identified?
5. Were costs and consequences measured accurately in appropriate physical units (e.g., hours of nursing time, number of physician visits, lost work days, gained life years)?
6. Were costs and consequences valued credibly?
7. Were costs and consequences adjusted for differential timing?
8. Was an incremental analysis of costs and consequences of alternatives performed?
9. Was allowance made for uncertainty in the estimates of costs and consequences?
10. Did the presentation and discussion of study results include all issues of concern to users?

Adapted with permission from Drummond et al. (2005).

---

## TYPES OF ECONOMIC EVALUATION

### Cost-Effectiveness Evaluation

As noted, CEA is a comparative evaluation of two or more interventions in which costs are calculated in dollars and outcomes are calculated in health-related units. Cost (the numerator) was discussed in the previous section. This section focuses on health-related units (the denominator), which represent the end points of interventions.

The conceptual models discussed in Chapter 3 and the types of measures described in Chapter 4 provide guidance in selecting appropriate outcome indicators. The primary criterion is that the effectiveness of the intervention has been established. Outcome indicators may be generic or specific to a disease; they may be midterm or long term; they may reference changes in morbidity or mortality. Depending upon the goal, a practitioner may use a number of indicators.

For example, a clinic establishes a program to improve the health status of patients with diabetes mellitus, which is a large segment of the patient population. Intermediate outcomes might be a decrease in blood glucose, decreased hospital admissions, or decreased absence from work. Long-term outcomes may be a decrease in the number of amputations and years of life gained in the patient population. Long-term outcomes are the preferred clinical end points but they may be difficult to obtain. When using intermediate end points, the analyst should establish the correlation between them and long-term end points to the extent possible (Drummond et al., 2005; Torrance et al., 1996).

CEAs are the type of analysis most frequently conducted by nurses (Lämås, Willman, Lindholm, & Jacobsson, 2009) and by other professionals in the health care field. CEAs have several advantages. The information they provide is useful to decision makers who must choose between two or more interventions or programs that have similar end points. Because the method has been so widely applied there are many cost-effectiveness studies that nurses will find useful in their practice.

A disadvantage is that while CEAs provide information about the change in the quantity of patient health status, they do not address the value to the patient of having achieved the change (Torrance et al., 1996). Currently, more health economic analyses are including both cost-effectiveness (quantity) and cost-utility (quantity and quality), and examples that use both types of denominators are described later in this chapter and presented in Table 5.3.

## Cost-Utility Analysis

A CUA is a comparative evaluation of two or more interventions in which costs are calculated in dollars and outcomes are calculated in quality of life units. This section focuses on quality of life units (the denominator of the ratio).

A CUA provides information to decision makers not only about the quantity of the outcome (e.g., years of life gained), but also provides information about how individuals perceive the quality of the life years that were gained (Elnitsky & Stone, 2005; Russell, Gold, et al., 1996). CUA has been described as a type of CEA in which the health unit considers both quantity and quality (Muennig, 2008; Russell, Gold, et al., 1996). There are a number of measures that can be used in a CUA. These include QALYs, disability adjusted life years (DALYs), years of healthy life (YHL), and healthy years equivalent (HYE). The focus of this section is on QALYs because they are the most widely applicable and frequently used measures (Drummond et al., 2005; Russell, Gold, et al., 1996).

The QALY was developed as an attempt to measure and evaluate the effect of a change in health status on quality of life. The value of QALYs generally range from 0 (death) to 1 (completely healthy) depending upon the adjustment made for disease or disability (Drummond et al., 2005; Muennig, 2008). There are a number of methodological issues inherent in measuring quality and each issue is open to debate. As an example, who should measure the quality of life after a bilateral mastectomy—a sample of the general community or a sample of individuals who have had or are deciding whether to have a mastectomy? The answer partly depends upon the nature of the question. If the issue is the allocation of resources to these interventions versus unrelated health care interventions, perhaps those selected to complete an instrument that measures quality should be drawn from the community because the objective is to obtain a societal preference. However, if the question deals with patients' choices among alternative interventions for breast cancer, measuring the impact of disease on quality of life would best be left to individuals who actually are affected by the disease or condition (Gold et al., 1996; Muennig, 2008; Nord, 1994).

There are a variety of economic methods available to measure a preference for one health state compared with another. In general, the methods were developed to calculate the utility of an outcome based on the probability that the outcome will occur (Drummond et al., 2005; Muennig, 2008). The standard gamble is a frequently used economic method that gauges an individual's preference for the certainty of chronic disease compared with a life and death alternative (Figure 5.1). In the standard gamble, the probability of the life and death alternatives are varied until the respondent is indifferent between the alternatives: (a) the uncertainty of a given probability of death or one minus that probability of living in perfect health, as opposed to (b) living in a chronic (but imperfect) health state with certainty.

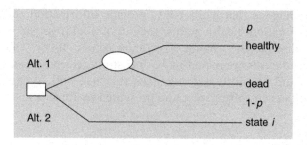

**Figure 5.1** Standard gamble.
Adapted with permission from Drummond et al. (2005).

For example, a patient with mitral valve disease must make a choice. Should the patient have surgery to repair the valve? If otherwise disease free, the surgery might return the patient to perfect health. On the other hand, all surgery has risks and the patient could die during the operation or from surgical complications. Perhaps the patient should elect to do nothing and live within the limitations of the condition? The patient decides that if the chance of dying during surgery is 30% or less, the patient will go ahead with the surgery. If the chance of dying is greater than 30%, then the patient will not have the surgery but will continue in the current health state. At this point, the patient has rated an acceptable quality of life as 70% of perfect health.

In addition to the standard gamble, another commonly used approach is the time trade-off method, in which participants are offered the choice of varying lengths of life in their current imperfect health state versus a shorter length of life in perfect health. Both the standard gamble and the time trade-off method have produced reliable QALY estimates.

There are also a variety of generic and disease-specific health-related quality of life (HRQL) measures that are currently used to calculate quality of life (McDowell & Newell, 1996). A discussion of each is beyond the scope of this chapter, but a few examples are: physical disability measurements (e.g., the Medical Outcomes Study Physical Functioning Measure), social health measurements (e.g., the Social Adjustment Scale), and general health status (e.g., the Short Form-36 Health Survey and the Short Form-12 Health Survey). During the last few decades, QALYs have gained international acceptance as the outcome of choice in economic CUA studies because they comprise a metric for effect and a preference for that effect (Iglehart, 2010). However, analyses using QALYs are often difficult and expensive.

While QALYs are not a perfect measure, they do represent systematically and objectively collected information from the perspective of affected individuals and societal members that can be used to help decision makers address difficult health care choices. In recent years, it has become common for the WTP approach to be applied to CUA, asking the question—what amount is society willing to pay per QALY saved?

For reasons that are not entirely clear, there has been a consensus among economists for decades that the benchmark for the cost of interventions should be around $50,000/QALY. Recently, some researchers have questioned that figure, noting that wealth in the United States has increased (Neumann, Cohen, & Weinstein, 2014). They recommended that the base QALY should reflect the increased income of our population and provided a range of between $50,000 and $200,000 per QALY. They also observed that, rationally, the amount of dollars spent per QALY should be determined by the nation's health care budget so that comparisons of alternative interventions might be made. However, the United States does not have a health care budget nor is it likely to have one in the foreseeable future. Even with a budget, there are currently not enough economic analyses of health care interventions upon which to base decisions. Sloan and Hsieh (2012) recommended that discussing a maximum WTP is an important conversation for our nation to hold. Using an alternate approach, Buyx, Friedrich, and Schone-Seifert (2011) advised that there needs to be a discussion about funding outcomes that have a minimum effect on health status.

An example of such a discussion is the cost of cancer treatment. Schickedanz (2010) reported on a symposium sponsored by the Institute of Medicine, the purpose of which was to discuss ways to optimize the value of cancer treatment. There was general agreement that money spent on cancer treatment in the United States far exceeds money spent by other nations, but that the outcomes obtained in this country are not appreciably better than those in countries spending much less. A survey of oncologists in one New England state revealed that an incremental cost utility of $300,000/QALY would meet their standards for a justifiable intervention. One reason given for this relatively high cost per QALY threshold was that oncologists do not have incentives to choose the less expensive of equally effective treatments, and that their choices do not always consider their patients' quality of life. Members of the symposium agreed that there were steps they could take to improve the value of treatment for their patients. They acknowledged the importance of cost and quality of life in making patient care decisions; and they developed outcome domains, care domains, and patient-centered domains to holistically improve patient health status.

### Application of Cost-Effectiveness and Cost-Utility Analyses

Following is a summary of economic evaluations, which is also presented in Table 5.3. Lal et al. (2012) used data from a randomized clinical trial of alternative treatment protocols (stereotactic radiosurgery [SRS] vs. SRS plus whole brain radiation therapy [WBRT]) for patients with brain metastases to conduct both a CEA and a CUA. They developed a decision analysis model and determined the incremental cost per life-years saved (LYS) and cost per QALY. Their institutional perspective costs included technical and professional costs. There was a statistically significant difference in the median survival between the two groups. The time trade-off method, using 10-year, 5-year, and 1-year time horizons, was used to determine patient utilities at baseline and at the last time of contact with each patient during the study. Results indicated that the cost for SRS plus WBRT ($74,000) was less than for SRS and observation alone ($119,000) but had a lower average effectiveness (0.60 LYS vs. 1.64 LYS, respectively). SRS alone had an ICER of $44,231 per LYS, or $41,783 per QALY. Sensitivity analyses showed robust results, indicating that SRS and observation was the more cost-effective intervention.

In another example, Schoenbaum, Denchev, Vitiello, and Kaltman (2012) examined the CEA and CUA of three alternatives for screening adolescent athletes for cardiac abnormalities to prevent sudden cardiac deaths (SCDs). The options were (a) history and physical (H & P) with referral to a cardiologist for abnormal findings, (b) H & P plus electrocardiogram (ECG) with referral for abnormal findings, and (c) ECG alone with referral for abnormal findings. The first option was considered

**TABLE 5.3  Examples of Economic Evaluations**

| Study | Method | Cost | Outcome | Result |
|-------|--------|------|---------|--------|
| Lal et al. (2012) compared SRS and SRS plus WBRT in a randomized controlled trial of patients being treated for brain metastases | CEA CUA | Collected data for 7 years, including data for both professional and technical costs | Reported LYS and QALYs; used the time trade-off method; conducted univariate sensitivity analysis for each probability point estimate | SRS had higher cost than SRS + WBRT ($119,000 vs. $74,000, respectively) 1.64 LYS for SRS and 0.60 LYS for WBRT were reported, resulting in an incremental cost-effectiveness ratio for SRS of $44,231 per LYS CUA revealed comparable results with $41,783 per QALY |
| Schoenbaum et al. (2012) examined three screening options for preventing sudden cardiac death in adolescent athletes | CEA CUA | Markov model | QALYs and deaths averted | Option 2 cost $68,800/QALY and averted 131 deaths. Option 3 cost $37,700/QALY and averted 127 deaths. Based on the assumptions and parameters of the study, screenings were not cost-effective. |
| Black et al. (2014) examined the cost of screening high-risk patients for lung cancer | CEA CUA | Personnel, supplies and equipment, and overhead. Direct and indirect costs | QALYs ICER | $81,000 per QALY $52,000 per life-year gained. Low-dose CT was cost-effective <$100,000/QALY but costs varied widely based on implementation |
| Siddharthan, Nelson, Tiesman, and Chen (2005) examined the VHA for a safe patient handling program versus no program | CBA | Capital costs, training costs, direct costs associated with treatment and productivity loss | Cost savings related to decreased incidence and severity of injuries | Net annualized benefit of $207,000 |

(continued)

**TABLE 5.3   Examples of Economic Evaluations (*continued*)**

| Study | Method | Cost | Outcome | Result |
|-------|--------|------|---------|--------|
| Bonafide et al. (2014) compared staffing options for medical emergency teams in a pediatric hospital | CBA | Cost of care used cost-to-charge ratio, staffing costs were modeled using various configurations. | Cost savings related to avoidance of CD | Net savings of $1,145,897 annually |

CBA, cost-benefit analysis; CD, critical deterioration; CEA, cost-effectiveness analysis; CUA, cost-utility analysis; LYS, life-years saved; QALY, quality adjusted life year; SRS, stereotactic radiosurgery; VHA, Veterans Health Administration; WBRT, whole brain radiation therapy.

standard care. Variables of interest included cost of screening and follow-up, QALYs, and deaths averted. A Markov modeling process, a type of analysis used to make estimations about the state of patients' health at defined periods of time, was used to calculate cost savings at selected end points (Muennig, 2008; Petitti, 1994). Variables entered into the model were selected on the basis of previous research and expert opinion. The study took a societal perspective, costs and effects were discounted at 3%, and sensitivity analysis was done on all variables. The authors used a WTP limit of $50,000/QALY. They determined that compared with the first option, option 2 cost $68,800/QALY and averted 131 deaths at a cost of $900,000 per person. Option 3 cost $37,700/QALY and averted 127 deaths at a cost of $600,000 per person. The authors concluded that based on the parameters of the study, screening was not cost-effective. Option 2 did not meet the $50,000/QALY threshold and option 3 was not practical because providers routinely include H & P's during office visits.

In the last example, Black et al. (2014) conducted an economic analysis to determine the cost-effectiveness and cost-utility of screening patients who were at high risk for lung cancer. They compared low-dose computed tomography (CT) versus chest radiography and a no screening alternative. Researchers had already determined that CT reduced mortality by 20%. Effectiveness measures included ICERs, cost per QALY, and cost per individual. The 7-year study involved 53,452 individuals between 55 and 74 years of age who had a smoking history. A societal perspective was used and both costs and effects were discounted. The researchers conducted sensitivity analysis that incorporated surgical mortality, chemotherapy and cost of future health care along with other variables. Base case results determined that radiographic screening was not beneficial when compared with the no screening alternative. Low-dose CT screening versus no screening was beneficial and had an additional cost of $1,631 for each individual. The ICER was $52,000 for each additional life year and $81,000 for each additional QALY. Sensitivity analysis indicated a large variation in cost when some of the variables, such as more costly screening and follow-up, were entered into the analysis. The authors concluded that while screening may be cost-effective when the cost per QALY remains below $100,000, this figure could vary widely based on how the processes of screening and follow up are implemented.

## Cost-Benefit Analysis

A CBA is a comparative evaluation of two or more interventions in which costs and outcomes are calculated in dollars. The results may be given in a ratio or as dollars saved or lost (Drummond et al., 2005). An advantage of CBAs is that comparisons can be made across disease states and interventions because both costs and outcomes are calculated in dollars. As such, only a CBA asks whether an intervention is worth undertaking. CEAs and CUAs make the implicit assumption that the best of the interventions will be undertaken. Assigning a monetary estimate to morbidity and mortality indicators is technically difficult; and it is not something with which many providers in the health care field are comfortable (Garber et al., 1996). While the number of WTP CBA calculations is growing in the health care field, they are far fewer in number than CEAs and CUAs (Sloan & Hsieh, 2012).

In an example of a CBA, Siddharthan et al. (2005) combined an observational study along with a CBA to determine the impact of a program designed to reduce the frequency and severity of staff injuries in the Veterans Health Administration (VHA) system (see Table 5.3). The 18-month study included 537 nursing personnel, and the perspective was the VHA hospital system. Costs included capital costs, training costs, and direct costs associated with treatment of injured nursing personnel and work time lost due to the injuries. The program significantly reduced the annual injury rate from 24 per 100 workers to 16.9 per 100 workers. The program resulted in a $207,000 (U.S. dollars) annualized net benefit stemming from a lower incidence and severity of injuries among nursing personnel. The authors noted that parts of the safety program had been integrated into national occupational health policy.

In another example, Bonafide et al. (2014) conducted a 5-year cohort study to determine the costs and benefits of alternate staffing options for medical emergency teams (METs) in a pediatric hospital. These teams provide timely assessment and initial treatment for seriously ill children who may or may not need more critical care. Staffing options included teams who did or did not have additional hospital responsibilities and were composed of two or more of the following health care professionals: registered nurses, registered therapists, nurse practitioners, fellows, and attending physicians. The outcome of treatment was avoidance of critical deterioration (CD) events, which included an unforeseen transfer to the ICU and ventilation within the first 12 hours of arrival in the unit. CD may result in an increased cost of $99,773 per patient ($185,051 for patients with CD events versus $85,278 for patients without CD events). Costs of care were established using a hospital cost-to-charge ratio. Costs of staffing were modeled using alternative staffing configurations of 2 to 3 member METs. A sensitivity analysis was conducted. In the base case analysis, an annual net savings of $1,145,897 was realized with an MET composed of a registered nurse, a respiratory therapist, and a critical care fellow who also had other duties.

## IMPACT OF THE ACA ON HEALTH CARE FINANCING

The saying "no margin, no mission" refers to all hospitals and clinics, whether they are for-profit, nonprofit, or public. To stay in business, they must remain financially solvent. Before the ACA, administrators could concern themselves with maintaining a threshold of quality that satisfied accrediting agencies and consumers while keeping the cost of quality improvement from becoming a burdensome budgetary item (Sadeghi, Barzi, Mikhail, & Shabot, 2013). Hospitals and providers did not need to overly concern themselves with the economic efficiency of individual interventions. If the goods and services they provided made a profit there was no need to establish their cost effectiveness. New equipment could be purchased and patients charged a sufficient amount to ensure that the hospital or clinic met their financial objectives without too much concern about whether the purchase improved care outcome.

The ACA provided the impetus for a national conversation on what value-based care means in the marketplace. Incentives encouraged the alignment of quality and financial performance. Payment incentives such as bundled price reimbursements and accountable care organizations prodded administrators to determine the most efficient way to provide effective health care.

Consumers are an important part of the conversation. Educated patients know that the price of a procedure is not always aligned with good outcomes. They are aware that as much as 30% of health care is not necessary (Colla, 2014). They realize that high costs for low-value interventions decrease the availability of high-value treatments and services (Porter, 2010; Ubel & Jagsi, 2014).

There are numerous opportunities for insurance companies to influence high-value care. They can encourage patients who need complex procedures to seek treatment at Centers of Excellence. This term refers to large hospitals and medical centers that have consistently better outcomes than small community hospitals where many complex interventions are infrequently performed. Insurance companies may further incentivize consumers by returning some of the savings realized from more cost-effective care to patients though mechanisms like decreased cost sharing (Robinson, 2010).

CER (discussed in Chapter 4) may be viewed as the logical corollary to CEA. Both compare treatment alternatives, both are concerned with patient preference, and both measure patient outcomes. However, federal legislation limits the Patient-Centered Outcomes Research Institute (PCORI) from funding economic research that uses QALYS or cost thresholds. The prohibition may be traced to conservative resistance to the ACA on the grounds that it would result in an expanded government role and rationed health care. However, the exclusion does not extend to many other public agencies. Nor does it affect providers and insurers who may decide that it is reasonable to provide consumers with health care options based on both effectiveness and financial considerations (Garber & Sox, 2010).

In 2011, the Centers for Medicare & Medicaid Services estimated that by 2015 per capita national health expenditures in the United States would be $10,928 and consume 18.9% of the GDP (Centers for Medicare & Medicaid Services, 2011). While the data are not yet available, there is some evidence that these projections may be too high, and that the steep climb in health care costs has slowed (Cohn, 2014; Roehrig, 2014). This would be welcome news because it would be one indication that the U.S. health care system has begun the transition from fee-for-service to value-based care. Whether that transition is quick or moves at a glacial pace depends, in large part, on the perceived benefit to providers, payers, and consumers.

## IMPLICATIONS FOR THE DNP

Nursing has assumed a limited responsibility in evaluating the efficiency of health care. In a review of nursing literature to determine the quantity and quality of economic evaluations of nursing care, Lämås et al. (2009) found that during a period of 23 years (1984–2007) nurses conducted 115 published studies. Most of the studies (53) related to prevention and treatment, with the greatest number (31) focused on wound care. In 78% of the studies, the economic method was not discussed, and in 75% the perspective was not provided. The authors attributed the paucity of studies to methodological problems including a lack of nursing outcome indicators.

Economic evaluations are complex and technically difficult. They require specialized knowledge in the disciplines of economics, statistics, epidemiology, and research. Nursing administrators, researchers, and educators have challenged nurses to assume a greater role in appraising the cost-effectiveness of care (AACN, 2006; Bensink et al., 2013; Newhouse, 2010; Siegel, 1998; Stone, 1998). The challenge may be addressed in three ways. First, educators must decide how much of an advanced practitioner program should be devoted to disciplines that enable nurses to conduct economic analyses. DNPs cannot be all things to all people. As a practical matter, nursing may need to focus on educating the very best practitioners and administrators, not on preparing health economists, statisticians, or epidemiologists. Nurses interested in greater participation in economic evaluation may want to take additional courses in economics. Second, nursing programs do need to provide sufficient content to ensure that DNPs have a good understanding of fundamental economic concepts and the skill to critique economic evaluations. These abilities will enable DNPs to choose the intervention that most effectively and efficiently meets the needs of their patients. Third, DNPs bring specialized knowledge to an interdisciplinary team and should collaborate with other health professionals in conducting economic evaluations. A basic grounding in economic concepts and methods will increase the likelihood that DNPs will be included in discussions that impact the health status of patients, the health care system, and health policy.

## REFERENCES

Adams, M. E., McCall, N. T., Gray, D. T., Orza, M. J., & Chalmers, T. C. (1992). Economic analysis in randomized control trials. *Medical Care, 30*(3), 231–243.

American Association of Colleges of Nursing. (2006). *The essentials of doctoral education for advanced nursing practice*. Washington, DC: Author.

Bensink, M. E., Eaton, L. H., Morrison, M., Cook, W. A., Randall Curtis, R., Gordon, D. B., Kundu, A., & Doorenbos, A. Z. (2013). Cost effectiveness analysis for nursing research. *Nursing Research, 62*(4), 279–284.

Black, W. C., Gareen, I. F., Soneji, S. S., Sicks, J. D., Keeler, E. B., Aberle, D. R., & National Lung Screening Trial Research Team. (2014). Cost-effectiveness of CT screening in the national lung screening trial. *New England Journal of Medicine, 371*(19), 1793–1801.

Bonafide, C. P., Localio, A. R., Song, L., Roberts, K. E., Nadkarni, V., Priestley, M., . . . Keren, R. (2014). Cost-benefit analysis of a medical emergency team in a children's hospital. *Pediatrics, 134*(2), 235–241.

Brook, R. H., & Lohr, K. N. (1985). Efficacy, effectiveness, variations, and quality. Boundary-crossing research. *Medical Care, 23*(5), 710–722.

Brosnan, C. A., & Swint, J. M. (2001). Cost analysis: Concepts and application. *Public Health Nursing, 18*(1), 13–18.

Buerhaus, P. I. (1998). Milton Weinstein's insights on the development, use, and methodologic problems in cost-effectiveness analysis. *Image: Journal of Nursing Scholarship, 30*(3), 223–228.

Buyx, A. M., Friedrich, D. R., & Schone-Seifert, B. (2011). Ethics and effectiveness: Rationing healthcare by thresholds of minimum effectiveness. *BMJ, 342*, d54. doi:10.1136/bmj.d54

Centers for Medicare and Medicaid Services. (2011). *National health expenditure projections 2008–2018.* Washington, DC: U.S. Social Security Administration.

Cohn, J. (2014). The paradox of reducing health care spending. *The Milbank Quarterly, 92*(4), 656–658.

Colla, C. H. (2014). Swimming against the current—What might work to reduce low-value care. *New England Journal of Medicine, 371*(14), 1280–1283.

Drummond, M. F., Sculpher, M. J., Torrance, G. W., O'Brien, B. J., & Stoddart, G. L. (2005). *Methods for the economic evaluation of health care programmes.* Oxford, UK: Oxford University Press.

Elnitsky, C. A., & Stone, P. (2005). Patient preferences and cost-utility analysis. *Applied Nursing Research, 18*(2), 74–76.

Finkler, S. A. (1982). The distinction between cost and charges. *Annals of Internal Medicine, 96*, 102–109.

Garber, A. M., & Sox, H. C. (2010). The role of costs in comparative effectiveness research. *Health Affairs, 29*(10), 1805–1811.

Garber, A. M., Weinstein, M. S., Torrance, G. W., & Kamlet, M. S. (1996). Theoretical foundations of cost-effectiveness analysis. In M. R. Gold, J. E. Siegel, L. B. Russell, & M. C. Weinstein (Eds.), *Cost-effectiveness in health and medicine* (pp. 25–53). New York, NY: Oxford University Press.

Gold, M. R., Patrick, D. L., Torrance, G. W., Fryback, D. G., Hadorn, D. C., Kamlet, M. S., . . . Weinstein, M. C. (1996). Identifying and valuing outcomes. In M. R. Gold, J. E. Siegel, L. B. Russell, & M. C. Weinstein (Eds.), *Cost-effectiveness in health and medicine* (pp. 25–53). New York, NY: Oxford University Press.

Hardin, G. (1968). The tragedy of the commons. *Science, 162*, 1243–1248.

Hiatt, H. (1975). Protecting the medical commons, who is responsible? *New England Journal of Medicine, 293*(5), 235–241.

Iglehart, J. K. (2010). The political fight over comparative effectiveness research. *Health Affairs, 29*(10), 1757–1760.

Lal, L. S., Byfield, S. D., Chang, E., Franzini, L., Miller, L. A., Arbuckle, R., . . . Swint, J. M. (2012). Cost-effectiveness analysis of a randomized study with stereotactic radiosurgery (SRS) versus SRS plus whole brain radiation therapy for patients with brain metastases. *American Journal of Clinical Oncology, 35*(1), 45–50. Advance online publication. doi:10.1097/COC.0b013e3182005a8f

Lämås, K., Willman, A., Lindholm, L., & Jacobsson, C. (2009). Economic evaluation of nursing practices: A review of literature. *International Nursing Review, 56*, 13–20.

Lipscomb, J., Weinstein, M. C., & Torrance, G. W. (1996). Time preference. In M. Gold, J. Siegel, L. B. Russell, & M. C. Weinstein (Eds.), *Cost-effectiveness in health and medicine* (pp. 214–246). New York, NY: Oxford University Press.

Luce, R. R., Manning, W. G., Siegel, J. E., & Lipscomb, J. (1996). Estimating costs in cost-effectiveness analysis. In M. Gold, J. Siegel, L. B. Russell, & M. C. Weinstein (Eds.), *Cost-effectiveness in health and medicine* (pp. 176–213). New York, NY: Oxford University Press.

Manning, W. G., Fryback, D. G., & Weinstein, M. C. (1996). Reflecting uncertainty in cost-effectiveness analysis. In M. Gold, J. Siegel, L. B. Russell, & M. C. Weinstein (Eds.), *Cost-effectiveness in health and medicine* (pp. 247–275). New York, NY: Oxford University Press.

McDowell, I., & Newell, C. (1996). *Measuring health.* New York, NY: Oxford University Press.

Muennig, P. (2008). *Cost effectiveness analyses in health: A practical approach.* San Francisco, CA: Jossey-Bass, a Wiley Imprint.

Muennig, P. A., & Glied, S. A. (2010). What changes in survival rates tell us about US health care. *Health Affairs, 29*(11), 1–9. doi:10.1377/hlthall.2010.0073

Neumann, P. J., Cohen, J. T., & Weinstein, M. C. (2014). Updating cost-effectiveness—The curious resilience of the $50,000-per-QALY threshold. *New England Journal of Medicine, 371*(9), 796–797.

Newhouse, R. P. (2010). Do we know how much the evidence-based intervention cost? *JONA, 40*(7/8), 296–299.

Nord, E. (1994). The QALY—A measure of social value rather than individual utility? *Economic Evaluation, 3,* 89–93.

Petitti, D. B. (1994). *Meta-analysis, decision analysis and cost-effectiveness analysis.* New York, NY: Oxford University Press.

Porter, M. E. (2010). What is value in health care? *New England Journal of Medicine, 363*(26), 2477–2481.

Robinson, J. C. (2010). Comparative effectiveness research: From clinical information to economic incentives. *Health Affairs, 29*(10), 1788–1795.

Roehrig, C. (2014). National health spending in 2014—Acceleration delayed. *New England Journal of Medicine, 371*(19), 1767–1769.

Russell, L. B., Gold, M. R., Siegel, J. E., Daniels, N., & Weinstein, M. C. (1996). The role of cost-effectiveness analysis in health and medicine. *JAMA, 276*(14), 1172–1180.

Russell, L. B., Siegel, J. E., Daniels, N., Gold, M. R., Luce, B. R., & Mandelblatt, J. S. (1996). Cost-efffectiveness analysis as a guide to resource allocation in health: Roles and limitations. In M. Gold, J. Siegel, L. B. Russell, & M. C. Weinstein (Eds.), *Cost-effectiveness in health and medicine* (pp. 3–24). New York, NY: Oxford University Press.

Sadeghi, S., Barzi, A., Mikhail, O., & Shabot, M. M. (2013). *Integrating quality and strategy in health care organizations.* New York, NY: Jones & Bartlett Learning.

Schickedanz, A. (2010). Of value: A discussion of cost, communication, and evidence to improve cancer care. *Oncologist, 15*(Suppl. 1), 73–79.

Schoenbaum, M., Denchev, P., Vitiello, B., & Kaltman, J. R. (2012). Economic evaluation of strategies to reduce sudden cardiac death in young athletes. *Pediatrics, 130*(2), e380–e389. doi:10.1542/peds.2011-3241

Siddharthan, K., Nelson, A., Tiesman, H., & Chen, F. (2005). Cost effectiveness of a multifaceted program for safe patient handling. In K. Henriksen, J. B. Battles, E. S. Marks, & D. I. Lewin (Eds.). *Advances in patient safety: From research to implementation* (Vol. 3, Implementation Issues). Rockville, MD: Agency for Healthcare Research and Quality.

Siegel, J. E. (1998). Cost-effectiveness analysis and nursing research—Is there a fit? *Image: Journal of Nursing Scholarship, 30*(3), 221–222.

Sloan, F. A., & Hsieh, C.-R. (2012). *Health economics.* Cambridge, MA: The MIT Press.

Stone, P. W. (1998). Methods for conducting and reporting cost-effectiveness analysis in nursing. *Image: Journal of Nursing Scholarship, 30*(3), 229–234.

Torrance, G. W., Siegel, J. E., & Luce, B. B. (1996). Framing and designing the cost-effectiveness analysis. In M. Gold, J. Siegel, L. B. Russell, & M. C. Weinstein (Eds.), *Cost-effectiveness in health and medicine* (pp. 54–81). New York, NY: Oxford University Press.

Ubel, P. A., & Jagsi, R. (2014). Promoting population health through financial stewardship. *New England Journal of Medicine, 370*(13), 1280–1281.

Weinstein, M. C., Siegel, J. E., Gold, M. R., Kamlet, M. S., & Russell, L. B. (1996). Recommendations of the panel on cost-effectiveness in health and medicine. *JAMA, 276*(15), 1253–1258.

Weinstein, M. C., & Stason, W. B. (1977). Foundations of cost-effectiveness analysis for health and medical practices. *New England Journal of Medicine, 296*(13), 716–721.

Williamson, J. W. (1978). *Assessing and improving health care and outcomes: The health accounting approach to quality assurance.* Cambridge, MA: Balinger Publishing Co.

World Bank. (2011). World Bank search. Retrieved from http://search.worldbank.org

World Health Organization. (2016a). Global Health Observatory data repository. Retrieved from http://apps.who.int/gho/data/node.main

World Health Organization. (2016b). Global Health Observatory country views. Retrieved from http://apps.who.int/gho/data/node.country

# SPECIAL AREAS OF EVALUATION IN HEALTH CARE

# CHAPTER SIX

# EVALUATION OF ORGANIZATIONS AND SYSTEMS

Nancy Manning Crider and Elizabeth Ulrich

*The hospital is altogether the most complex human organization ever devised.*
—Peter Drucker

Whether the goal is to assess an organization for benchmarking purposes, to select a new practice setting, or to better understand one's current organization in order to successfully lead organizational improvements, it is important for nurses to know how to assess and evaluate health care organizations and systems. Evaluation of an organization or system requires a systematic review of key indicators, much like performing a systematic physical assessment of an individual patient. Like a patient, organizations have a structure (anatomy), ways of functioning that require all parts to work together for success (physiology), and the need for resources and support systems.

Organizations are social structures created by individuals to support collaboration and the pursuit of specific goals (Scott & Davis, 2015). Organizations have defined objectives and, in order to provide and dispense products and services, must induce participants to provide services, garner resources from the environment, and work with their neighbors (Scott & Davis, 2015).

Using the approach developed by Donabedian (1978) for assessing a health care organization's performance relative to structure, process, and outcome, the intent of this chapter is to provide a framework to assess health care organizations and health care systems. Structure refers to the resources dedicated to provide patient care services. Structure is a key driver of organizational culture that influences institutional processes and ultimately determines clinical outcomes. Leadership skills, human resource management, nurse staffing, and the use of advanced practice nurses (APNs) and other nurses with advanced degrees such as doctor of nursing practice (DNP) graduates also influence the culture of the organization, practice models, and clinical outcomes (Glickman, Baggett, Krubert, Peterson, & Schulman, 2007). Other factors including patient care technology, information management systems, and support services, as well as special designations provided by external organizations, all reflect the comprehensiveness

---

**TABLE 6.1  Key Components of Organization and System Evaluations**

- History and overview
- Type of organization
- Sources of funding and revenue
- Size and scope of services
- Governance
- Mission, vision, and values
- Strategy, goals, and strategic culture
- Organizational structure
- Authority and decision making
- Culture
- Reputation
- Outcomes, quality, and patient satisfaction
- The role of nursing in the organization

---

and quality of care delivered. Process addresses the organization's reputation and ability to sustain systems of care that are of the highest quality and that are recognized by peers through benchmarking databases. Outcomes data on care effectiveness compare an institution's morbidity and mortality with comparable institutions and other threshold targets set by national organizations.

Performing a comprehensive organizational assessment and evaluation requires knowledge of the structure and mission of the organization, understanding how the organization functions in its current environment, knowledge of sources of relevant information, openness to see the organization as others see it (whether they are inside or outside the organization), and the ability to evaluate organizational performance in relation to other organizations. This chapter provides a framework that can be used to perform an evaluation of health care organizations and systems (see Table 6.1).

## HISTORY AND OVERVIEW OF THE ORGANIZATION

Similar to a physical assessment, the first step of an organizational assessment is to complete a history and overview of the organization or system. Widespread Internet access makes this fairly simple, as most health care organizations maintain a robust website to engage customers. The first question to ask is, when was the health care organization established and by whom? Generally, hospitals were established to meet the health needs of the community or a specific population (e.g., company employees, active military personnel, or veterans). The organization may be privately owned by individuals or investors, or publicly owned by a local, state, or federal agency. Many health care organizations were established by a religious order or have an affiliation with an established religious denomination (e.g., the Roman Catholic church or a local Protestant or Jewish congregation). The ownership and purpose for establishing the enterprise strongly influences the current mission, vision, and values of the system. Ownership and purpose also, at least partially, determine an organization's tax status.

## TYPE OF ORGANIZATION

The type of the organization—not-for-profit, for-profit, or governmental—can offer information on the mission of the organization as well as on resources that may be available and restrictions that may apply to the use of "profit" or revenue over expenses. Key characteristics of a not-for-profit organization include an exemption from paying state and federal taxes on income and property, the obligation to reinvest all profits back into the organization, and required reporting of the community benefits offered by the organization (The Advisory Board Company, 2015). Tax-exempt organizations are also able to issue tax-exempt bonds that allow them to secure money at a lower interest rate and reduce their financing costs (Burns, Bradley, & Weiner, 2012). There is, however, a lack of consensus on what constitutes a community benefit, but such benefits typically include the provision of uncompensated care and Medicaid-covered services, and the provision of certain specialized services (such as emergency care, labor and delivery, etc.) that have been identified as generally unprofitable (Congressional Budget Office [CBO]. The Congress of the United States, 2006). Key characteristics of a for-profit organization include the ability to distribute profits to its investors and to raise capital through investors, as well as the obligation to pay income and property taxes (The Advisory Board Company, 2015). The third type of organization is governmental organizations, such as the military, Veterans Administration, and county hospitals. They are financially supported by designated governmental agencies, often as a result of legislation with accompanying rules and regulations, and provide specific services to a designated population.

## SOURCES OF FUNDING AND REVENUE

All organizations must have sources of funding and revenue or they will not be able to continue to provide services. Health care organizations are no different. Public hospitals and health care systems designed as safety net providers for the poor are, at least in part, funded by local, state, and/or federal tax dollars that must be approved by elected officials (e.g., city council, a state legislature, or the U.S. Congress). Public hospital systems and private health care organizations may receive funds from publicly sponsored programs such as Medicare and Medicaid for services provided to patients. Operating revenue is also generated from fees for service or payments from private insurance companies or contractual agreements with major employers or managed care organizations. Payors may also negotiate with providers for bundled services or negotiate a risk-based per-member per-month contract to manage health care services. Revenue may also be generated from designated grants and cash payments.

Health care organizations frequently have a separate philanthropic fundraising organization to secure donations to provide services and support strategic initiatives and capital improvements. Many also generate revenue through investments and other nonpatient care services like parking, gift shops, or retail pharmacies in a professional office building.

## SIZE AND SCOPE OF SERVICES

The size and location of the health care organization will impact on the type and scope of services that the organization provides as well as the available resources. Multiple questions must be answered to understand the organization. What is the size of the organization? Is the organization located in an urban or a rural area? Is the organization a large health care system, a 600-bed urban tertiary care center, an acute care community hospital, or a primary care practice? What types of services are provided? Are specialty services available on site or are patients referred to another provider? Does the organization provide pediatric and obstetrical care? Is the institution a teaching hospital? Are there academic or research affiliations? Is the organization an accountable care organization (ACO)? The organization's website and annual report are good sources for this type of general information.

The American Hospital Association (AHA) annual survey is another source of information that describes the organizational structure and scope of hospitals and health systems. In 2014, this self-report survey was completed by 6,400 hospitals and includes detailed financials, bed size, and services offered (AHA, 2014). It also provides detailed staffing and physician data as part of the overall organizational structure. The AHA survey data, which has been collected since 1980, is used extensively for research and benchmarking purposes.

## GOVERNANCE

Both for-profit and not-for-profit hospitals and health care systems are governed by a board of directors (BOD) or board of trustees (BOT). The BOD/BOT is responsible and accountable for the performance of the organization and has ultimate authority for the financial stability and quality of care provided by the institution. Boards are composed of a specified number of members and include health care professionals and executives as well as business representatives and lay members from the community served by the organization. When completing an organizational assessment, one should examine the composition of the board and determine if all stakeholders are represented. Specifically, the evaluator should determine if the chief nurse executive or another nurse is a member of the board.

## MISSION, VISION, AND VALUES

The mission, vision, and values of an organization or system flow from the original purpose for establishing the organization. Simply stated, the mission is the purpose or reason the organization exists. An organization's mission statement should be distinct, long enough to guide strategy and short enough for staff to understand and apply (Burns et al., 2012).

The vision is what the organization wants to achieve or look like in the future. Vision statements should stretch and challenge an organization. The ideal vision statement will resonate with those involved with the organization and create a feeling of pride about being part of something much larger than themselves (Burns et al., 2012).

The values of the organization determine how decisions are made. An organization's values are a visible guide for employees to follow and serve as an ethical compass for decision making at all levels of the organization. Values should not be contingent upon circumstances. Rather, values should be constant and endure over time. In reviewing the values of the organization, it is important to consider not only the published values, but also what values are manifested in the actions of the organization.

## STRATEGY, GOALS, AND STRATEGIC CULTURE

Strategy refers to the choices that the organization makes about who it will serve, where services will be provided, and how services will be delivered. Goals are specific outcome measures that are established to carry out the strategy and meet the mission and vision of the organization. Many organizations target specific segments (niches) in the health care market such as women and children, cancer care, orthopedics, cardiovascular surgery, and transplantation.

Miles and Snow (1978) describe four types of strategic culture: prospectors, defenders, analyzers, and reactors. Prospectors are the most aggressive with their strategy. They tend to focus on creating innovative products and services and expanding services into new markets. Often they create change and uncertainty that requires their competitors to respond. Defenders, on the other hand, prefer a rather narrow product line and maintain a secure and stable market. They focus more on internal efficiency and tend not to search for new opportunities. Analyzers maintain a combination strategy. They take less risk than a prospector but are less committed to stability than defenders. Analyzers maintain a combination of established products and services and regularly update their business with new offerings that have been proven effective. The final group, known as reactors, often lack focus and respond to external changes only when forced to respond. Some organizations demonstrate characteristics of a mixed strategy by choosing to be a leader and innovator in one area and an analyzer in other areas.

## ORGANIZATIONAL STRUCTURE

The organizational structure formalizes the governance of an organization and provides rational direction to coordinate the activities required for an organization to survive and deal with the external environment. Factors that influence organizational structure include:

- The product
- The complexity and uncertainty of the work
- The environment in which the work is performed
- Skills and knowledge of the workers
- Characteristics of the objectives on which the work is performed
- Technical systems used to produce the work
- Use of information technology (IT) in the production process (Bolman & Deal, 2013; Burns et al., 2012; Scott & Davis, 2015)

Organizational structure may be conveyed by an organizational chart, a diagram that depicts how different parts of the health care organization/system relate to one another and who reports to whom. Organizational charts are typically shaped like a pyramid. A hierarchical organization has an organizational structure with many layers, where every entity in the organization—except the top one—is subordinate to another entity.

In recent years, to improve communication and respond more rapidly to consumer preferences and environmental changes, some health care organizations have moved from the traditional hierarchal structure to a flatter, more horizontal structure with fewer layers. A flat organization has an organizational structure in which a number of middle-management levels have been eliminated. The result is an organizational structure with fewer layers that fosters communication by bringing top management in closer contact with the frontline employees and customers.

Organizational charts are useful in understanding the rational, formal nature of an organization; however, the organizational chart is often out of date and it does not convey the informal behavioral structures that impact employee performance and patient outcomes. The informal structure of the organization reflects the culture, norms, values, and social networks that exist within the organization.

## AUTHORITY AND DECISION MAKING

Rational–legal authority generally serves as the foundation of a permanent administrative structure. In a rational–legal organization, the position of authority is held because the leaders are either elected or hired (Scott & Davis, 2015). In the case of a health care organization, the final authority rests with the BOD who hire the chief executive officer (CEO) to run the operations of the organization.

Depending on the organizational structure, leadership style of the executive team, and the culture of the system, decision making may be centralized or decentralized. In less hierarchal and bureaucratic organizations, decision making may be delegated and shared among leaders and employees at various levels of the organization.

## CULTURE

Culture is "the set of shared attitudes, values, goals, and practices that characterizes an institution or organization" ("Culture," 2016). There are many cultures and subcultures within an organization, reflecting the written and unwritten "rules" of the organization, the norms, and what is acceptable behavior. There is a culture of the organization as a whole, which may be influenced by such things as the organization's history, ownership, mission, and executive leadership. Different parts of the organization (e.g., nursing, physician services, housekeeping/environmental services) may also have their own subcultures.

Two important aspects of culture are the patient safety culture and the work environment. While there is overlap, patient safety culture focuses primarily on the care of patients while the work environment focuses primarily on the health of the environment in which employees work.

## Patient Safety Culture

Patient safety culture has been described as "the values shared among organization members about what is important, their beliefs about how things operate in the organization, and the interaction of these with work unit and organizational structures and systems, which together produce behavioral norms in the organization that promote safety" (Singer, Lin, Falwell, Gaba, & Baker, 2009, p. 400). The three main components of a safety culture are a just culture, a reporting culture, and a learning culture (Reason & Hobbs, 2003). In a just culture, there is trust; what is acceptable and what is not acceptable are clear; and fairness and accountability are consistent. In a reporting culture, reporting errors and safety issues is the norm. Reporting is encouraged and facilitated, and the organization has a commitment to fix what has been found to be unsafe. A learning culture is a culture in which the organization learns from errors, near misses, and other safety issues.

The Agency for Healthcare Research and Quality (AHRQ, 2014) has identified the dimensions of a patient safety culture and created survey instruments to measure those dimensions in various patient care settings. The dimensions of patient safety culture for hospitals are shown in Table 6.2.

## Work Environment

The environment and culture in which people in health care organizations work impact patient and employee outcomes. Poor work environments have been associated with negative outcomes for patients (e.g., lower quality of care, not prepared for discharge, increased falls, increased readmissions) and nurses (e.g., burnout,

---

**TABLE 6.2  AHRQ Patient Safety Culture Dimensions—Hospitals**

- Communication openness
- Feedback and communication about error
- Frequency of events reported
- Handoffs and transitions
- Management support for patient safety
- Nonpunitive response to error
- Organizational learning—continuous improvement
- Overall perceptions of patient safety
- Staffing
- Supervisor/manager expectations and actions promoting safety
- Teamwork across units
- Teamwork within units

*Source:* AHRQ (2014).

job dissatisfaction, high turnover; Aiken et al., 2011; Blake, Leach, Robbins, Pike, & Needleman, 2013; Institute of Medicine [IOM], 2004; McHugh & Chenjuan, 2013). There is also evidence that the quality of nurse work environments is significantly related to patient satisfaction, a key Hospital Consumer Assessment of Healthcare Providers and System (HCAHPS) measure (McHugh, Kutney-Lee, Cimiotti, Sloane, & Aiken, 2011) so important to any organization.

Components of healthy and positive work environments have been identified by the IOM (2004), the Magnet® program (American Nurses Credentialing Center [ANCC], 2015b), the Nursing Organizations Alliance (NOA) (2004), the American Association of Critical-Care Nurses (AACN, 2014), and many others. Key components of a healthy and positive work environment include: physical safety and mental safety; respect, communication, and collaboration; adequate staffing (number of staff, competency of staff) to meet patient care needs; effective and authentic leadership; engagement and involvement of staff and, where applicable, patients and families in decision making; a learning culture that supports professional development; and meaningful recognition.

## REPUTATION

Reputation reflects how the organization is viewed. For health care organizations, there are two main views of reputation—how the organization is viewed by the health care community (e.g., other health care organizations, health care professionals) and how the organization is viewed by the lay community. Both views are important to the success of the organization.

A variety of external reference groups provide summary data related to excellence in clinical performance that can be used to benchmark an organization against other health care organizations. Examples of sources that one might review when assessing the reputation of a particular organization include hospital rankings by *U.S. News and World Report* and *Fortune*, as well as websites, patient portals, and social media sites.

### U.S. News and World Report Rankings

In 1990, *U.S. News and World Report* introduced "Best Hospitals" as a resource to help individuals select those hospitals that might provide the best level of care for their specific medical issues and concerns (*U.S. News and World Report* LP, 2013). The annual *U.S. News and World Report* Best Hospitals list, prepared by the Research Triangle Institute (RTI) International (2015), ranks hospitals in 16 specialties. Hospital rankings are primarily based on quality data as well as physician survey information. Metrics such as nurse staffing, use of technologies, and external recognition by organizations such as the ANCC are also factored into the hospital rankings (*U.S. News and World Report* LP, 2015). These hospital rankings provide information on specialty services as well as on reputation.

### Fortune 100 Best Companies to Work For®

On an annual basis, the Great Place to Work Institute (2015) publishes the list of the *Fortune* 100 Best Companies to Work For. In addition to other businesses, this list contains a list of and details on health care organizations that, via random employee survey, have indicated their work environment is one that reflects a partnership between employer and employee and provides employees with unique and innovative programming reflective of common values.

## Websites, Patient Portals, and Social Media

Social media sites such as Facebook (www.facebook.com), Twitter (www.twitter.com), and Yelp (www.yelp.com) have become a popular means for the lay public to use to rate and comment on their experience and interactions with health care organizations and other local businesses. Many organizations provide links to these social media sites from their home page. There are also sites on which employees provide information and opinions about their employing organization.

## OUTCOMES, QUALITY, AND PATIENT SATISFACTION

Quality care, according to the IOM (2001), must be safe, effective, patient centered, timely, efficient, and equitable. In the current age of transparency, there is no shortage of data for an objective review of an organization's performance. Magnet designation from the ANCC (2015a) and accreditation and/or certification by The Joint Commission (TJC, 2015c), or Det Norske Veritas (DNV) Healthcare, Inc. (DNV-GL Healthcare, 2015) are examples of ways an organization can be recognized for achieving gold standards.

According to The Commonwealth Fund, transparency and better public information on cost and quality are essential for three reasons: (a) to help providers improve by benchmarking their performance against others, (b) to encourage private insurers and public programs to reward quality and efficiency, and (c) to help patients make informed choices about their care (Collins & Davis, 2006). Transparency is also important to level the playing field through disclosure of accurate and comparable information on how all components of patient care are addressed. Accurate information is critical for the expected level of transparency related to health care.

Some of the outcomes and process measures collected in health care organizations are abstracted from databases that are used by payors, and many of these data are routinely published for review by both practitioners and the general public. Although there are far more options for inpatient comparisons, data on the outpatient environment are improving. In recent years, a number of states have developed extensive data collection requirements and are publicly reporting clinical and quality outcomes. Payors, including Centers for Medicare & Medicaid Services (CMS), managed care, and fee-for-service organizations, also have additional reporting capabilities that are often utilized by employers to make choices for their employee health care needs. The Hospital Compare website provides the data for public review as does the Leapfrog Group. Sources for quality and reputation data are shown in Table 6.3.

| TABLE 6.3   Sources for Quality Data |
| --- |
| Hospital Compare<br>    www.hospitalcompare.hhs.gov<br>American Hospital Association<br>    www.ahadataviewer.com/about/hospital-database/<br>*U.S. News & World Report* on Best Hospitals<br>    www.rti.org/besthospitals<br>*Fortune* 100 Best Companies to Work For<br>    www.greatplacetowork.com/best-companies/100-best-companies-to-work-for<br>    archive.fortune.com/magazines/fortune/best-companies/2014/list/<br>American Nurses Credentialing Center Magnet<br>    www.nursecredentialing.org/Magnet/FindaMagnetFacility<br>Leapfrog Group<br>    www.leapfroggroup.org/<br>Health Grades<br>    www.healthgrades.com/business/services/ |

## Core Measure Sets

In 1998, TJC began the ORYX initiative to measure hospital quality. By 2001, TJC announced four initial core measures for hospitals: acute myocardial infarction, heart failure, pneumonia, and pregnancy. Beginning in 2002, TJC required hospitals to collect and report data on two of the four core measure sets. TJC released the quality outcome data to the public starting in 2004 (Chassin, Loeb, Schmaltz, & Wachter, 2010). Since 2004, TJC and the CMS have worked together to align these and other common measures and create one set of specifications and documentation with a common (i.e., identical) data dictionary, measurement information forms, and algorithms (TJC, 2015b). Common terminology and reporting methods minimize data collection efforts and allow hospitals to focus efforts on the use of data to improve the health care delivery processes.

There are currently 14 core measure sets: acute myocardial infarction, children's asthma care, heart failure, hospital-based inpatient psychiatric services, substance use, tobacco treatment, hospital outpatient department measures, perinatal care, immunizations, pneumonia, stroke, venous thromboembolism, emergency department measures, and surgical care improvement project (TJC, 2015a). These measures are based on approved evidence-based guidelines adopted by TJC, the National Quality Forum (NQF), and CMS. The success of core measures requires a multimodal approach with a major focus on a collaborative practice model, the nursing process, and excellent technological support. Centers for Medicare and Medicaid Services (CMS, 2015a) reports data on the comparative effectiveness of health care organizations on core measures at its hospital compare website.

## Hospital-Acquired Conditions

Hospital-acquired conditions (HACs) are serious conditions that patients may acquire during an inpatient hospital stay. If hospitals follow proper procedures and use evidence-based guidelines to treat and care for patients, patients are less likely to acquire these conditions. Nurse leaders may wish to collect information for several organizations to determine if the organization being evaluated has a disproportionate share of poor outcomes (CMS, 2014a). Organizations that are outliers may have different processes from best practices or significant process failures. A review of these findings provides information that nurse leaders may use to determine the organization's approach to evidence-based practice and effective deployment of those practices.

## Healthcare-Associated Infections

Healthcare-associated infections (HAIs) are infections caused by a wide variety of both common and unusual bacteria, fungi, and viruses that patients acquire during the course of receiving treatment for other conditions within a health care setting (Centers for Disease Control and Prevention [CDC], 2014). Medical advances have brought lifesaving care to patients, yet many of those advances come with a risk of HAIs. These infections can be debilitating and even deadly. Currently, the infections that are being publicly reported are bloodstream infections, urinary tract infections, and ventilator-associated pneumonias (CDC, 2014). These infections all carry a significant morbidity and mortality risk.

## Hospital Value-Based Purchasing

Value-based purchasing (VBP) is part of CMS's long-standing effort to link Medicare's payment system to a value-based system to improve health care quality. Beginning in 2015, the program attaches VBP to the Medicare payment system, including the quality of care provided in the inpatient hospital setting. Under the program, CMS will make value-based incentive payments (or reduce expected payments) to acute care hospitals, based either on how the hospitals perform on certain quality measures or how much the hospitals' performance changes on certain quality measures from their performance during a baseline period (CMS, 2015b). An example of a value-based incentive is 30-day readmissions (readmission within 30 days of discharge). If a hospital's 30-day readmission rate is excessive, the hospital's payments from CMS will be reduced.

## Magnet Designation

Of the 15 hospitals identified in *U.S. News and World Report's* "Best Hospitals" list in 2015, 14 were Magnet-designated hospitals (ANCC, 2015c). Magnet criteria identify five domains and over 60 sources of evidence that are essential for creating an environment in which nurses thrive and innovate (ANCC, 2015b), Leading these domains is transformational leadership, which addresses the quality of nursing leadership in an organization. A transformational nurse leader (e.g., chief nurse executive) is one who establishes a strategy that outlines the direction of nursing and effectively communicates the vision and the role of nursing in transforming health care processes in ways that can influence program innovation and quality outcomes for patients and families. Effective Magnet-designated organizations have nursing strategic plans that address the following elements: collaborative patient care delivery; workplace environment; community presence; evidence-based practice and research; innovation and technology; and financial stewardship (ANCC, 2015b).

Magnet designation and the Pathway to Excellence Program offered by the ANCC are indicators of a nursing enterprise that is focused on nurses, quality, service, and innovation in care. The initial designation is preceded by what has been referred to as the "Magnet Journey," which is when an organization engages in a rigorous self-assessment to determine if it meets Magnet criteria and pursues the Magnet designation. For successful organizations, Magnet designation is awarded for a period of 4 years; annual reports are submitted to demonstrate the sustainability of the Magnet culture and high-quality outcomes. A documentation system that tracks performance on nurse-sensitive indicators (e.g., pressure ulcers) with corrective action plans must be demonstrated for a 4-year period prior to every redesignation (ANCC, 2015a). The rigors of this process account for the fact that only about 7% of the nation's hospitals achieve Magnet designation (ANCC, 2015d).

## Consumer Assessment of Healthcare Providers and Systems

The HCAHPS survey is the first national, standardized, publicly reported survey of patients' perspectives of hospital care (CMS, 2014b). HCAHPS is a survey instrument and data collection methodology for measuring patients' perceptions of their hospital experience. While many hospitals have collected information on patient satisfaction for their own internal use, until HCAHPS, there was no national standard for collecting and publicly reporting information about patients' experience of care that allowed valid comparisons to be made across hospitals locally, regionally, and nationally. For many nonhospital health care entities (such as hemodialysis units, health plans, clinician and group practices, and surgical care centers), the Consumer Assessment of Healthcare Providers and Systems (CAHPS) surveys, their results, and comparative data are available from AHRQ (2015). Like the HCAHPS surveys, the CAHPS surveys ask consumers and patients to report on and evaluate their experiences with health care.

## Information From Other Organizations

Private organizations such as Healthgrades (2015) and Truven Healthcare Analytics (2015) have developed proprietary methodologies to analyze public datasets to evaluate the quality of health care providers. Nurse leaders can gather the most recently published information on hospitals related to clinical quality outcomes for employers from these sources.

## THE ROLE OF NURSING IN THE ORGANIZATION

The role of nursing in the organization is an important part of the organizational assessment. Where is the chief nurse executive positioned in organizational structure in relation to other executives? Is nursing a part of critical committees and task forces? What is nursing's role in quality improvement? What leadership roles do nurses with advanced degrees hold in the organization? How does a new registered nurse (RN) or a nurse with an advanced degree move from a novice to an expert in this organization? How are APNs and nurses with DNPs integrated into the organization and what purposeful actions do they take to advance patient outcomes and use their knowledge and skills? If nurses and leaders in the organization do not have a credible answer to these questions, it might not be a good fit for a nurse leader with an advanced degree and aspirations for advancement and professional development.

With the passage of the Patient Protection and Affordable Care Act (PPACA) of 2010, several new models of patient care delivery have emerged that are consistent with the holistic, patient-centered approach which is the backbone of professional nursing. The PPACA addresses three emerging care delivery models: the ACO; the medical or health home; and the nurse-managed health center. The elements of the holistic, patient-centered approach, promoted and incentivized by PPACA, include the family and community; prevention and wellness care; chronic disease management; care continuity; coordination and integration across settings and providers; patient education; and information management (PPACA, 2010). Registered nurses are fundamental to the success of all of these models. APNs and clinical nurse specialists have the chance to provide significant organizational leadership within the ACO and Health Home models, which rely on an interdisciplinary, interprofessional team of providers comprised of medical specialists, nurses, pharmacists, nutritionists, dieticians, social workers, behavioral and mental health providers, and other licensed and unlicensed health care providers (American Nurses Association [ANA], 2010).

When assessing an organization, one should look for an organizational commitment to collaborative, interprofessional, and evidence-based practice that includes the development of specific goals that are measured and shared with both the individual and the organization. Nurses who are the first APN or the first nurse with a DNP to be employed in a facility will have opportunities to educate administrators, employees, nurse leaders, executive colleagues, and collaborating physicians about their preparation, abilities, and scope of practice. Frequent communications and collaboration will offer the best opportunities for meeting expectations, achieving professional goals, and meeting organizational needs.

## SUMMARY

Health care organizations and systems are complex structures that are frequently evaluated based on limited information and anecdotal data. The purpose of this chapter is to provide nurse leaders with a systematic approach to complete a comprehensive organizational assessment. The approach was compared with a "head to toe" physical assessment of an individual patient and began with a history and overview of the institution. Structure, process, and outcome measures were discussed. The impact of the internal and external environment, leadership style and abilities, organizational culture, and the role of nursing in the enterprise were also identified as key factors that influence both clinical operations and patient care outcomes of an organization. The methodology presented by the authors provides nurses with advance degrees a framework to evaluate an organization that can be used for a variety of purposes—to select a new practice setting; benchmark an organization among competitors; or to better understand one's current organization when planning and implementing a change in practice. Whatever the motivation, the consistent use of a systematic approach to organizational assessment will provide a better understanding of both the formal and informal structure of the health care organization or system being evaluated.

# REFERENCES

The Advisory Board Company. (2015). *Daily briefing primer: What's the difference between for profit and not-for-profit hospitals?* Washington, DC: Author. Retrieved from https://www.advisory.com/daily-briefing/resources/primers/whats-the-difference-between-for-profit-and-not-for-profit-hospitals

Agency for Healthcare Research and Quality. (2014). *Hospital survey on patient safety culture: Items and dimensions.* Rockville, MD: Author. Retrieved from http://www.ahrq.gov/professionals/quality-patient-safety/patientsafetyculture/hospital/userguide/hospdim.html

Agency for Healthcare Research and Quality. (2015). *CAPHS: Surveys and tools to advance patient-centered care.* Rockville, MD: Author. Retrieved from https://www.cahps.ahrq.gov/index.html

Aiken, L. H., Sloane, D. M., Clarke, S., Poghosyan, L., Cho, E., You, L., . . . Aungsuroch, Y. (2011). Importance of work environments on hospital outcomes in nine countries. *Quality in Health Care,* 23(4), 357–364.

American Association of Critical-Care Nurses. (2014). *AACN's healthy work environment initiative.* Aliso Viejo, CA: Author. Retrieved from http://www.aacn.org/WD/HWE/Content/hwehome.content?menu=hwe

American Hospital Association. (2014). *AHA annual survey database™ fiscal year 2014.* Chicago, IL: Author. Retrieved from www.ahadataviewer.com/book-cd-products/aha-survey/

American Nurses Association. (2010). *New care delivery models in health system reform: Opportunities for nurses and their patients.* Silver Spring, MD: Author.

American Nurses Credentialing Center. (2015a). *ANCC Magnet Recognition Program®.* Silver Spring, MD: Author. Retrieved from http://www.nursecredentialing.org/Magnet.aspx

American Nurses Credentialing Center. (2015b). *Announcing a new model for ANCC's Magnet Recognition Program®.* Silver Spring, MD: Author. Retrieved from http://www.nursecredentialing.org/MagnetModel

American Nurses Credentialing Center. (2015c). *Find a Magnet Hospital.* Silver Spring, MD: Author. Retrieved from http://www.nursecredentialing.org/Magnet/FindaMagnetFacility

American Nurses Credentialing Center. (2015d). *Growth of the program.* Silver Spring, MD: Author. Retrieved from http://nursecredentialing.org/Magnet/ProgramOverview/HistoryoftheMagnetProgram/GrowthoftheProgram

Blake, N., Leach, L. S., Robbins, W., Pike, N., & Needleman, J. (2013). Healthy work environments and staff nurse retention: The relationship between communication, collaboration, and leadership in the pediatric intensive care unit. *Nursing Administration Quarterly,* 37(4), 356–370.

Bolman, L. G., & Deal, T. E. (2013). *Reframing organizations: Artistry, choice, and leadership* (5th ed.). San Francisco, CA: Jossey-Bass.

Burns, L. R., Bradley, E. H., & Weiner, B. J. (2012). *Shortell and Kaluzny's health care management organization design and behavior* (6th ed.). New York, NY: Delmar.

Centers for Disease Control and Prevention. (2014). *Healthcare-associated infections.* Atlanta, GA: Author. Retrieved from http://www.cdc.gov/HAI/infectionTypes.html

Centers for Medicare and Medicaid Services. (2014a). *HCAHPS: Patients' perspectives of care survey.* Baltimore, MD: Author. Retrieved from https://www.cms.gov/Medicare/Quality-Initiatives-Patient-Assessment-Instruments/HospitalQualityInits/HospitalHCAHPS.html

Centers for Medicare and Medicaid Services. (2014b). *Hospital-acquired condition (HAC) reduction program.* Retrieved from https://www.cms.gov/Medicare/Medicare-Fee-for-Service-Payment/AcuteInpatientPPS/HAC-Reduction-Program.html

Centers for Medicare and Medicaid Services. (2015a). *Hospital compare.* Baltimore, MD: Author. Retrieved from http://www.hospitalcompare.hhs.gov/

Centers for Medicare and Medicaid Services. (2015b). *Hospital value-based purchasing.* Baltimore, MD: Author. Retrieved from https://www.cms.gov/Medicare/Quality-Initiatives-Patient-Assessment-Instruments/hospital-value-based-purchasing/index.html?redirect=/hospital-value-based-purchasing/

Chassin, M. R., Loeb, J. M., Schmaltz, S. P., & Wachter, R. M. (2010). Accountability measures—Using measurement to promote quality improvement. *New England Journal of Medicine, 363*(7), 683–688. doi:10.1056/NEJMsb1002320

Collins, S. R., & Davis, K. (2006). *Transparency in health care: The time has come.* New York, NY: The Commonwealth Fund. Retrieved from http://www.commonwealthfund.org/publications/testimonies/2006/mar/transparency-in-health-care–the-time-has-come

Congressional Budget Office. The Congress of the United States. (2006). *Nonprofit hospitals and the provision of community benefits.* Washington, DC: Author. Retrieved from https://www.cbo.gov/publication/18256

Culture. (2016). In *The Merriam-Webster Dictionary* Online. Retrieved from http://www.merriam-webster.com/dictionary/culture

DNV-GL Healthcare. (2015). *Hospital accreditation.* Milfred, OH: Author. Retrieved from http://dnvglhealthcare.com/accreditations/hospital-accreditation

Donabedian, A. (1978). The quality of medical care. *Science, 200*(4344), 856–864.

Glickman, S. W., Baggett, K. A., Krubert, C. G., Peterson, E. D., & Schulman, K. A. (2007). Promoting quality: The health-care organization from a management perspective. *International Journal for Quality in Health Care, 19*(6), 341–348.

Great Place to Work Institute. (2015). *Fortune 100 great places to work for.* San Francisco, CA: Author. Retrieved from https://clients.greatplacetowork.com/list-calendar/fortune-100-best-companies-to-work-for

Healthgrades. (2015). *How America finds a doctor.* Orlando, FL: Healthgrades Operating Company, Inc. Retrieved from www.healthgrades.com/

Institute of Medicine. (2001). *Crossing the quality chasm: A new health system for the 21st century.* Washington, DC: National Academies Press. Retrieved from http://iom.edu/Reports/2001/Crossing-the-Quality-Chasm-A-New-Health-System-for-the-21st-Century.aspx

Institute of Medicine. (2004). *Keeping patients safe. Transforming the work environments of nurses.* Washington, DC: The National Academies Press. Retrieved from http://www.iom.edu/Reports/2003/Keeping-Patients-Safe-Transforming-the-Work-Environment-of-Nurses.aspx

The Joint Commission. (2015a). *Core measure sets.* Chicago, IL: Author. Retrieved from http://www.jointcommission.org/core_measure_sets.aspx

The Joint Commission. (2015b). *Specifications manual for national hospital inpatient quality measures.* Chicago, IL: Author. Retrieved from http://www.jointcommission.org/specifications_manual_for_national_hospital_inpatient_quality_measures.aspx

The Joint Commission. (2015c). *What is accreditation?* Chicago, IL: Author. Retrieved from http://www.jointcommission.org/accreditation/accreditation_main.aspx

McHugh, M. D., & Chenjuan, M. (2013). Hospital nursing and 30-day readmissions among Medicare patients with heart failure, acute myocardial infarction, and pneumonia. *Medical Care, 51*(1), 52–59.

McHugh, M. D., Kutney-Lee, A., Cimiotti, J. P., Sloane, D. M., & Aiken, L. H. (2011). Nurses' widespread job dissatisfaction, burnout, and frustration with health benefits signal problems for patient care. *Health Affairs, 30*(2), 202–210.

Miles, R. E., & Snow, C. C. (1978). *Organizational strategy, structure, and process.* New York, NY: McGraw-Hill.

Nursing Organizations Alliance. (2004). *Principles and elements of a healthful practice/work environment*. Retrieved from www.aone.org/resources/leadership%20tools/PDFs/PrinciplesandElements HealthfulWorkPractice.pdf

Patient Protection and Affordable Care Act. (2010). P. L. 111–148. Sec. 3502.

Reason, J., & Hobbs, A. (2003). *Managing maintenance error*. Farnham, Surrey, England: Ashgate.

Research Triangle Institute International. (2015). U.S. News and World Report's *annual ranking of best hospitals*. Research Triangle Park, NC: Author. Retrieved from http://www.rti.org/BestHospitals

Scott, W. R., & Davis, G. F. (2015). *Organizations and organizing: Rational, natural and open systems perspectives*. London, NY: Routledge.

Singer, S., Lin, S., Falwell, A., Gaba, D., & Baker, L. (2009). Relationship of safety climate and safety performance in hospitals. *Health Services Research, 44*(2), 399–421.

Truven Healthcare Analytics. (2015). *100 top hospitals*. Ann Arbor, MI: Author. Retrieved from http://100tophospitals.com/

U.S. News and World Report LP. (2013). *Celebrating 80 years: A timeline of events in the life of* U.S. News and World Report, *1933–2013*. Washington, DC: Author. Retrieved from http://www.usnews.com/info/articles/2013/05/17/celebrating-80-years?page=2

U.S. News and World Report LP. (2015). *Best hospitals*. Washington, DC: Author. Retrieved from http://health.usnews.com/best-hospitals

# CHAPTER SEVEN

# EVALUATION OF HEALTH CARE INFORMATION SYSTEMS AND PATIENT CARE TECHNOLOGY

Sharon McLane and Juliana J. Brixey

*The problems that exist in the world today cannot be solved by the same level of thinking that created them.*
*—Albert Einstein*

This chapter discusses the role of the advanced practice nurse (APN) in the assessment of various types of technologies and information systems used by health care providers and patients. The purpose of this chapter is to equip the APN with increased knowledge of: (a) the tenets of information technology evaluation; and (b) effective partnerships and collaborations with informaticians and other members of the information systems team.

The first section addresses the framework of informatics and informaticians within the context of the clinical environment. It includes the following topics:

- Informatics and the role of the advanced practice informatician
- The collaborative relationship of the APN and informaticians
- The national mandate for electronic health records (EHR) and implications of reimbursement for eligible hospitals and providers
- The scope of the term *information technology* (IT)

The second part of the chapter discusses the specific areas in which DNPs can make effective contributions in the evaluation of health care and information technologies, including:

- Unintended and unexpected consequences of the introduction of information technologies
- Information technology as a communication tool and the emergence and implications of personal mobile devices in health care
- Informatics competency as a basic tenet of effective use and evaluation of information technology and information systems
- Electronic personal health records (ePHRs) and recommended evaluation criteria

- Recommended guidelines to support patients' searches for authentic health care information on the Internet
- Ergonomic and human factors evaluation of the work environment with respect to information technologies
- Evaluation of computerized patient care equipment

## INFORMATICS AND ADVANCED PRACTICE INFORMATICIANS

Adding informatics to the discussion of evaluation inserts an interesting and important domain of consideration. The discussion begins by defining informatics, specifically nursing informatics (NI), and the relationship between APNs and informatics practitioners. The American Nurses Association (ANA) defines *NI* as "the specialty that integrates nursing science with multiple information and analytical sciences to identify, define, manage and communicate data, information, knowledge, and wisdom in nursing practice," with the goal of improving the "health of populations, communities, groups, families, and individuals" through the "identification of issues and the design, development and implementation of effective informatics solutions and technologies within the clinical, administrative, educational, and research domains of practice" (ANA, 2015, pp. 1–2). The key concept of the ANA definition is the *management and communication of data, information, knowledge, and wisdom to improve health.* Informatics embraces IT in its multiple facets as a *tool* that is purposed to enhance information management and knowledge discovery. Much of the practice of informatics is devoted to the design of an information system. Advanced practice informaticians are also involved in informatics research including "design, development, implementation, and evaluation of informatics solutions, models, and theories" (ANA, 2015, p. 32) using "systematic methods of inquiry to identify, retrieve, represent, and evaluate data, information, and knowledge within informatics solutions and data repositories" (ANA, 2015, p. 32). The discovery of knowledge and understanding gleaned from the research findings will lead to models of health care delivery that are more effective, seamless, and transparent in the delivery of quality patient care and improvement of patient outcomes.

Preparation for informatics practice has not been standardized to date. Nurses may begin informatics practice through on-the-job training, completion of an informatics certificate program, and/or completion of a degree-granting program at the bachelor's, master's, or doctoral degree level. Degree domains include health informatics, health care informatics, clinical informatics, NI, and similar informatics domains. The common thread between these entry-to-practice levels is the creation of tools that practitioners can use to promote patient safety, enhance the quality of care delivery, promote health maintenance and disease prevention, and improve outcomes for individuals and populations.

The ANA classifies nurses working in informatics based on interest, experience, and academic preparation. The informatics nurse (IN) "is a registered nurse with an interest or experience in an informatics field." In contrast, the informatics nurse specialist (INS) "is a registered nurse with formal graduate-level education in informatics or an informatics-related field" (ANA, 2015, p. 7).

Frequently, the role of the informatician focuses on the configuration and design of the clinical information system (CIS) in preparation for system implementation. Informaticians who have completed an undergraduate or graduate program are prepared to embrace other important dimensions that are fundamental to developing an information system that effectively supports critical thinking and decision making. These dimensions include:

- Assessment of the socio-technical (e.g., the convergence of people, relationships, systems, and organizational culture) facets of an IT implementation, and the transformations that are deeply embedded in the implementation process.
- Awakening, promoting, and supporting innovative problem solving, appropriately employing the tools of information technology (Cassano, 2014).
- Assessment and management of the human–computer interface; that is, creating positive, intuitive, "error-free" experiences for practitioners as they use the technology.
- Assessment of current workflow, identifying opportunities for streamlining processes, for standardizing practice, and for development of new workflows in the context of the IT system.
- Application of informatics science to align application design with the cognitive needs of practitioners.
- System assessment that assures clinical staff are active, informed participants in evaluation, and quality improvement decisions regarding information technology systems (Jones et al., 2011).
- Establish, maintain, and update policies, processes, workflows, and/or technology designs that address EHR-related problems and issues (Jones et al., 2011).
- Strategic planning that anticipates and positions the organization for the cultural and practice transformation that is associated with the implementation of IT and information systems.
- System design that is aligned with the information management and knowledge management needs and characteristics of the organization (Greenes & Shortliffe, 2009; Gruber, Cummings, Leblanc, & Smith, 2009; Jones et al., 2011; Koppel & Gordon, 2012; Koppel, Wetterneck, Telles, & Karsh, 2008; McLane & Turley, 2011).

## NATIONAL MANDATE FOR EHR

We are living in the digital information age. Health care adopted IT to support the financial imperatives of the organization in the 1970s. However, the complexities of patient care, the multiple environments in which health care is delivered, the diverse patient populations, and the variability of resources of the health care industry resulted in a much more tentative approach to embracing IT for documentation, display, and storage of clinical data. A few intrepid early adopters began the journey to digital CIS in the late 1960s, and the number of hospitals and health care systems using IT for clinical documentation increased very slowly over the next 4 decades. By 2009, less than 4% of the nation's hospitals had "closed-loop medication administration"; that is, the seamless alignment of computerized provider order entry (CPOE), pharmacy review, electronic medication administration record (eMAR), and positive patient identification with bar code or radio frequency (RFID) technology (Health Information Management Systems Society [HIMSS] Analytics, 2013).

The stimulus of the American Recovery and Reinvestment Act (ARRA) of 2009 provided incentives to health care organizations to implement EHR. Between 2008 and 2013, 59% of the nation's hospitals adopted at least a basic EHR (patient demographics; problem lists; medication lists; discharge summaries; CPOE for medications; and lab, radiology, and diagnostic test results). While the rate of adoption is impressive, representing a fivefold increase between 2008 and 2013, it is interesting to note that adoption is highly variable across the individual states, ranging between 26% and 83% (Dustin, Gabriel, & Furukawa, 2014). Adoption of EHR technology is greater among urban hospitals. The adoption of EHR and IT in small and critical access hospitals lags behind their urban counterparts due to capital and infrastructure challenges, as well as limited access to a qualified workforce to support implementation (Adler-Milstein et al., 2014; Altarum Institute, 2011).

National health care policy, as established by ARRA, provided direction to the Centers for Medicare and Medicaid Services (CMS) to responsively create meaningful use rules and criteria for eligible providers and eligible hospitals. CMS also issued criteria for certification of EHRs, and eligible providers and eligible hospitals were required to report meaningful use of data from a certified EHR by 2015 (Obama, 2009). Due to the lack of meaningful use reporting functionality by several certified EHR systems, meaningful use reporting requirements were modified during the third quarter of 2014 (Centers for Medicare & Medicaid Services [CMS], 2014; U.S. Government Publishing Office, 2015). Under the new rules, the timeline for Stage 2 reporting is extended to 2016. Stage 3 rules of meaningful use will not be finalized until mid-2015, and implementation is scheduled in 2017 (CMS, 2013a, 2015b; HiTech Answers, 2015).

Design of the stages of meaningful use is intended to assist eligible hospitals and providers to move beyond data capture and storage to the next level of improved quality of care for patient populations. The goal is to transform health care organizations into continual learning environments that iteratively improve outcomes and processes based on their performance as measured by the data. Table 7.1 provides a high-level summary of the purpose of each stage of meaningful use and the expected outcomes of each stage.

Beginning in 2015, Medicare payments to eligible providers and eligible hospitals that do not demonstrate meaningful use were reduced, and the level of reimbursement will continue to decline in subsequent years. Recognizing the significant cost associated with implementation of EHR systems, CMS offered incentive payments to eligible providers and eligible hospitals, beginning in 2011 and running through 2015. Eligible providers and eligible hospitals that do not successfully demonstrate meaningful use by 2015 will experience payment adjustments to their Medicare reimbursement. These reimbursement changes have created a compelling inducement to reluctant or uncertain health care organizations and eligible providers to embrace IT, specifically the EHR. Since mid-2010, eligible providers and eligible hospitals have accelerated plans for implementation of an EHR, with an initial focus on achieving meaningful use. As of January 2105, more than $29 billion in EHR incentives has been paid to eligible hospitals and providers (CMS, 2015a).

**TABLE 7.1 Meaningful Use Stages**

|  | Stage 1 | Stage 2 | Stage 3 |
|---|---|---|---|
| Outcome | Data capture and sharing | Advanced clinical processes | Improved outcomes |
| Criteria for success | Standardize electronic data capture | Increase rigor of health information exchange | Improve quality, safety, and efficiency, leading to improved outcomes |
|  | Track key clinical conditions using electronic health record (EHR) data | Increase requirements for e-prescribing and reporting of lab data | Clinician decision support (CDS) linked to quality measures and drug–drug and drug–allergy alerts for entire reporting period |
|  | Improve care coordination processes | Electronic transmission of care summaries across multiple settings | Patient access to self-management tools |
|  | Begin reporting of clinical quality measures and public health data | More patient-controlled data | Health information exchange (HIE) provides access to comprehensive patient-centered data |
|  | Engage patients and families |  | Evidence of improved population health through public health and clinical data registry reporting |

*Source:* HealthIT.gov (2013b).

Collaboration between DNPs and nurse informaticians creates an ideal partnership for the effective use of and design of a CIS. The nursing knowledge, clinical expertise, and experience of APNs, in combination with the nursing knowledge, informatics knowledge, and CIS experience of nurse informaticians, merge to inform the design of a database that collects the information necessary to provide excellent patient care. The synergy of clinical subject matter experts and informatics subject matter experts establishes a harmony of design and function. The APN's expert clinical knowledge and understanding of the data necessary to support clinical assessment, critical thinking, ongoing modification of the plan of care, and patient education are essential to the design of an effective CIS that will be useful to and usable by practitioners. The nurse informatician carefully evaluates the knowledge and information needs defined by the APN in the context of factors such as future workflow, data visualization, cognition, system navigation, information management, terminology and taxonomy, training, practitioner adoption of the system, and data reporting needs.

An interesting and important dimension of the design of an EHR information system is the duality of purpose. The primary focus of an EHR is the individual patient and the information that is necessary to provide effective and efficacious care for that individual. The second, yet still very powerful, purpose of an EHR system is related to the data stored by the system, which can be used to evaluate practice, quality of care, outcomes, and many other dimensions for patient populations. Careful design of the system and thoughtful, intentional data input will create a database that can inform evidence-based practice and provide highly powered data regarding quality of care and patient outcomes. While the quality of care for the individual who has presented for care is the primary focus of the moment, a system that is thoughtfully designed to support data input and data visualization by practitioners who understand and respect the importance and value of the prescribed data input has the potential to create a robust evidence-based database.

## UNEXPECTED AND UNINTENDED CONSEQUENCES

Unexpected and unintended consequences have been persistent topics of interest to society. For example, Merton attributes unintended consequences to ignorance, error, fixation with immediacy, basic values that entail or block action, and self-defeating prophecy (Merton, 1936). Furthermore, history has recorded a number of memorable quotations regarding unexpected and unintended consequences regarding technology. For example, Reilly's Law and Murphy's Law each point out that the unexpected and unintended can and will occur (Murphy, 1949; Reilly, 1931). Tenner comments that "Americans believe that things can be contrary by nature" (Tenner, 1997, p. 4), and "whenever we try to take advantage of some new technology, we may discover that it induces behavior which appears to cancel out the very reason for using it" (Tenner, 1997, p. 7). Therefore, from a historical perspective of "laws" regarding not only the perception but also the actual performance of technology, it should not be astonishing that unexpected and unintended consequences should extend to EHRs and health information technology (HIT).

Unexpected and unintended consequences in health care began to receive attention as the early adopters of HIT began to implement various patient care information systems (PCISs) (Ash, Berg, & Coiera, 2004; Bloomrosen et al., 2011; Campbell, Sittig, Ash, Guappone, & Dykstra, 2006; Harrison, Koppel, & Bar-Lev, 2007; Jones et al., 2011; Middleton et al., 2013). Ash, Berg, and Coiera noted that "PCISs might not be as successful in preventing errors as generally hoped but could actually generate new errors," and "that PCIS applications seemed to foster errors rather than reduce their likelihood" (Ash et al., 2004, p. 105). The findings from their review of the literature and a series of qualitative studies identified that errors occurred in the process of data entry and retrieval as well as in the communication and coordination processes. Interest in unexpected and unintended consequences has continued with additional research studies and reports (Bloomrosen et al., 2011) with computerized order entry (CPOE), clinician decision support (CDS), and bar code medication administration technology at the forefront of attention. In 2011, the RAND Corporation, under contract with the Agency for Healthcare Research and Quality (AHRQ), released the *Guide to Reducing Unintended Consequences of Electronic Health Records* (Jones et al., 2011). Clinicians should be well-informed about the weaknesses as well as the benefits of technology (Kuperman & McGowan, 2013, p. 1666).

## IT AS A COMMUNICATION TOOL

IT refers to the tools—software, hardware, and communication devices—that support the communication and management of data and information. Computers and computer software are central to IT, and it is important to recognize that the presence of the computer and the software may not be immediately apparent to the user. IT extends beyond the traditional computer to include smart IV pumps, text messaging, and e-mail; social networking systems such as Facebook, Twitter, LinkedIn, Pinterest, Google Plus, Tumblr, Instagram, VK, Flickr, Vine, Meetup, Tagged, AskFM, Meetme (eBizMBA, 2015, September); point of care testing and data collection devices; patient education databases; online procedure manuals; scheduling and productivity management systems; and voice communication systems such as smartphones and mobile wireless communication systems.

Pen and paper are also a form of IT, as are the signal flags used by naval ships, and Morse code. Each of these examples is a form of communication, and it is important to ensure that the communication of information is the focus of attention, rather than the tools used to convey that information. By reframing the concept of IT as tools used for the purpose of communication of data and information, new horizons are disclosed. The perception of IT as a *tool* rather than as a goal is important. IT projects require a significant focus on the technology development and implementation process. However, the purpose of the tool must be the outcome of the project or we have failed our practitioner customers.

## MOBILE TECHNOLOGY: BACKGROUND AND SIGNIFICANCE

Mobile wireless communication technology has become ubiquitous. The concept of the cell phone emerged in the late 1940s (*Washington Post*, 2014). Dr. Martin Cooper is recognized as the inventor of the modern cell phone and, in 1973, he was the first person to place a call from a mobile phone (Hopkins, 2013). The first smartphone, Simon, was introduced in 1992 and included advanced functions that extended beyond making a telephone call. Simon's features included a pager, fax machine, computer, and touch screen with icons that could be tapped or activated with a stylus. Most importantly, Simon had apps for a camera, maps, and music (Sager, 2012). Apple launched the first iPhone in 2007 (Ritchie, 2014), and was soon followed by other smartphones such as those from Samsung (Segan, 2013). Smartphones with multiple apps and easy access to the Internet have rapidly become commonplace. Organizations were challenged to keep pace with rapidly changing mobile technology, and before long, bring your own device (BYOD) surfaced. The term BYOD was introduced in 2009, but the full impact was not realized until 2010 (Laird, 2014).

## BYOD/BYOX

BYOD evolved as employees began to utilize their personal mobile devices, such as smartphones and tablets, to complete job-related tasks. Employees frequently make the choice because of familiarity and skill with their personal device. Further, personal devices are often more technologically advanced than what is provided by the organization. Moreover, employers receive cost savings as the cost of the device shifts to the employee. For example the employee more often has purchased state of the art technology and a service provider, relieving the employer of the expense of purchasing the technology. Laird (2014) argues that BYOD has been replaced by even more diverse technologies and that the preferred term is bring your own everything (BYOx), as this is more inclusive and encompasses wearables as well as future technologies.

## BYOD IN THE HEALTH CARE ORGANIZATION

Health care organizations are not exempt from the BYOD movement. Currently, 73% of hospitals permit some use of BYOD, and more than 50% have a specific BYOD policy (Spok, 2015). Clinicians are using their own devices, with physicians leading the charge. Approximately 96% of practicing physicians use personal smart devices for clinical communication (Spyglass Consulting Group, 2014a). Furthermore, 67% of hospitals report that nurses use their own devices (Spyglass Consulting Group, 2014a); however, many hospitals prevent or discourage the use of smartphones, leaving nurses to use voice-only phones, multiple pagers, and/or wearable voice-activated two-way communication devices (Parker, 2014). A recently released report indicates that physician use of BYOD continues to outnumber BYOD use by nurses (Spok, 2015). Although health care organizations have lagged in providing technologies to improve communication processes for nurses, more than 50% of hospitals in the survey plan to acquire or consider smartphones within the upcoming 18 months, perhaps as early as late 2015 (Spyglass Consulting Group, 2014b).

Employer policies regarding BYOD need to be carefully crafted to avoid standard of care issues. Some employees may be unwilling, financially or for other reasons, to use personal communication devices to support patient care communication activities. Employers need to assure that these employees are provided with appropriate communication technology so that patient care is not delayed or impeded due to ineffective or inefficient communication technology.

## BYOD AND CHALLENGES

The term *BYOD* presents unique challenges to the health care organization. The IT department must maintain a secure network to protect the privacy and security of health and personal information. The IT department not only has to support the operating system for the health care organization, but is charged with supporting additional operating systems such as iOS, Android, Bada, MeeGo, Windows Mobile, and Blackberry, to name a few. Furthermore, the use of the mobile device may not be exclusive to the owner. Family members and coworkers cannot and should not be excluded as possible users of the device.

Moreover, the health care organization needs to consider infection control, as a mobile device may become a vector for the dissemination of disease. In BYOD, the mobile device travels from one clinical setting to the next, most likely without disinfection. Employer-owned mobile devices are a similar source of disease dissemination and just as unlikely to be disinfected as proscribed by policy.

Microorganisms and fungi are known to survive on various surfaces including plastics and fabrics and are easily transferred to other surfaces and objects, including by human hand contact (Sittig & Ash, 2011, pp. 203–210).

## RECOMMENDATIONS FOR MANAGEMENT OF BYOD

Data security and HIPAA compliance are a major concern for health care organizations. HealthIT.gov (HealthIT.gov, 2014) offers tips to guide health care organizations as they decide if BYOD is the right solution for the organization. The organization must assess the risks, threat, and vulnerabilities, and subsequently develop appropriate policies and procedures to protect health information. It is imperative to educate and train health care providers and professionals in strategies to protect the privacy and security of health information.

Health IT.gov (HealthIT.gov, 2013a, 2013d, 2014) offers recommendations to health care providers and professionals regarding BYOD in the clinical setting. Before using a personal device, a health care provider or professional should consult with the IT department or privacy and security officers concerning the organization's BYOD policies and procedures. It is paramount the device owner maintain physical control of the device at all times. Furthermore, the mobile device must be protected from breach and theft through encryption, security software, and user authentication, as well as securing and maintaining tracking software. It is obligatory that the most current security software and patches be installed upon release when personal devices are used in a clinical setting. Definitely, any and all stored health information must be purged before discarding or reusing the mobile device.

## INFORMATICS COMPETENCY

The health care agenda of the United States ensures that nearly all clinical information will be digitally recorded and stored (Office of the National Coordinator for Health Information Technology, 2014, 2015). CMS's meaningful use rules signal possible new characterizations and understanding of evidence-based practice. The dominance of digital information has been characterized as an information tsunami (Vastag, 2011). Research has established that as recently as 2007, nearly 94% of available information was digitally stored (Hilbert & Lopez, 2011). These concepts and facts illustrate that the development and maintenance of basic computer skills is no longer a choice and has become a basic life skill, similar to the use of an ATM or paying for groceries with the use of a debit card. Developing and maintaining computer skills is foundational to informatics competency but cannot be equated with informatics competency (Hersh et al., 2014).

The digitization of information demands that health care practitioners develop the ability to recognize the need for information, locate the information, and effectively evaluate, manipulate, and use the information; and it requires computer literacy and information literacy skills (Association of College and Research Libraries, 2000). Computer literacy and information literacy skills are generally referred to as informatics competencies. Informatics competencies are new or significantly revised skills for care providers who were born prior to 1980. Those earlier generations are often referred to as digital immigrants in comparison to those born after 1980, who are characterized as digital natives (Prensky, 2001).

Integration of informatics competencies into education has been recommended since the mid-1990s (Hersh et al., 2014; Staggers, Gassert, & Curran, 2001); however, implementation and adoption of these recommendations has occurred slower than anticipated. The growing importance of informatics competency served as the catalyst for an invitational summit of nursing leaders in practice, education, informatics, technology, information system vendors, government, and other key stakeholder entities from across the United States in the fall of 2006. The focus of the summit was the development of a vision for the nursing profession that embraces IT to improve practice, patient safety, and patient outcomes. The outcomes of the summit are included in the Technology Informatics Guiding Education Reform (TIGER) report. As the work of the summit evolved, a 10-year vision and a 3-year action plan were developed (Technology Informatics Guiding Education Reform [TIGER], 2007, 2009). In 2007, nine action items were defined and subsequently assigned to one of nine collaboratives. The development of computer literacy skills and information literacy skills by nurses is the focus of one of these nine collaboratives. The outcome of informatics competency is the preparation of nurses to understand and competently use the EHR to improve the health care of each patient and, ultimately, the health care of our nation. A brief summary of the collaboratives and their purposes is presented in Table 7.2.

**TABLE 7.2  TIGER Collaboratives**

| Collaborative | Purpose |
| --- | --- |
| Standards and interoperability | Improve patient care by promoting standardized nursing data, which will enable data mining and will facilitate measurement and comparison of nursing interventions and patient outcomes. Interoperability will assist in communication and data sharing between disparate information systems. |
| National health IT agenda | Increase nursing visibility and participation in the development of national health care policies. |
| Informatics competencies | Identify the skills necessary for nurses to effectively use an electronic health record (EHR), to use and contribute to evidence-based practice, and to efficiently access and use information. Recommended competencies include basic computer competency, information literacy, and information management. |
| Education and faculty development | Embed informatics competencies, theories, and research throughout the nursing curriculum and at all educational levels. Encourage funding of informatics curriculum development by foundations. Increase the informatics competency of faculty. |
| Staff development | Promote development of cost-effective resources and programs that foster IT innovation, and that promote development of the informatics competency of the practicing nurse. |

(continued)

| TABLE 7.2  TIGER Collaboratives (*continued*) | |
|---|---|
| **Collaborative** | **Purpose** |
| Leadership development | Heighten awareness and understanding of nurse leaders regarding the value of information technology and the importance of developing their personal informatics competency to lead the drive for improved patient safety, care delivery, and patient outcomes. |
| Usability and clinical application design | Promote user-focused system design and adoption of proven system integration, usability, and application design principles in the development of clinical information systems. |
| Virtual demonstration center | Two virtual conferences were held to increase visibility of the actual and potential benefits to be realized from IT, which will: enhance practice and improve patient care; demonstrate best practices; and improve quality and safety. |
| | One outcome of this collaborative is the TIGER Virtual Learning Environment (VLE). Under the auspices of HIMSS, the VLE provides a one-stop learning environment to assist educators, students, and adult learners in acquiring competencies that reflect international core computing standards (TIGER, 2015). |
| Consumer empowerment and personal health records | Empower patients to increase understanding of their health, to effectively prevent disease, and to manage their chronic diseases. Nurses need to understand ePHR tools so that they can knowledgeably discuss the ePHR options and benefits with the patient and his or her family or caregiver. |

Adapted from TIGER (2009).

DNPs are in an excellent position to observe the computer competency skills of the nurses with whom they work. TIGER recommends that all practicing nurses demonstrate basic skills, such as the ability to:

- Access, send, and add attachments to e-mail
- Use the Microsoft Windows operating system, such as starting applications, opening files, saving files, use of the taskbar and desktop, etc.
- Prepare, modify, and print a document in a word processing software application
- Copy and paste functions in various applications
- Prepare a simple spreadsheet and use simple formulas, filter data, manipulate data, and prepare a simple graph or chart

When informatics skills are inadequate or missing, APNs may wish to champion informatics skill acquisition, thus positioning the staff for future success. Often there are computer and information management continuing education program options available within the community at local high schools, vocational schools, colleges, or universities. A wide variety of distance education programs are available online, which can generally be completed at the learner's pace. The TIGER Initiative suggested several options for the development of informatics competency, including the Virtual Learning Environment (VLE; TIGER, 2015), European Computer Driving License (ECDL) Foundation (European Computer Driving License [ECDL], 2015), HIMSS, and the American Library Association (TIGER, 2009). Development of informatics competency self-assessment tools is an active research focus (Choi & Bakken, 2013; Choi & Zucker, 2013; Hunter, McGonigle, & Hebda, 2013)

Informatics competencies for the chief nurse executive (CNE) are equally important. Nursing leadership organizations, such as the American Organization of Nurse Executives (AONE), have established baseline competencies for nurses in the executive and leadership roles, and research is emerging to define the nature and application of informatics competency for nurse leaders (Collins, Kennedy, Phillips, & Yen, 2015; Simpson, 2013). Basic knowledge of information technology is necessary for the CNE and nurse leaders to effectively support nursing practice and envision how technology can be leveraged to enhance nursing practice and the collection of nursing and related data. Information technology can be a crucial strategic decision-making tool for the knowledgeable CNE. Further, a knowledge-able CNE is prepared to communicate and advocate for the tools and budget necessary to train staff, as well as effectively and safely use new or upgraded HIT. Understanding workflow and process mapping tools will provide the CNE with the tools and rationale for appropriate application of the principles of practice standardization (Simpson, 2013).

## PHR FOR PATIENTS

ePHRs or PHRs, are a more recent entry in the electronic health record field and, relatively speaking, have received much less attention than the development and installation of EHR systems. A generally accepted definition of PHR, as well as agreement regarding standards for the content, functionality, and interoperability of the PHR, have not been established to date (Halamka et al., 2005; HealthIT. gov, 2013c; Kaelber, Jha, Johnston, Middleton, & Bates, 2008; Reti, Feldman, & Safran, 2009). It is likely, however, that some patients/clients may have already adopted a PHR, or have made the decision to create a PHR. Those interested patients who do not have a PHR may seek advice from the APN on how to select a PHR.

PHRs generally assume one of three configurations (Tang, Ash, Bates, Overhage, & Sands, 2006). One configuration is the stand-alone PHR. PHRs offered by health care plans and a number of commercial vendors offer a stand-alone PHR. The choice of a stand-alone PHR is solely within the control of the patient. Additionally, information entry and maintenance of stand-alone PHRs are the responsibility of the patient or designated surrogate. It is the choice of the patient to grant access of his or her PHR to family members, primary care providers, and other care providers. Standalone PHRs have limitations: first, the ongoing commitment necessary to maintain accuracy by ensuring that the PHR is regularly reviewed and updated; and second, regardless of the diligence of the patient, providers may suspect the authenticity, accuracy, and completeness of the PHR.

Another available PHR configuration is a hybrid model in which web access is provided for the patient to view a portion or all of the health data that is stored by his or her health provider's EHR. Additionally, the patient is able to update or enter selected information in the PHR. Some providers are reluctant to enable data entry by the patient due to concerns regarding accuracy and the patient's health literacy.

The third PHR option is one in which patients are granted web-based access to selected portions of their EHR record without the ability to amend or add data. The view-only and limited-data-entry EHRs maintained by the individual's health care providers are often referred to as "patient portals" or porthole views into the patient's comprehensive health care record. The advantages to the patient of the view-only and limited-data-entry PHR options include the availability of more robust content as compared with the stand-alone PHR, and the inclusion of data backup systems in the event of computer failure or natural disasters (Tang et al., 2006).

A variety of added services may be available with patient portals depending upon the services the health care provider is able to support. For example, patient portals may include one- or two-way e-mail communication with the provider. Online appointment scheduling and medication refill requests are features attractive to many patients. In addition to direct communication with the nurse or physician primary care provider, robust PHRs may support communication with the pharmacies used by the patient, thus enabling a more comprehensive list of current medication therapies and drug–drug or drug–allergy clinical decision support to the health provider. More comprehensive resources for PHR assessment may be accessed at the CMS (2013b) and the American Health Information Management Association (AHIMA, 2016) websites.

The PHR marketplace is changing rapidly. Patients who elect to develop and maintain a stand-alone PHR would be wise to carefully assess the features of the products that they are considering. Significant considerations include privacy, security, encryption, and whether the PHR offer is free or fee based (AHIMA, 2016; H360ventures, 2015; HealthIT.gov, 2013c; U.S. Department of Health & Human Services [HHS], 2015). Health care practitioners who wish to knowledgeably advise their patients may find the AHIMA website a helpful guide (AHIMA, 2016).

In addition to PHRs, patients are beginning to embrace another new marketplace entrant, fitness trackers. At the time of this writing, fitness trackers are evolving quickly and vary widely in price and feature/function. Many trackers monitor heart rate, sleep patterns, step counters, GPS, and other features, and several models have sport-specific designs. Patients may present data from their fitness tracker, and it behooves the APN to develop familiarity with this quickly evolving phenomenon.

## GUIDING PATIENT DISCERNMENT OF HEALTH CARE INFORMATION ON THE INTERNET

As patients become increasingly adept in the use of information technology and the Internet, the APN may notice a change in the questions patients ask, and in their patients' knowledge about their health and self-care. They may also seek advice about the veracity of various websites. The APN must equip the patient with information and tools that will guide him or her to make informed choices and feel confident that he or she is able to discern credible health care websites containing authentic, accurate, and useful information.

The proliferation of health and health care information available on the Internet can be difficult to comprehend. To gain an appreciation of the pervasiveness of websites on the Internet that address health or health issues, you need only "Google" the search term "health." A search conducted on June 5, 2015, disclosed nearly 3.2 trillion sites, an increase of 33% since the same search was conducted in April 2011. The available information is overwhelming, and many patients need some assistance to determine the validity of the information present on these websites.

A 2013 survey disclosed that 72% of the American population searched the Internet for health and health-related information in the previous year, and that one in three Americans have used the web to determine the cause of the medical problems they or someone else were experiencing (Fox & Duggan, 2013). The authenticity of information that patients find on the Internet is highly variable. Authenticity and accuracy concerns increase with the realization that the content of the Internet is not regulated. Consequently, health care information on the Internet should be carefully evaluated for accuracy and reliability prior to developing a level of confidence in the website content (Baildon & Baildon, 2012; Cornell University Library, 2015; Kent State University Libraries, 2016; Weber, Derrico, Yoon, & Sherwill-Navarro, 2009).

Two important indicators of authenticity and accuracy of data on an Internet site are the source of the data and the date the site was last updated. Interestingly, 75% of people who search for health information on the Internet do not check the data source (e.g., author, credentials, affiliation) or the date that the website was last updated (Fox, 2006). Patients need to understand that virtually anyone can publish information on the Internet and that quality control is nominal at best (Ramsey Library at UNC Ashville, 2013). Consequently, health care professionals provide a critical service to their patients—and the patients' family members—by equipping them with criteria that empowers them to effectively cull their search results.

Health care websites vary in quality and accuracy of information, and patients seeking information are often vulnerable and not in the best position to discriminate among advice offered on health care websites. Researchers from the University of Florida (summarized in Exhibit 7.1), and Michigan State University (summarized in Table 7.3) provide guidelines to assist care providers and patients to more effectively evaluate website content on the Internet.

Proactive introduction of the subject of health care information available on the Internet and exploration of the patient's experiences when seeking such information on the Internet may assist the APN to determine the patient's readiness for education about effective use of the Internet. Empowering patients with knowledge of how to evaluate the information on the Internet provides the opportunity for patients to openly discuss information they may have discovered, and may promote a greater sense of partnership and accountability for managing their health status. Once the APN understands the information and sources the patient is consulting, the APN can continue the patient's education by exploring when and where such new knowledge is complementary to the medical plan of care. Table 7.4 is a selected sample of current resources that can assist the APN to become more knowledgeable regarding Internet evaluation.

---

**EXHIBIT 7.1**

**GATOR Website Assessment Criteria**

---

**G**enuineness of information can be assessed by exploring the stated goals and purpose of the site. For example, Internet addresses ending with ".com" are commercial websites that are usually selling a product or service; information provided by commercial websites should be independently verified with a credible resource. Care should also be taken to examine logos and website names, which may be ingeniously designed to closely resemble highly trusted and credible sites.

**A**ccuracy of the information is a second consideration. Look for a date to determine the last time the website was updated, which is often at the bottom of the page. Also look for indications of peer review. Consider seeking verification of information on other credible websites, particularly if the content is different from other credible sites.

**T**rustworthiness helps to ensure the veracity and reliability of the information. Check for references from credible sources, the credentials of site authors, and whether the authors are affiliated with established and respected organizations. The presence of contact information, such as telephone numbers and mail and e-mail addresses, is another indication of trustworthiness.

**O**rigin or source of the site content is an additional indicator of trustworthiness. In most cases authorship or sponsorship by a governmental (.gov in the United States), academic (.edu in the United States), research, or health care organization lends some assurance that the content is trustworthy.

**R**eadability is an indicator of how well the average consumer will be able to read and understand the website content. Patients need to recognize that some sites are designed for use by health care professionals and, therefore, seek sites that are created and maintained for use by the lay information consumer.

*Source:* Weber et al. (2009).

---

**TABLE 7.3   Telehealth Website Evaluation**

| | |
|---|---|
| Design | Links within the site or to other reference sources are recognizable and working. The site can be accessed from multiple browsers (e.g., Internet Explorer, Firefox, Safari). |
| Literacy | The site provides information that helps the user evaluate the credibility and trustworthiness of the site. |
| Information | Readability is demonstrated through the limited use of jargon; tables and charts are clear and well labeled; less common terminology is clearly explained. |
| Content | The site guides the readers' evaluation and understanding of the information presented, suggests questions they may direct to health care providers, directs users to other credible sources, and so on. Advertising, if present, should be clearly distinguished from the content of the site. |

*Source:* Whitten, Holtz, Cornacchione, and Wirth (2011).

TABLE 7.4   Additional Health Website Evaluation Resources

Health on the Net Foundation: *The HON Code of Conduct for Medical and Health Web Sites* (Health on the Internet Foundation [HON], 2013)

Medical Library Association: *Find Good Health Information* (Medical Library Association [MLA], 2016) Retrieved from http://www.mlanet.org/resources/userguide.html

MedLine Plus: *Evaluating Internet Health Information: A Tutorial From the National Library of Medicine* (MedlinePlus, 2012)

National Cancer Institute: *Using Trusted Resources* (NIH: National Cancer Institute, 2015)

National Library of Medicine: *Guide to Finding Health Information* (National Library of Medicine [NLM], 2014)

National Network of Libraries of Medicine (NN/LM): *Evaluating Health Websites* (National Network of Libraries of Medicine [NN/LM], 2014)

## HUMAN FACTORS AND ERGONOMICS

Human factors, or ergonomics, focus on the relationship of the worker with the work systems with which the worker interacts. In health care, human factors examine the systems that health care practitioners employ in the process of gathering data, assessing information related directly or indirectly to the care of the patient, and the actual delivery of care. Increasingly, technology is integral to the work processes of health care practitioners and, consequently, much of human factors research and engineering centers on patient safety and reduction of medical error.

Technology changes the way in which individuals perform and complete their work, the task itself, and the workplace in general. Despite goals such as enhanced efficiency, improved quality, and reduced medical errors, the introduction of technology presents unique challenges that are not always immediately discernible by the health care practitioner (Carayon & Wood, 2010). Without careful attention to human factors, technologies intended to improve the quality of care can introduce new risks and negative consequences (Jones et al., 2011; Koppel & Gordon, 2012; Koppel et al., 2008; Norman, 1991; Patterson, Rogers, Chapman, & Render, 2006).

Ergonomics is an applied science that defines the physical, cognitive, and organization requirements of the work environment. Ergonomics is an important consideration when designing tools or configuring the spaces in which practitioners work; one important goal is to promote effective and safe use of the tools (Harrison et al., 2007; Prensky, 2001). Ergonomics is an overarching principle embedded within informatics practice, is woven throughout each ANA NI practice standard, and recognizes the criticality of promoting a safe practice environment that minimizes the likelihood of injury (ANA, 2015). Incorporating ergonomic principles in the design of new environments or the retrofit of older work environments can reduce the risk of musculoskeletal injuries or other related injuries that often occur as the result of a poorly designed setting (Nielsen & Trinkoff, 2003).

An important ergonomic consideration is the computer workstation, which must be designed to enable the user to work with the computer without strain or risk of temporary or permanent injury. The duration of sustained use of a computer workstation and the number of people who will use a workstation influence the necessary space modifications that will promote safe use. Design of workstations that are to be used by multiple individuals requires flexibility that enables each user to adjust the station to the best position for his or her physical and task needs.

Expert resources are available to guide objective purchase decisions for furniture and equipment, as well as to guide workstation design. The Occupational Safety and Health Administration (OSHA) offers evidence-based checklists for evaluation of workstations and to guide purchasing decisions. The consultative services of certified ergonomic professionals are also available as another expert consideration when planning computer workstations (Board of Certification in Professional Ergonomics, 2015). Given the personal anguish, lost productivity, and costs associated with ergonomic work-related injuries, some organizations choose to have a certified professional ergonomics engineer as a permanent part of the staff (Columbia University, 2008; Occupational Safety & Health Administration, 2015a, 2015b, 2015c).

## USABILITY AS AN EVALUATION TOOL

Usability is a dimension of the interface between people and technology. Zhang and Walji define *usability* as "how useful, usable, and satisfying a system is for its intended users to accomplish goals in a work domain" (Zhang & Walji, 2014, p. 27). The World Health Organization articulates an important nuance of usability in that good usability makes "it easier to do the work in the right way" (World Health Organization, 2008).

*User-friendly* is a term often used to convey the concept of usability. However, user-friendly is a subjective descriptor and is absent objective and measurable qualities or criteria. Zhang and Walji and their colleagues at the University of Texas, School of Biomedical Informatics, developed TURF, a unified conceptual framework to quantify usability. TURF, or *Task, User, Representation,* and *Function*, is "a theory for describing, explaining, and predicting usability differences; an objective method for defining, evaluating, and measuring usability; a process for designing in good usability; and a potential principle for developing EHR usability guidelines and standards" (Zhang & Walji, 2014, p. 29). Developers and clinicians can employ TURF as a framework for redesign or enhancement of an existing EHR system. Careful discernment of the TURF framework will equip the advanced practitioner to be a much more knowledgeable participant and consumer throughout information technology acquisition and implementation.

Patient safety is a fundamental consideration when purchase decisions are made for equipment that will be used in the direct or indirect care of patients. A critical facet of equipment evaluation is assessment of the usability of that equipment. Usability addresses the design of devices with attention to how the device will be used, the ways in which people may abuse the device, the types of errors people could make while using the device, and the outcomes people wish to achieve through use of the device (Norman, 2002; Phansalkar et al., 2010; Zhang, Johnson, Patel, Paige, & Kubose, 2003). Poor usability is a significant contributor to unexpected and unintended consequences of information technology.

A respected means of evaluating the usability of equipment or software is to examine and observe how the system or equipment is used. An APN can apply some of the basic principles of usability that are embodied in a process called heuristic testing, the principles of which are described in Table 7.5. These principles may prove useful to evaluate patient care technologies in APN practice. They are applicable when evaluating equipment, software, EHR designs, and other information technology equipment. Heuristic evaluation principles are not difficult to apply and can support objective comparative information based on the usability characteristics of equipment, information systems, communication systems, and so forth.

**TABLE 7.5  Usability Evaluation Using Heuristic Principles**

| Heuristic Principle | Example |
|---|---|
| 1. Consistency and standards | Does the application use color consistently and do the colors make sense? Are terms clear to the user and are they used consistently? Are buttons consistently used for the same purpose? Is there consistency in general layout between screens? |
| 2. Visibility of the system state | Can the user tell when the system is working? Is the next action to be taken clear to the user? |
| 3. Match between the system and the world | Does use of the equipment match what the user would generally expect? Does pressing buttons or turning knobs result in expected outcomes? Does the user see what is expected? |
| 4. Minimalist | Is the information present on the screen only what is needed to inform the user? Is superfluous information on the screen? Is there a logical and sequential level of detail and action? |
| 5. Memory load is minimized | Does the system require the user to rely on memory to use the equipment, or is the user appropriately prompted? Are examples for data entry expectations offered (e.g., YYYY/MM/DD or YY/MM/DD)? Does the system progress through a logical hierarchy? |
| 6. Feedback that is informative | Does the system offer immediate and understandable feedback to user actions, particularly incorrect actions? Is the feedback specific, providing clear direction regarding the next step to be taken? |
| 7. Flexibility and efficiency | Does the system support shortcuts for the experienced user? Are the information needs of the novice distinguished from those of the expert? |
| 8. Good error messages | When the user makes an error, does the system provide a meaningful and understandable feedback message, enabling the user to learn from the error? Does the system avoid the use of error "codes" (e.g., "Error 147")? Are error messages polite and helpful (e.g., "fatal error," "illegal action")? |
| 9. Preventing error | Is the system designed to help the user avoid mistakes? Does the system prevent egregious errors? Are audible or pop-up messages present when the user is about to perform an incorrect action? |

(*continued*)

**TABLE 7.5   Usability Evaluation Using Heuristic Principles (*continued*)**

| Heuristic Principle | Example |
|---|---|
| 10.  Clear closure | Is it clear when a user is at the beginning, middle, or end of a task? Is it clear when a task, or required sequence of tasks, is completed? |
| 11.  Reversible actions | Does the system allow the user to recover from mistakes? Does the system prevent serious errors? Does the system allow the user to explore the system and back out without consequences? |
| 12.  User language | Does the system use language familiar to the user? Do the terms used by the system have a standard meaning? |
| 13.  User in control | Is the user in control of the system? Does the user, not the system, initiate action? |
| 14.  Help and documentation | Does the system provide context-sensitive help? Is the help embedded in the system? Is help available when needed? |

*Sources:* Graham et al. (2004); Nielsen (1995); Norman (2002); Zhang et al. (2003); and Zhang & Walji (2014).

Usability evaluation of patient care equipment is an important measure in reducing risk, increasing safety, and minimizing human error in the delivery of patient care. Cost, return on investment, functionality, and compatibility with the current clinical environment are important considerations in selection of patient care equipment from various vendor options. Equally important are the usability characteristics of each vendor's product. It is important to select equipment that is easy to use and that actively promotes the avoidance of error. The usability characteristics demonstrated by the equipment options under consideration for purchase should have at least equal weight with the other considerations in making the purchase decision. Zhang et al. (2003) suggest a rating scale to assist in assigning weights to the evaluation outcomes, which may be helpful when comparing the same equipment from different vendors.

A properly conducted heuristic evaluation is very unlikely to find no usability problems—the sophistication of human factors engineering has not attained that level of refinement to date. The primary intent of usability evaluation is to identify the product that is most appropriate for the target clinical environment. Additionally, usability evaluation will shed light on usability problems so that users can be informed of the risks and policies can be established to reduce and mitigate the identified risks.

## SUMMARY

This discussion has established the role of an informatician and the criticality of developing and maintaining an ongoing partnership between nurse informaticians and APNs. This partnership can provide significant guidance to IT project design and implementation. The scope and variety of IT and how deeply it is embedded in practice and in personal and professional lives is briefly addressed. The national mandate for EHRs was discussed along with why EHR selection and implementation is such a central focus at this time.

The DNP is in an excellent position to influence nursing practice, technology implementation, and the integration of practice and technology. The APN can influence and participate in BYOD/BYOx decisions by knowledgeably articulating the benefits, challenges, and risks of personal mobile devices. As a respected member of the health care team, the APN can identify the informatics competency needs of colleagues and staff and can influence understanding of the power of this essential skill, advocating for resources that will support skill building. The DNP can empower patients to become more knowledgeable and involved in health maintenance, disease prevention, and management of chronic diseases through an understanding of the PHR and can identify the patients in his or her practice that would benefit from the PHR. Such understanding will inform the patient-teaching process and assist patients to discern authentic, accurate information on the Internet.

The DNP can be a powerful advocate for practice and patient safety through promoting and participating in usability evaluation as an integral part of the information system purchase decision. Also considered was the role of the DNP in the influence of technology-driven patient care equipment purchase decisions though a constructive heuristic evaluation. The heuristic evaluation metrics presented can serve as important and objective criteria to evaluate patient care equipment. Design of computer workstations is important to avoid or minimize user injury. We established basic workflow design issues and, more importantly, directed readers to several evidence-based websites that described ergonomically appropriate computer design.

---

## CASE STUDY

Anywhere Hospital has been using IV pumps for the past 20 years. Over the years, models from various vendors were researched and purchased. The complexity of the pumps increased with each subsequent purchasing cycle. The hospital currently maintains IV pumps from 10 different vendors to meet the needs of critical care, trauma, anesthesiology, and the medical/surgical patient care units; five of these pumps are used on the medical/surgical units. The decision to purchase each brand of pump was based on new and enhanced patient safety features. The last model was purchased nearly 5 years ago, and each of the other brands received feature/function upgrades in the past 4 years.

While each of the pumps was purchased with the intent of increasing patient safety, Anywhere Hospital has also experienced unintended consequences. First, each pump has a different user interface, which has lengthened orientation for newly hired medical/surgical nurses. Second, the different interfaces have resulted in programming errors that have compromised patient safety. Because the demand for IV pumps is high, a nurse may be responsible for several IV pump brands in his or her patient care assignment. Third, the expense to inventory replacement parts and ensure biomedical engineering competency to repair the ten pump brands was not anticipated in the original cost of ownership projections.

Anywhere Hospital recently completed an analysis intended to "right size" the number and types of IV pumps necessary to provide safe, evidence-based IV therapy to the patients who entrust their lives to this health care organization. In addition to establishing the appropriate number and type of IV pumps that will meet the needs of the patient demographic mix cared for at Anywhere

*(continued)*

---

**CASE STUDY (continued)**

Hospital, several criteria were established to guide future decisions about information technology related to IV therapy.

- Anywhere Hospital recognized that a single pump brand/model most likely would not meet the needs of critical care, the Level I trauma center, anesthesiology, and the inpatient medical/surgical units. The primary goal was to identify a single pump brand to serve the medical/surgical clinical care areas of the hospital with the intent of reduced user interface confusion issues and reduced parts inventory and biomedical competency costs.
- A request for information (RFI) containing the requisite functions and safety features required by Anywhere Hospital would be issued to IV pump vendors. Biomedical engineering, pharmacy, and nursing would collaborate to create multiple clinical scenarios to address usability (heuristic) in various clinical test situations in which an IV pump would be used, such as: (a) hang an initial bag of fluid; (b) initiate an IV bag with medication using the pump drug library; (c) titrate a medication drip; (d) titrate multiple drips through the same site/catheter; and (e) clear the pump for a new patient.
- All pump vendors that submit a successful response to the RFI will be invited to demonstrate their product in strict accordance with the clinical scenarios defined by Anywhere Hospital. Vendors with successful demonstrations will be required to leave a sample pump with Anywhere Hospital for 3 weeks to allow further usability testing, employing the heuristic evaluation principles.
- Two to three practicing nurses will be solicited to complete each usability (heuristic) clinical scenario after appropriate orientation to the use of the IV pump. Each scenario will be filmed to enable effective analysis of usability.
- Usability (heuristic) functionality will be scored in accordance with Zhang et al.'s (2003) methodology.
- Purchase decisions will be heavily weighted by the scored usability (heuristic) test outcomes.

# REFERENCES

Adler-Milstein, J., DesRoches, C. M., Furukawa, M. F., Worzala, C., Charles, D., Kralovec, P., . . . Jha, A. K. (2014). More than half of US hospitals have at least a basic EHR, but stage 2 criteria remain challenging for most. *Health Affairs, 33,* 1664–1671. doi:10.1377/hlthaff.2014.0453

AHIMA. (2016). *What is a personal health record (PHR)?*. Retrieved from http://www.myphr.com/StartaPHR/what_is_a_phr.asp

Altarum Institute. (2011). *Overcoming challenges to health IT adoption in small, rural hospitals.* Retrieved from http://www.healthit.gov/sites/default/files/pdf/OvercomingChallenges_in_SmallRuralHospitals.pdf

American Nurses Association. (2015). *Nursing informatics: Scope & standards of practice* (2nd ed.). Silver Spring, MD: Author.

AHIMA. (2016). *What is a Personal Health Record (PHR)?* Retrieved from http://www.myphr.com/StartaPHR/what_is_a_phr.aspx

Ash, J. S., Berg, M., & Coiera, E. (2004). Some unintended consequences of informtion technology in health care: The nature of patient care information system-related errors. *Journal of the American Medical Informatics Association, 11*(2), 104–112. doi:10.1197/jamia.M1471

Association of College and Research Libraries. (2000). *Information literacy competency standards for higher education.* Retrieved from http://www.ala.org/acrl/standards/information literacycompetency

Baildon, M., & Baildon, R. (2012). Evaluating online sources: Helping students determine trustworthiness, readability, and usefulness. *Social Studies and the Young Learner, 24*(4), 11–14.

Bloomrosen, M., Starren, J., Lorenzi, N. M., Ash, J. S., Patel, V. L., & Shortliffe, E. H. (2011). Anticipating and addressing the unintended consequences of health IT and policy: A report from the AMIA 2009 health policy meeting. *Journal of the American Medical Association, 18*(1), 82–90. doi:10.1136/jamia.2010.007567

Board of Certification in Professional Ergonomics. (2015). Retrieved from http://www.bcpe.org

Campbell, E. M., Sittig, D. F., Ash, J. S., Guappone, K. P., & Dykstra, R. H. (2006). Types of unintended consequences related to computerized provider order entry. *Journal of the American Medical Informatics Association, 13*(5), 547–556. doi:10.1197/jamia.M2042

Carayon, P., & Wood, K. E. (2010). Patient safety: The role of human factors and systems engineering. *Studies Health Technology and Informatics, 153,* 23–46. Retrieved from http://www.ncbi.nlm.nih.gov/pmc/articles/PMC3057365/pdf/nihms274759.pdf

Cassano, C. (2014). The right balance—Technology and patient care. *Online Journal of Nursing Informatics, 18*(3). Retrieved from http://www.himss.org/ResourceLibrary/GenResourceDetail.aspx?ItemNumber=33541

Centers for Medicare & Medicaid Services. (2013a). *Progress on adoption of electronic health records.* Retrieved from http://www.cms.gov/eHealth/ListServ_Stage3Implementation.html

Centers for Medicare & Medicaid Services. (2013b). *Summary of responses to an industry RFI regarding a role for CMS with personal health records.* Retrieved from https://www.cms.gov/Medicare/E-Health/PerHealthRecords/downloads/SummaryofPersonalHealthRecord.pdf

Centers for Medicare & Medicaid Services. (2014b). *Medicare and Medicaid programs; Modifications to the Medicare and Medicaid electronic health record (EHR) incentive program for 2014 and other changes to the EHR incentive program; and health information technology: Revisions to the certified EHR technology definition and EHR certification changes related to standards (45 CFR Part 170; 52910).* Retrieved from http://www.gpo.gov/fdsys/pkg/FR-2014-09-04/pdf/2014-21021.pdf

Centers for Medicare & Medicaid Services. (2015a). *Medicare & Medicaid EHR incentive programs. HIT Policy Committee.* Retrieved from http://www.healthit.gov/FACAS/sites/faca/files/HITPC_CMS_Presentation_2015-03-10.pdf

Centers for Medicare & Medicaid Services. (2015b). *The official web site for the Medicare and Medicaid electronic health records (EHR) incentive programs.* Retrieved from http://www.cms.gov/Regulations-and-Guidance/Legislation/EHRIncentivePrograms/index.html?redirect=/EHRIncentivePrograms/

Choi, J., & Bakken, S. (2013). Validation of the self-assessment of nursing informatics competency scale among undergraduate and graduate nursing students. *Journal of Nursing Education, 52*(5), 275–282. doi:10.3928/01484834-20130412-01

Choi, J., & Zucker, D. M. (2013). Self-assessment of nursing informatics competencies for doctor of nursing practice students. *Journal of Professional Nursing, 29*(6), 381–387. doi:10.1016/j.profnurs.2012.05.014

Collins, S., Kennedy, M. K., Phillips, A., & Yen, P. Y. (2015). *Nursing informatics competencies for nurse leaders/managers: A delphi study.* Paper presented at the AONE 2015 Annual Conference, Phoenix, AZ.

Columbia University. (2008). *Ergonomic self-evaluation tool.* Retrieved from http://www.ehs.columbia.edu/ErgoEvaluateTool.html

Cornell University Library. (2015, May 17). *Evaluating web pages: Questions to consider.* Retrieved from http://guides.library.cornell.edu/evaluating_Web_pages

Dustin, C., Gabriel, M., & Furukawa, M. F. (2014, May 14). *Adoption of electronic health record systems among U.S. non-federal acute care hospitals: 2008–2013.* Retrieved from http://www.healthit.gov/sites/default/files/oncdatabrief16.pdf

eBizMBA. (2015, September). *Top 15 most popular social networking sites.* Retrieved from http://www.ebizmba.com/articles/social-networking-websites

European Computer Driving License. (2015). *New ECDL: Digital skills to get ahead.* Retrieved from http://www.ecdl.org/programmes/ecdl_icdl

Fox, S. (2006). *Online health search 2006.* Retrieved from http://www.pewinternet.org/2006/10/29/online-health-search-2006/

Fox, S., & Duggan, M. (2013, January 13). *Health online 2013.* Retrieved from http://www.pewinternet.org/files/old-media/Files/Reports/PIP_HealthOnline.pdf

Graham, M. J., Kubose, T. K., Jordan, D., Zhang, J., Johnson, T. R., & Patel, V. L. (2004). Heuristic evaluation of infusion pumps: Implications for patient safety in intensive care units. *International Journal of Medical Informatics, 73*(11–12), 773–779. doi:10.1016/j.ijmedinf.2004.08.002

Greenes, R. A., & Shortliffe, E. H. (2009). Informatics in biomedicine and health care. *Academic Medicine, 84*(7), 818–820. doi:10.1097/ACM.0b013e3181a81f94

Gruber, D., Cummings, G. G., Leblanc, L., & Smith, D. L. (2009). Factors influencing outcomes of clinical information systems implementation. *Computers Informatics Nursing, 27*(3), 151–163. doi:10.1097/NCN.0b013e31819f7c07

H360ventures. (2015). *PHRs today: Resources to manage your health.* Retrieved from http://www.phrstoday.com/index.html

Halamka, J., Overhage, J. M., Ricciardi, L., Rishel, W., Shirky, C., & Diamond, C. (2005). Exchanging health information: Local distribution, national coordination. *Health Affairs, 24*(5), 1170–1179. doi:10.1377/hlthaff.24.5.1170

Harrison, M. I., Koppel, R., & Bar-Lev, S. (2007). Unintended consequences of information technologies in healthcare—An interactive sociotechnical analysis. *Journal of the American Medical Informatics Association, 14*(5), 542–549. doi:10.1197/jamia.M2384

Health on the Internet Foundation. (2013). *The HON code of conduct for medical and health web sites.* Retrieved from http://www.hon.ch/HONcode/Conduct.html

HealthIT.gov. (2013a). *How can you protect and secure health information when using a mobile device?* Retrieved from https://www.healthit.gov/providers-professionals/how-can-you-protect-and-secure-health-information-when-using-mobile-device

HealthIT.gov. (2013b). *How to attain meaningful use.* Retrieved from http://www.healthit.gov/providers-professionals/how-attain-meaningful-use

HealthIT.gov. (2013c). *What is a personal health record?* Retrieved from http://www.healthit.gov/providers-professionals/faqs/what-personal-health-record

HealthIT.gov. (2013d). *You, your organization, and your mobile device.* Retrieved from http://www.healthit.gov/providers-professionals/you-your-organization-and-your-mobile-device

HealthIT.gov. (2014). *Your mobile device and health information privacy and security.* Retrieved from https://www.healthit.gov/providers-professionals/your-mobile-device-and-health-information-privacy-and-security

Hersh, W. R., Gorman, P. N., Biagioli, F. E., Mohan, V., Gold, J. A., & Mejicano, G. C. (2014). Beyond information retrieval and electronic health record use: Competencies in clinical informatics for medical education. *Journal of Advances in Medical Education and Practice, 5,* 205–212. doi:10.2147/AMEP.S63903

Hilbert, M., & Lopez, P. (2011). The world's technological capacity to store, communicate, and compute information. *Science, 332*(6025), 60–65. doi:10.1126/science.1200970

HIMSS Analytics. (2013). *Electronic medical record adoption model: Closed loop medication administration.* Retrieved from http://www.himssanalytics.org/emram/

HiTech Answers. (2015). *The stages of meaningful use.* Retrieved from http://www.hitechanswers.net/ehr-adoption-2/meaningful-use/

Hopkins, C. S. (2013, February 20). *5 Inventors of the cell phone honored for wiring the world.* Retrieved from http://www.nationaljournal.com/daily/5-inventors-of-the-cell-phone-honored-for-wiring-the-world-20130220

Hunter, K. M., McGonigle, D. M., & Hebda, T. L. (2013). TIGER-based measurement of nursing informatics competencies: The development and implementation of an online tool for self-assessment. *Journal of Nursing Education and Practice, 3*(12), 70–80.

Jones, S. S., Koppel, R., Ridegely, M. S., Wu, S., Palen, T. E., & Harrison, M. I. (2011). *Guide to reducing unintended consequences of electronic health records.* Retrieved from AHRQ Publication No. 11-0105-EF: https://healthit.ahrq.gov/sites/default/files/docs/publication/guide-to-reducing-unintended-consequences-of-electronic-health-records.pdf

Kaelber, D. C., Jha, A., Johnston, D., Middleton, B., & Bates, D. W. (2008). A research agenda for personal health records (PHRs). *Journal of the American Medical Informatics Association, 15*(6), 729–736. doi:10.1197/jamia.M2547

Kent State University Libraries. (2016). *Criteria for evaluating web resources.* Retrieved from http://www.library.kent.edu/criteria-evaluating-web-resources

Koppel, R., & Gordon, S. (Eds.). (2012). *First, do less harm: Confronting the inconvenient problems of patient safety.* Ithaca, NY: Cornell University Press.

Koppel, R., Wetterneck, T., Telles, J. L., & Karsh, B. T. (2008). Workarounds to barcode medication administration systems: Their occurrences, causes, and threats to patient safety. *Journal of the American Medical Association, 15*(4), 408–423. doi:10.1197/jamia.M2616

Kuperman, G., & McGowan, J. (2013). Potential unintended consequences of health information exchange. *Journal of General Internal Medicine, 28*(12), 1663–1666. doi:10.1007/s11606-012-2313-0

Laird, J. (2014, November 7). *A brief history of BYOD and why it doesn't exist anymore.* Retrieved from http://www.lifehacker.co.uk/2014/11/07/brief-history-byod-doesnt-actually-exist-anymore

McLane, S., & Turley, J. P. (2011). Informaticians: How they may benefit your healthcare organization. *Journal of Nursing Administration, 41*(1), 29–35. doi:10.1097/NNA.0b013e3181fc19d6

Medical Library Association (2016). Find good health information. Retrieved from http://www.mlanet.org/resources/userguide.html

MedlinePlus. (2012, April 19). *Evaluating Internet health information: A tutorial from the National Library of Medicine.* Retrieved from http://www.nlm.nih.gov/medlineplus/webeval/webeval.html

Merton, R. K. (1936). The unanticipated consequences of purposive social action. *American Sociological Review, 1*(6), 894–904. Retrieved from http://www.d.umn.edu/cla/faculty/jhamlin/4111/Readings/MertonSocialAction.pdf

Middleton, B., Bloomrosen, M., Dente, M. A., Hashmat, B., Koppel, R., Overhage, J. M., . . . Zhang, J. (2013). Enhancing patient safety and quality of care by improving the usability of electronic health record systems: Recommendations from AMIA. *Journal of the American Medical Informatics Association, 20*(e1), e2–e8. doi:10.1136/amiajnl-2012-001458

Murphy, E. A. (1949). *Murphy's law.* Retrieved from http://www.murphys-laws.com/murphy/murphy-true.html

NIH: National Cancer Institute. (2015). *Using trusted resources.* Retrieved from http://www.cancer.gov/about-cancer/managing-care/using-trusted-resources

National Library of Medicine (NLM). (2014, November 3). *Guide to finding health information.* Retrieved from http://www.nlm.nih.gov/services/guide.html

National Network of Libraries of Medicine (NN/LM). (2014, November 10). *Evaluating health websites.* Retrieved from http://nnlm.gov/outreach/consumer/evalsite.html

Nielsen, J. (1995/2005). *10 usability heuristics for user interface design*. Retrieved from http://www .nngroup.com/articles/ten-usability-heuristics/

Nielsen, K., & Trinkoff, A. (2003). Applying ergonomics to nurse computer workstations: Review and recommendations. *CIN: Computers, Informatics, Nursing, 21*(3), 150–157.

NIH: National Cancer Institute. (2015, March 10). *Using trusted resources*. Retrieved from http:// www.cancer.gov/about-cancer/managing-care/using-trusted-resources

Norman, D. A. (1991). Cognitive artifacts. In J. M. Carroll (Ed.), *Designing interaction: Psychology at the human–computer interface*. Cambridge, UK: Cambridge University Press.

Norman, D. A. (2002). *The design of everyday things*. New York, NY: Basic Books.

Obama, B. (2009, February 9). Obama's prime-time press briefing. *The New York Times*. Retrieved from http://www.nytimes.com/2009/02/09/us/politics/09text-obama.html?_r=0

Occupational Safety & Health Administration. (2015a). *Computer workstation etools*. Retrieved from https://www.osha.gov/SLTC/etools/computerworkstations/

Occupational Safety & Health Administration. (2015b). *Computer workstation: Evaluation checklist*. Retrieved from https://www.osha.gov/SLTC/etools/computerworkstations/checklist_evaluation .html

Occupational Safety & Health Administration. (2015c). *Computer workstation: Purchase checklist*. Retrieved from https://www.osha.gov/SLTC/etools/computerworkstations/checklist_purchasing_ guide.html

Office of the National Coordinator for Health Information Technology. (2014, October). *Report to Congress: Update on the adoption of health information technology and related efforts to facilitate the electronic use and exchange of health information*. Retrieved from http://www.healthit.gov/sites/ default/files/rtc_adoption_and_exchange9302014.pdf

Office of the National Coordinator for Health Information Technology. (2015, January 28). *Federal health IT strategic plan 2015-2020*. Retrieved from http://www.healthit.gov/sites/default/files/ FederalHealthIT_Strategic_Plan.pdf

Parker, C. D. (2014, November 20). *Evolution of revolution? Smartphone use in nursing practice*. Retrieved from http://www.americannursetoday.com/evolution-revolution-smartphone-use-nursing-practice/

Patterson, E. S., Rogers, M. L., Chapman, R. J., & Render, M. L. (2006). Compliance with intended use of bar code medication administration in acute and long-term care: An observational study. *Human Factors, 48*(1), 15–22.

Phansalkar, S., Edworthy, J., Hellier, E., Seger, D. L., Schedlbauer, A., Avery, A. J., & Bates, D. W. (2010). A review of human factors principles for the design and implementation of medication safety alerts in clinical information systems. *Journal of the American Medical Informatics Association, 17*(5), 493–501. doi:10.1136/jamia.2010.005264

Prensky, M. (2001). Digital natives, digital immigrants. *On the Horizon (Lincoln, NCB University Press), 9*(5), 1–6.

Reilly, W. J. (1931). *The law of retail gravitation*. New York, NY: Knickerbocker Press.

Reti, S. R., Feldman, H. J., & Safran, C. (2009). Governance for personal health records. *Journal of the American Medical Informatics Association, 16*, 14–17. doi:10.1197/jamia.M2854

Ritchie, R. (2014, August 22). *History of iPhone: Apple reinvents the phone*. Retrieved from http://www .imore.com/history-iphone-2g

Sager, I. (2012). *Before iPhone and Android came Simon, the first smartphone*. Retrieved from http:// www.bloomberg.com/news/articles/2012-06-29/before-iphone-and-android-came- simon-the-first-smartphone

Segan, S. (2013, March 12). *Samsung's smartphone history: From zero to Galaxy S4*. Retrieved from http://www.pcmag.com/slideshow/story/309047/samsung-s-smartphone-history-from-zero-to-galaxy-s4

Simpson, R. L. (2013). Chief nurse executives need contemporary informatics competencies. *Nursing Economic$*, *31*(6), 277–287; quiz 288. Retrieved from http://www.ncbi.nlm.nih.gov/pubmed/24592532

Sittig, D. F., & Ash, J. S. (Eds.). (2011). *Clinical information systems: Overcoming adverse consequences.* Sudbury, MA: Jones and Bartlett Publishers.

Spok. (2015). *BYOD trends in healthcare: An industry snapshot.* Retrieved from http://www.healthcare-informatics.com/whitepaper/2015-survey-report-byod-trends-healthcare-industry-snapshot

Spyglass Consulting Group. (2014a). *Healthcare without bounds: Point of care communications for physicians 2014.* Retrieved from http://www.spyglass-consulting.com/Abstracts/Spyglass_PCOM_Physician2014_abstract.pdf

Spyglass Consulting Group. (2014b). *Healthcare without bounds: Point of care communications for nursing 2014.* Retrieved from http://spyglass-consulting.com/wp_PCOMM_Nursing_2014.html

Staggers, N., Gassert, C. A., & Curran, C. (2001). Informatics competencies for nurses at four levels of practice. *Journal of Nursing Education, 40*(7), 303–316.

Tang, P., Ash, J. S., Bates, D. W., Overhage, J. M., & Sands, D. Z. (2006). Personal health records: Definitions, benefits, and strategies for overcoming barriers to adoption. *Journal of the American Medical Informatics Association, 13*(2), 121–126. doi:10.1197/jamia.M2025

Technology Informatics Guiding Education Reform. (2007). *Informatics competencies for every practicing nurse: Recommendations from the TIGER collaborative.* Retrieved from http://docplayer.net/1884922-Overview-informatics-competencies-for-every-practicing-nurse-recommendations-from-the-tiger-collaborative.html

Technology Informatics Guiding Education Reform. (2009). *Collaborating to integrate evidence and informatics into nursing practice and education: An executive summary.* Retrieved from http://www.himss.org/resourcelibrary/Topiclist.aspx?MetaDataID=4132

Technology Informatics Guiding Education Reform. (2015, August 20). *TIGER virtual learning environment (VLE).* Retrieved from http://www.himss.org/professional-development/tiger-initiative/virtual-learning-environment

Tenner, E. (1997). *Why things bite back: Technology and the revenge of unintended consequences.* New York, NY: Vintage Books.

U.S. Department of Health & Human Services (HHS). (2015, April 27). *Personal health records and the HIPAA privacy rule.* Retrieved from http://www.hhs.gov/sites/default/files/ocr/privacy/hipaa/understanding/special/healthit/phrs.pdf

U.S. Government Publishing Office. (2015, September 9). Health information technology standards, implementation specifications, and certification criteria and certification programs for health information technology. *Electronic code of federal regulations.* Retrieved from http://www.ecfr.gov/cgi-bin/retrieveECFR?gp=&SID=c494467846b7f32b4bf2ee8526b425a3&r=PART&n=pt45.1.170

Vastag, B. (2011, February 10). Exabytes: Documenting the "digital age" and huge growth in computing capacity. *The Washington Post.* Retrieved from http://www.washingtonpost.com/wp-dyn/content/article/2011/02/10/AR2011021004916.html

*Washington Post.* (2014, September 9). The history of the mobile phone. Retrieved from https://www.washingtonpost.com/news/the-switch/wp/2014/09/09/the-history-of-the-mobile-phone/

Weber, B. A., Derrico, D. J., Yoon, S. L., & Sherwill-Navarro, P. (2009). Educating patients to evaluate web-based health care information: The GATOR approach to healthy surfing. *Journal of Clinical Nursing, 19*, 1371–1377. doi:10.1111/j.1365-2702.2008.02762.x

Whitten, P., Holtz, B., Cornacchione, J., & Wirth, C. (2011). An evaluation of telehealth websites for design, literacy, information and content. *Journal of Telemedicine and Telecare, 17,* 31–35. doi:10.1258/jtt.2010.091208

World Health Organization. (2008, June). *What is human factors and why is it important to patient safety?* Retrieved from http://www.who.int/patientsafety/education/curriculum/who_mc_topic-2.pdf

Zhang, J., Johnson, T. R., Patel, V. L., Paige, D. L., & Kubose, T. (2003). Using usability heuristics to evaluate patient safety of medical devices. *Journal of Biomedical Informatics, 36*(1–2), 23–30.

Zhang, J., & Walji, M. (2014). TURF unified framework of EHR usability. In J. Zhang & M. Walji (Eds.), *Better EHR: Usability, workflow and cognitive support in electronic health records.* Houston, TX: UTHealth.

# CHAPTER EIGHT

# PROGRAM EVALUATION

Joanne V. Hickey and Christine A. Brosnan

> *One of the great mistakes is to judge policies and programs by their*
> *intentions rather than their results.*
> —*Milton Friedman*

## INTRODUCTION

The historical roots of systematic evaluation go back to the 17th century while its contemporary interpretation coalesced in the 20th century. Social research methods for program evaluation evolved parallel to the growth and refinement of general evaluation research methods, which in turn followed ideological, political, and demographic trends (Rossi et al., 2014, p. 8). Following World War II, a number of major federal and privately funded programs in housing, hospital, and health care were launched. This naturally led to a need to judge the effectiveness and value of these programs. The methodologies and the information acquired through program evaluation have developed to a point where evaluation is an intrinsic component of most programs. Doctor of nursing practice (DNP) graduates are often enlisted to conduct program evaluations either as the leader and/or as a member of a team. The program evaluated may be small, such as for comprehensive management of a diabetic patient population in a particular clinic, or large, such as a palliative care program offered by interprofessional teams at multiple facilities within a major health care system. Program evaluation is an important competency for DNP graduates to develop so that they can influence health care delivery decision making and enhance cost-effective high-quality outcomes for populations. Much has been written about program evaluation with many different views expressed. This chapter addresses the planning, designing, implementing, and use of comprehensive program evaluation with the DNP evaluator in mind. It discusses the types of evaluations they will most likely conduct. The information is designed to be practical and useful. We begin by defining the term *program* and program evaluation.

## PROGRAM AND PROGRAM EVALUATION DEFINED

Program evaluation is a special subset of evaluation that utilizes the same general principles of evaluation, but with a focus on programs. A *program* is "a set of resources and activities directed toward one or more common goals, typically under

171

the direction of a single manager or management team. A program may consist of a limited set of activities in one agency or a complex set of activities implemented at many sites by two or more levels of an organization and by a set of public, nonprofit, and even private providers" (Wholey, Hatrey, & Newcomer, 2010, p. 5). *Program evaluation* is the application of systematic methods to address questions about program operations and results. It may include ongoing monitoring of a program as well as a one-time study of program processes or program impact. It is the systematic assessment of the processes and/or outcomes of a program with the intent of furthering its development and improvement. The approaches used for program evaluation are based on social science research methodologies and professional standards. The methods of program evaluation provide processes and tools that any evaluator or agency can utilize to acquire valid, reliable, and credible data to address a variety of questions about the performance of programs (Wholey et al., 2010, p. 6). Good evaluations should provide useful information about program functioning that can contribute to program improvement (Kellogg, 2004). Successful program planning and implementation require an evaluator who knows not only what the program expects to achieve, but also how it plans to achieve those outcomes. The evaluator must understand the principles on which a program is based (Weiss, 1998). Discussion about *how* and *why* a program is successful (or not) requires credible evidence and attention to the means by which outcomes and impacts are produced. An evaluation serves two purposes. It elucidates how a program is working now, and provides direction on how it can be improved in the future.

Program evaluations are initiated for many reasons. The intent may be to help improve a program or to compare its value with other programs competing for resources. The evaluation of a program should gain knowledge about its effect, and should help sponsors understand the relative contributions of its components. In general, program evaluation not only focuses on identifying the merits of the program, but also gives stakeholders information that will help them to decide what to do next. To be most useful, program evaluation needs to equip stakeholders with knowledge of those program elements that are working well and those that are not. Program evaluation should facilitate stakeholders' search for appropriate actions to take in addressing problems and improving programs (Chen, 2005, p. 6).

Previous chapters discussed the difference between evaluation and research. You will recall that research seeks generalizable knowledge independent of specific applications (e.g., does treatment A cure disease B). Evaluation examines specific programs or interventions, proposed or in place, to measure their effectiveness in achieving agreed upon goals (e.g., does our clinic's A treatment program reduce disease B deaths). Evaluators employ many of the same qualitative and quantitative methodologies used by researchers, and there is comparable rigor in evaluation. Evaluation is more client-focused than research, and evaluators work closely with program staff to create and execute an evaluation plan that addresses the particular needs of the program. By its very nature, evaluation requires judgments to be made. The purpose of evaluation is to facilitate a program's development, implementation, and improvement by examining its processes and/or outcomes.

Differentiation can also be made between evaluation and assessment, primarily regarding focus. Evaluation tends to look at a program's structure and process in relation to an outcome. Assessment is focused more on measuring the performance of component individuals or groups by appraising their skill levels on a variable of interest such as compliance with guidelines.

## TYPES OF PROGRAM EVALUATION

Experts categorize types of evaluation in a variety of ways. Although terminology may differ, the fundamental concepts are similar, and much of the difference in terminology relates to the maturity of the program under scrutiny. Programs move through various stages of development. Program evaluation can address the performance of a program at any stage. The type of program evaluation conducted should align with the program's maturity (e.g., developmental, implementation, or completion), the purpose of conducting the evaluation, and the questions that it seeks to answer. The purpose of the evaluation points to the type of evaluation that is needed, and helps the evaluator craft the appropriate design. Rossi, Lipsey, and Freeman (2004) suggest that evaluation typically involves one or more of five program domains as a program matures through a sequence of developmental stages:

- The need for the program
- The design of the program
- Program implementation and services delivery
- Program impact or outcomes
- Program cost and efficiency

The following are common types of evaluation described by the Environmental Protection Agency (EPA). One may wonder how an evaluation model employed by such a huge agency such as the EPA is useful to the smaller scale projects that a DNP might conduct. The answer is that the principles are similar regardless if one is conducting a large or small evaluation. There are many other similar classifications. Most evaluations may fall in more than one category (EPA, 2016):

- Design evaluation—conducted early in the planning stages or implementation phase of a program to define the scope of a program or project and to identify appropriate goals and objectives. Design evaluations can also be used to pretest ideas and strategies.
- Process evaluation—examines whether a program or process is implemented as designed or operating as intended, and identifies opportunities for improvement. Process evaluations often begin with an analysis of how a program currently operates. Process evaluations may also assess whether program activities and outputs conform to statutory and regulatory requirements, policies, program designs, or customer expectations.
- Outcome evaluation—examines the results of a program (intended or unintended) to determine the reasons for any differences between the outcomes and the program's stated goals and objectives. Outcome evaluations often examine program processes and activities to better understand how outcomes are achieved and how quality and productivity could be improved.
- Impact evaluation—a subset of an outcome evaluation. It assesses the causal links between program activities and outcomes by comparing the observed outcomes with an estimate of what would have happened if the program had not existed.
- Cost-effectiveness evaluation—identifies program benefits, outputs or outcomes and calculates the internal and external costs of the program.

Evaluations can also be classified as formative or summative (Chen, 2005, p. 47; Wholey et al., 2010, pp. 8–9), ongoing or stand-alone, objective observer or participatory, goal based or goal free, quantitative or qualitative, problem oriented or nonproblem oriented. One point to bear in mind is that an evaluation must be tailored to the political and organizational context of the program being examined.

## MODELS AND FRAMEWORKS FOR EVALUATION

General models for evaluation were discussed in the previous chapters of this book. In this chapter, three specific models with particular relevance to program evaluation are reviewed. They were selected from many because of their practicality and relevance to the work of DNP graduates. They are not presented in exhaustive detail, but are designed to introduce useful concepts. Actual application will require intense contact with the original literature. They are the systems model; the context, input, process, and product (CIPP) model; and the Centers for Disease Control and Prevention (CDC) model, including systems model. Each addresses program evaluation from a unique perspective.

## Systems Model

The systems model employs concepts of systems theory and complexity science to illustrate the anatomy of the programs studied (Chen, 2005, pp. 3–5). For success and survival, a program has an internal and external functionality. Internal functionality is the smooth transformation of program inputs into desirable outputs. External functionality is the program's continuous interaction with its environment in order to obtain the resources and support required for its survival. Since programs are open to the influence of their environments, a program can be thought of as an open system. The principles of complexity science which build on systems theory are also relevant. In complexity science, systems are dynamic and adaptive as a result of interactions with the environment so that a small change in one part of the system can have a large impact on other parts of the system.

There are five components of programs identified in systems theory: input, transformation, output, feedback, and environment. These components are viewed as an open system and can be applied to program evaluation. *Inputs* are resources of all kinds coming from the environment and include personnel, capital, technology, equipment, structures (e.g., offices, building), and clients. They must be organized and managed in some harmonious way within a program. *Transformation* is the process by which a program converts inputs into outputs. It is the organized and sequential step in implementation of a program through which services are provided to the recipient. *Output* refers to the anticipated and unanticipated results of that transformation, including achievement of the goals of the program. The *environment* refers to any entity lying outside the program that can positively or negatively influence the program's implementation and outcomes. These factors include social/cultural norms, regulatory practices, special interest groups, funding, political agendas, and perception of the value of the program. All open systems must have a feedback component to respond and adjust in a dynamic way to information from other parts of the system. This information is defined as *feedback*, and is the essence of evaluation. Chen (2005, p. 5) explains that programs need information to gauge whether inputs are adequate and organized, interventions are implemented appropriately, target groups are reached, clients receive quality services, and output goals are achieved according to the expectations of funding agencies and decision makers. What is emphasized in this systems model is the dynamic interrelationship of the various components.

## CIPP Model of Evaluation

The CIPP model of evaluations was developed by Stufflebeam et al. in the 1960s. It is a comprehensive and systematic model that links evaluation and decision making for improvement purposes. The model judges the value of a program by examining its CIPP. *Context* evaluation addresses the program's needs, problems, assets, and opportunities to help decision makers define goals, priorities, and outcomes. *Input* evaluation examines alternative approaches, competing action plans, staffing plans, and budget for their feasibility and potential cost-effectiveness to meet targeted needs and achieve goals (Alkins, 2004). With this information, decision makers can choose among alternate plans, funding proposals, allocation of resources, and other aspects of the program. At a later time, it can also assist others in judging the overall quality of the plan. *Process* evaluations investigate the implementation plan so that decision makers can evaluate feasibility and flow as well as to later judge program performance. *Product* evaluations focus on the identification and evaluation of outcomes. Outcomes are classified broadly as intended and unintended, short term, intermediate, and long term. The evaluation helps staff to judge the success of the program in meeting its target needs (Alkins, 2004).

The CIPP model is designed to assist decision makers in deciding to maintain, improve, or discontinue the program under review. The model is useful in examining a program at different stages of development. It can help evaluators establish the need for a program before the process begins and determine its effect when the program is completed. The purpose of evaluation is not to prove, but to improve (Stufflebeam et al., 1971). The model is applicable to both formative and summative program evaluation.

## CDC Model

The CDC provides a generic framework for evaluating large programs such as community- or population-based systems (see Figure 8.1). According to the CDC, the following framework is a practical nonprescriptive tool that summarizes in a logical order the important elements of program evaluation. It contains two related dimensions of steps in the evaluation process and sets standards for "good" evaluation. The following six connected steps of the framework are components of any evaluation, large or small. There are many options at each step and a large number of potential ways to gather evidence.

- Engage stakeholders—to include those involved in program operations, those served or affected by the program, and primary users of the evaluation.
- Describe the program—to include the need, expected effects (outcomes), activities, resources, stage, context, and logic model.

- Focus the evaluation design—to assess the issues of greatest concern to stakeholders while using time and resources as efficiently as possible. Consider the purpose, users, uses, questions, methods, and agreements.
- Gather credible evidence—to strengthen evaluation judgments and the recommendations that follow. These aspects of evidence gathering typically affect perceptions of credibility: indicators, sources, quality, quantity, and logistics.
- Justify conclusions—to link conclusions to the evidence gathered and judging those against agreed-upon values or standards set by the stakeholders. Justify conclusions on the basis of evidence (data) using these five elements: standards, analysis/synthesis, interpretation, judgment, and recommendations.
- Ensure use and share lessons learned—developing evaluation reports requires design, preparation, feedback, follow-up, and dissemination.

In general, activities flow according to a sequence of logical activities, although in practice the steps may be encountered slightly out of order. Following the sequence is useful because earlier steps provide the foundation for subsequent progress, although the built-in flexibility is acknowledged. Decisions about conduct of a given step should not be finalized until prior steps have been thoroughly addressed (CDC, 2011).

### Standards

Intrinsic to the framework is the application of each of four groups of evaluation standards that are used as a "lens" to help isolate the best approaches at each step. The CDC offers 30 standards that are organized into the four groups. These standards help answer the question, "Will this evaluation be a 'good' evaluation?"

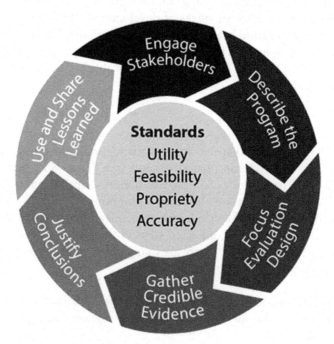

**Figure 8.1** CDC evaluation model.
*Source:* CDC (2016).

The set of 30 standards assesses the quality of evaluation activities, determining whether a set of evaluative activities are well-designed and working to their potential. These standards, adopted from the Joint Committee on Standards for Educational Evaluation, answer the question, Will this evaluation be effective? The standards are recommended as criteria for judging the quality of program evaluation efforts in public health.

The four groups of standards are:

- Utility standards—ensure that an evaluation will serve the information needs of intended users.
- Feasibility standards—ensure that an evaluation will be realistic, prudent, diplomatic, and frugal.
- Propriety standards—ensure that an evaluation will be conducted legally, ethically, and with due regard for the welfare of those involved in the evaluation, as well as those affected by its results.
- Accuracy standards—ensure that an evaluation will reveal and convey technically adequate information about the features that determine worth or merit of the program being evaluated.

The steps (www.cdc.gov/eval/steps/index.htm) and standards are used together throughout the evaluation process. For each step, there is a subset of standards that are most relevant to that aspect of the appraisal.

## STAGES IN PROGRAM EVALUATION

Before one commits to conducting an evaluation, five basic questions should be answered (Wholey et al., 2010, pp. 7–8). First, can the results of the evaluation influence decisions about the program? Second, can the evaluation be conducted in time to be useful? Third, is the program significant enough to merit evaluation? Fourth, is the program performance viewed as problematic? Fifth, where is the program in its development?

An evaluation can answer many questions and assume many forms, not all of which are useful. Tailoring the evaluation to the needs of the stakeholders is perhaps the most important work of the project. The evaluator collaborates with those requesting the evaluation and the recipients of the information to identify questions that the evaluation needs to answer about the program. This is critical because if the evaluation does not address what is truly important to the decision makers, the evaluation will have little or no value (Grembowski, 2001, p. 17).

There are many reasons to conduct a program evaluation and many types of programs. Frameworks, designs, and methods vary and some are more congruent to one type of evaluation than another. As a result, the stages in program evaluation can be approached in a variety of ways; however, they generally fall into three categories: planning, implementation, and dissemination.

### Planning a Program Evaluation

As noted previously, an evaluation is usually a collaborative process and brings together professionals with the expertise required to appraise a health care program. Forming an effective team is often the key determinant of success. An evaluation team that spends time to carefully plan and individualize the study to the needs of stakeholders is more likely to conduct a meaningful appraisal. Components of the planning phase include purpose, perspective, framework, design, and methodology. Each of the components is briefly reviewed in the following.

### Purpose

All members of the team should participate in determining and clarifying the purpose of the evaluation. Following are questions that can guide the discussion. Who requested the evaluation? Is the evaluation for internal and/or external use? Is the evaluation the result of an adverse event or is it being made in response to an accrediting agency? What aspect of the program are we going to evaluate? What questions does the evaluation hope to answer? Who will use this evaluation? How will they use it?

### Perspective

Perspective determines the scope and depth of an evaluation. Will the evaluation take the viewpoint of an organization (such as a hospital, clinic, continuous care, residential, community, or school of nursing) or will it take a more societal approach (city, county, state, nation, or international)? The purpose and perspective will influence the design and methods. Perspective will also affect the resources required, the cost, and the timeline for completion of the evaluation.

### Model or Framework

The framework provides a roadmap for the evaluation and must be congruent with its purpose and perspective. As part of the planning process, the team reviews models and frameworks to determine the best fit for evaluating the program under study. For example, the effectiveness–efficiency–equity framework is frequently used for evaluating health policy, but would not be appropriate for studying an educational program. The CIPP model, which is often applied in educational settings, would be a good choice in appraising a service learning program (Zhang et al., 2011). Logic models are often employed by public and nonprofit organizations concerned with mission-motivated rather than revenue-motivated outcomes (Chen, 2005; Fitzpatrick, Sanders, & Worthen, 2004; McLaughlin & Jordan, 1999).

### Design and Methodology

The decisions made about the purpose, perspective, and framework guide the selection of the study design and methods (Wholey et al., 2010). *Design* refers to how the evaluation's questions, methods, and overall processes are constructed and organized. An organization with a clear focus helps those who will conduct the evaluation determine who will do what, and what will be done with the findings. Furthermore, the process of creating and expressing a clear design will highlight ways that stakeholders can improve the evaluation and facilitate the use of the results. A series of questions such as those in the following list can help shape the design:

- For what purpose(s) is the evaluation being conducted, that is, what do you want to be able to decide as a result of the evaluation?

- Who is the intended audience (policy makers, chief nursing officers [CNO], chief executive officer; program directors, physicians, nurses)?
- What kinds of information are needed to make the decisions you need to make and/or to inform your intended audiences? With the varied intended audiences in mind, what kind of information does each group need to understand (its inputs, activities, and outputs): the product or program, strengths and weaknesses of the product or program, benefits to customers or clients (outcomes), or how the product or program failed and why?
- What are the sources from which the information should be collected (e.g., employees, providers, administrators, patients/clients, family members; program documentation, registries, and databases)?
- How can that information be collected efficiently (e.g., using questionnaires or interviews, examining documentation, observing patients or providers, focus groups)?
- What is the timeline (When is the information needed)?
- What resources are available to collect the information?

## Study Design

The following discussion provides an overview of some of the more frequently used research designs for program evaluation. An *experimental design* can establish causality, that is, a cause-and-effect relationship between the program and attainment of program objectives. This is possible because of three characteristics inherent in an experimental design: random assignment, control, and manipulation. Well-conducted experimental studies provide solid evidence that a program made a significant difference to a population. DNPs should keep in mind, however, that these studies have several drawbacks. They are conducted under ideal conditions and not in actual settings. They may be expensive and difficult to implement. They also may not be feasible because of ethical considerations. Health care studies that include experimental designs are frequently referred to as randomized controlled trials (RCTs).

A *quasi-experimental design* is less robust than an experimental design, and cannot establish causality because it lacks one or more of the characteristics of an experimental design. Quasi-experimental studies are frequently used in health care evaluation because they are more feasible, less expensive, and usually easier to conduct in a real world setting. A well-conducted quasi-experimental study will provide evidence that there is a significant association between a program and an outcome.

Observational designs are *nonexperimental* but they may still offer important information if they are congruent with the purpose, perspective, and framework of the evaluation. Observational designs include descriptive studies, surveys, correlational studies, and case studies (Centers for Disease Control and Prevention, 2011; LoBiondo-Wood & Haber, 2010, p. 178, 197).

DNPs may also want to consider using a *goal-based evaluation* (Centers for Disease Control and Prevention, 2011). This design is constructed to measure the success of a program's goals as they were initially described by the program's developers. Closely related is the *objectives-oriented evaluation*, which is widely used in education (Fitzpatrick et al., 2004, p. 80). Both designs may incorporate evidence-based criteria, standards, and benchmarks into the development of program goals and objectives.

### Data Collection

After selecting a design, the evaluation team may proceed to making decisions about data collection. Each method has pros and cons. The team should base their selection on relevance to the program under scrutiny, the reliability and validity of the method, and the amount of resources available for the evaluation. Selected data collection methods along with their strengths and limitations are presented in Table 8.1 (Centers for Disease Control and Prevention, 2011).

**TABLE 8.1  Selected Categories of Data and Sources**

| Type of Data | Data Sources | Strengths | Limitations |
|---|---|---|---|
| Observation | Meetings and conferences Site visits | Allows for direct examination | Requires trained observer Complex and expensive |
| Surveys | Interviews Questionnaires | Directly gathers data about client characteristics, satisfaction, and behavior | Cannot be certain client's statements are accurate May be complex and expensive |
| Discussion | Focus groups | Obtains a variety of opinions and suggestions | Requires a trained moderator May be difficult to interpret |
| Record review | Hospitals, clinics, meeting minutes, logs | Contains primary information Data have already been collected | Data may be missing or not pertinent May be difficult and expensive to access data |
| Vital statistics | State health departments | Large available database with extensive health information | May not have needed data |
| Registries | Centers for Disease Control State and local public health departments Registries for selected diseases and programs | Contains epidemiologic data about many diseases and conditions Data have already been collected | May not have needed data May be difficult to access data |
| Population data | U.S. Census Bureau | Large available database with extensive demographic information | May not have needed data |
| National data sets | Centers for Disease Control | Appropriate for evaluating large public health programs Data have already been collected | May not have needed data Complicated statistical analysis Often relies on individual self-reporting which may not be accurate |

Adapted from Centers for Disease Control and Prevention (2011) and Wholey et al. (2010).

### Analysis and Interpretation

Decisions about data analysis are largely based on the design of the study and the level of data collected (nominal, ordinal, interval, and ratio). Program evaluation commonly uses one or a combination of analyses—descriptive, bivariable, and multivariable (Grembowski, 2001, pp. 246–252). Descriptive analysis produces measures of means, medians, frequencies, and percentages that are sufficient for many evaluations. Bivariable analysis constructs associations (or differences) between two items; for example, a handwashing program and nosocomial infections. Multivariable analysis employs more complex statistical techniques, such as multiple regressions, in order to determine the effect of a program, the direction of the effect, and how variables act separately and together. It is a good idea to consult with a statistician or epidemiologist during the planning phase so that the analytical techniques used produce the most meaningful results.

## Implementing a Program Evaluation

There are always surprises that crop up during an evaluation. Some are good and some can drastically disrupt the procedure. Most evaluators prefer a smooth and predictable experience; a good way to accomplish this is by using a well-written management plan and carefully following protocol. The management plan contains the study protocol, a timeline, a projected cost estimate, resources needed, and potential barriers. Evaluators should refer to the management plan frequently for guidance and direction as they move through the stages of the evaluation.

The management plan clearly establishes what will be done, when it will be done, and who is responsible for doing it. Each stage in the evaluation is linked to the person(s) responsible for the process. For example, one team member is accountable for supervising the ethical status of the study and seeking approval from the institutional review board, if approval is recommended. During data analysis, two members of the team are responsible for assigning each variable a code name and value, checking the integrity of each value, and accurately entering data into a data set. Another member creates a data manual that contains management protocols (Grady, Newman, & Vittinghoff, 2001, p. 247).

## DISSEMINATING THE RESULTS

No evaluation is complete until the results of the evaluation have been provided to the intended audience in a form that is meaningful and useful to the target audience. Many forms of dissemination can be used to report results, but the most common forms are a written report and an oral report. Both forms of communications will be briefly addressed in this section as methods of dissemination.

## Written Report of the Program Evaluation

Multiple sources of models to write an effective evaluation report are available on the Internet and publications. What is available can be overwhelming to both the novice and experienced evaluator. In providing the reader with practical information, a few resources are cited as a beginning point. One excellent source published by the CDC (CDC, National Center for Chronic Disease Preventions and Health

Promotion, 2013) is titled *Developing an Effective Evaluation Report*, which is available at the CDC website. (See pages 62–64 for sample outlines for writing an evaluation report.) Other resources are found in textbooks (Wholey et al., 2010) and other publications. These and other resources provide advice about writing an effective report. The intent of this section is to provide a generic outline of the content to be included in an evaluation report along with some suggestions to keep in mind in writing the report. Standards of utility, feasibility, propriety, and accuracy discussed previously in this chapter should be incorporated into the writing of the report. Your goal is to produce a compelling evaluation report that convinces readers of the credibility of the findings, logical recommendations based on collected data and thoughtful analysis, and prompts for action based on the data and recommendations. The report must be practical and useful to the receiver.

### Audience

Before putting fingers to the keyboard, think about the intended audience. The intended audience is who asked for the evaluation and what their reasons were for that request. Have a clear picture in your mind of these individuals or group because this is who you are addressing through the written word. Craft the report to the intended audience, providing the kind of information that they need and in a format that will be understandable and useful.

### Message

Connecting with the intended audience and establishing and maintaining credibility are critical. Your approach, style, and language must convey that you have a clear understanding of the questions that they wanted to be answered and that you have approached the evaluation in a respectful and unbiased manner. The evaluation report is not a term paper for a course. The report must be well written, concise, and substantive, and conform to professional standards of a written report. Tell the readers something that they do not already know, not a rehash of known facts. Considerable time is required to prepare a report for high impact and usability.

### Format

The report must have the earmarks of a polished and professional product. Font type and font size should be easily readable. Trying to cram a lot of information into the report by using single spacing and a small font should be avoided. Formatting of the pages should include one inch margins, page numbers, and clear headings. Consider the best way to present information. Judicious use of tables, graphs, and charts can be very effective in helping the reader to rapidly grasp the information. Paper quality and placing the report into a professional looking folder is expected, if you are providing a hard copy. Be concise and clear. As a general guideline, the body of the report should be about 10 pages.

### Outline

As noted previously, multiple models are available to structure the report. Whatever form is chosen, it should follow a logical flow of information as the reader is taken through the process followed in the conduct of the evaluation. Exhibit 8.1 provides

---

> **EXHIBIT 8.1**
> **Components of an Evaluation Report**
>
> - Title page
> - Executive summary
> - Purposes and intended users
> - Program description
> - Evaluation focus and design
> - Data sources and methods
> - Results, interpretations, and conclusions
> - Recommendations
> - Appendix
> - References

a basic outline for content to be included. Areas can be enhanced or deleted, as appropriate for your project.

## Components of the Report

The following briefly describes each component of the report.

### Title Page

Provide the title of the project and the date submitted center in the middle to upper third of the page. Do not include a page number on the title page.

### Executive Summary

This is a very important component because some people may only read the executive summary. It should include the program description, evaluation questions or focus, design description, key findings, and recommendations. The executive summary should take no more than two to three pages.

### Purposes and Intended Users

In this section, the purposes of the evaluation and the intended uses of the evaluation report are identified and described. In addition, the primary intended users and the evaluation stakeholder workgroup are identified. This section fosters transparency about the purposes of the evaluation, who is involved, and who will have access to the evaluation results.

### Program Description

A brief overview of the program including background, program resources, program activities, stage of development, environmental context, statement of need, and any other key characteristics of the program that influence the evaluation are described (CDC, National Center for Chronic Disease Preventions and Health Promotion, 2013, p. 12). This description helps to focus the evaluation and leads to a common and shared understanding of the program as well as frames the evaluation questions and how they are prioritized. It is important to know the stage of development (e.g., planning, implementation, maintenance) of the program because programs are dynamic systems and change over time. The change in developmental stage will suggest different questions, priorities, and needs.

### Evaluation Focus and Design

In this section, the focus of the evaluation is identified and clearly delineated. If there is more than one focus for the evaluation, the priorities assigned to each question by the evaluator should be based on stakeholder priorities and intended users of the evaluation. This is an important section because of the many areas that could be evaluated. Therefore, the specific focus must be identified so that an appropriate design can match the questions being addressed in the evaluation. The questions help to identify the data needed to answer the questions.

### Data Sources and Methods

Several elements related to data and data collection processes are described in this section. With knowledge of the questions to be answered, the design of the evaluation process emerges with a clear notion of what data needs to be collected. The evaluator must briefly describe the sources of the data, location of the data, and how it was collected. In addition, the rationale for selection of the data as well as data acquisition, management, analysis, and credibility of data sources are addressed to support reliability and validity.

### Results, Interpretations, and Conclusions

This section discusses both processes and outcomes. The analysis processes are briefly described and interpreted in an understandable way for the intended audience. Using the results along with the interpretation, conclusions are described in relation to the questions that were the focus of the evaluation. Connecting the findings and interpretations with the questions being addressed is an important step that requires careful attention in the writing process. Conclusions must be justified. Guiding the reader from results to interpretations to conclusions in a logical format informs the reader of the process and supports transparency and credibility. As noted in the CDC, National Center for Chronic Disease Preventions and Health Promotion (2013) discussion of standards, the propriety standard plays a role in guiding the evaluator's decisions in how to analyze and interpret data to assure that all stakeholders' values are respected in the process of drawing conclusions.

### Recommendations

The final narrative section of the report is recommendations. Based on the data collected, results, interpretation, and conclusion, what recommendations are offered in relation to the purpose and questions that were the focus of the evaluation? The recommendations should be clear directions with a timeline for action or the next steps to be taken. Take into consideration the resources needed to implement each recommendation. In presenting recommendations, give options with a brief analysis of consequences of action or no action.

### Appendix

Place items into the appendix that provide more data and information addressed in the report. Tables, charts, and graphs may be included here or in the body of the report.

### References

List the sources of information that were used in conducting the evaluation including journal articles, external and internal reports, databases, websites, interviews, and other sources of information. The list of references helps to support transparency and credibility of the evaluation process.

In summary, a winning narrative report should be clear, concise, accurate, logical, and provide answers to the questions important to the individual or group requesting the evaluation. It should follow best practices and standards of high quality (Sanders & The Joint Commission on Standards for Educational Evaluation, 1994). A compelling report is useful to build awareness, facilitate growth and program improvement, and inform decision making of the stakeholders. The evaluation report is the property of the person or group sponsoring the evaluation and should be treated as confidential by the evaluator. Any requests from the outside for information about the report is directed to the sponsoring person or group.

## Oral Report of the Program Evaluation

In addition to a written report of the program evaluation, an oral report may be requested as a means of communicating results. The oral presentation can take many forms and requires crafting for the particular audience, message to be delivered, and format. Audience, message, and format are intertwined and require careful consideration.

### Audience

Knowing who the intended audience is critical in planning the oral presentation. There are often a variety of audiences such as the C-suite, program directors or managers, program staff, and program recipients, all of which will have different perspectives and information needs. The person or group who sponsored the evaluation should be consulted on who will be in the audience, when the presentation will take place, and what format will be used.

### Message

The area of particular interest regarding the program evaluation for each group is often quite different. For example, members of the C-suite may have a particular interest of the program's market share, cost, profit margin, return on investment, and potential for growth. The program director or manager may be interested in the efficiency of delivery and program outcomes in relation to program objectives. The program staff may be interested in ongoing funding of the program, expansion, and increasing the number of personnel. Therefore, the message needs to be crafted to the needs and interests of the target group.

### Format

The third intertwined consideration is the format or how the information is delivered. In addition to an oral presentation, PowerPoint slides, flip charts, handout material of PowerPoint slides, graphs, tables, executive summary, or other handout material may be used to augment the oral presentation. These are important decisions for the evaluator to make.

It is beyond the scope of this chapter to address the fine points of oral presentations, but suffice it to say it is a very important final step in coming to closure with the program evaluation.

---

### CASE STUDY

The following is intended to provide a brief overview of key elements of an evaluation to illustrate the operationalization of an evaluation project. The details of any project are specific to the particular evaluation.

A DNP graduate who is the director of cardiovascular clinical services at a major academic center is asked to evaluate the need for an outpatient cardiovascular program at one of the smaller community-based facilities of this large system. She begins with a clear understanding of the *purpose* of the evaluation and who is requesting the evaluation. A point person is identified as the person she can contact for any questions or if there is a need for assistance. A conversation also ensues regarding what the deliverables will be at the conclusion of the project as well as the timeline and resources available to complete the project. It is agreed that an oral presentation to the leadership of both the academic medical center and community facility will be provided in addition to a written report. The DNP uses a planning, implementation, and dissemination format to conduct her evaluation.

#### Planning

She begins by identifying the stakeholders. This includes the clinical facility (leadership, staff, resources, current cardiovascular services provided, etc.), the community it serves (demographics, socioeconomic profile, other cardiovascular services currently available in that community, etc.), and the relationship of this facility with the primary facility in the academic medical center. The point person is someone with whom to establish a working relationship because she will communicate progress of the project and be available for assistance to help with any barriers encountered. The next step in planning is to determine the subobjectives of the project and what data are needed to answer the questions. Based on these considerations, the design for the evaluation can be determined. Data elements and data sources need to be identified, as well as how and by whom these data will be collected and stored. This step may include plans for interviews with stakeholders and key personnel, review of a variety of documents and databases, review of the literature, and review of other data sources. Critical to any evaluation is a communication plan. This means that the DNP needs to plan with whom she will need to communicate, what messages need to be conveyed, and the timeline. Many tools are available to assist the evaluator in conducting an evaluation, such as a logic model. The DNP created a detailed logic model and used it not only for planning, but also to evaluate the success of the evaluation process base on identified outcomes. She also created a communication plan that included the person(s) with whom to communicate, as well as the key message and frequency of the communications. It is important to think through the project carefully in the planning phase to be efficient and effective in answering the questions posed by the evaluation purpose.

#### Implementation

Thoughtful and detailed planning leads to a smoother implementation. However, the DNP recognized that she needed to conduct an ongoing environmental scan to assess how things were

*(continued)*

---

**CASE STUDY (*continued*)**

progressing. Barriers are identified and a new plan is devised to address the barrier. For example, the CNO at the community facility is reluctant to give the DNP access to quality metrics for the facility. The DNP was able to communicate with the point person, who discusses this matter with the CNO; the CNO now feels comfortable providing the information. The implementation of the evaluation plan continues. Frequent formative evaluations are conducted by the DNP to assess progress as well as any need for change in the process. The DNP spends time assessing the community needs for cardiovascular services, current resources available along with gaps, and the relationship of both clinical facilities. She determines that a business plan is needed to plan the outpatient program that can be used by the leadership for decision making about creating this new service. (Preparing a business plan is beyond the scope of this case study, but it is necessary when expenditure of capital funds is at stake. There are many resources available to the DNP to prepare a business plan that includes working with the finance/business department.)

**Dissemination**

A written report is prepared. See the section on writing a report for models. The DNP completes the project and meets with the point person at the sponsoring facility to deliver the written report and plan for an oral presentation. She verifies who will be in attendance so that she can tailor her presentation to the intended audience. She plans to keep it short, focused, and connected to the purpose of the evaluation. A few (about 6–8) slides are prepared to guide the discussion, and photocopies of the slides are distributed at the presentation.

## Coming to Closure

The DNP comes to closure by meeting with the point person, thanking him or her for the opportunity to conduct this evaluation and point person's assistance, and returning any written or other material that is the property of the facility. She bears in mind that this was confidential work. That means that she is not at liberty to discuss the evaluation or disseminate any information about the project (in any form) without clear permission from the facility.

## SUMMARY

Program evaluation is a common focus in health care organizations, and DNP graduates are perfectly positioned and knowledgeable about the framework, process, and methods for conducting an credible and effective evaluation. In this chapter, an overview of the principles, processes, and methods has been presented to guide the DNP graduate in the conduct of program evaluation.

In summary, this chapter has addressed program evaluation as a special form of evaluation by the DNP graduate. Conceptual models and specific information related to program evaluation were addressed, including the steps to guide an evaluator through the planning, implementation, and evaluation phases of the project. In addition, a brief overview of preparing both a written and oral report of a program evaluation for dissemination has been given. It is clear from the evolving role of the DNP graduate and the increasing focus in health care on the requirement for evaluation to determine the value of programs that the DNP graduates will be engaged as leaders or team members in the evaluation of programs.

# REFERENCES

Alkin, M. C. (Ed.). (2004). *Evaluation roots: Tracing theorists' views and influences.* Thousand Oaks, CA: Sage.

Centers for Disease Control and Prevention. (2016). *A framework for program evaluation.* Retrieved from http://www.cdc.gov/eval/framework/

Centers for Disease Control and Prevention. (2011). *Introduction to program evaluation for public health programs: A self-study guide.* Atlanta, GA: CDC.

Centers for Disease Control and Prevention, National Center for Chronic Disease Preventions and Health Promotion. (2013). *Developing an effective evaluation report: Setting the course for effective program evaluation.* Atlanta, GA: CDC.

Chen, H. T. (2005). *Practical program evaluation.* Thousand Oaks, CA: Sage Publications, Inc.

Environmental Protection Agency. (2016). Evaluating EPA's programs. Retrieved from www.epa.gov/evaluate/basicinfo/index.htm

Fitzpatrick, J. A., Sanders, J. R., & Worthen, B. R. (2004). *Program evaluation: Alternative approaches and practical guidelines* (3rd ed.). Boston, MA: Pearson Education, Inc.

Grady, D., Newman, T. B., & Vittinghoff, E. (2001). Data management. In S. B. Hulley, S. R. Cummings, W. S. Browner, D. Grady, N. Hearst, & T. B. Newman (Eds.), *Designing clinical research* (2nd ed., pp. 247–257). Philadelphia, PA: Lippincott Williams & Wilkins.

Grembowski, D. (2001). *The practice of health program evaluation.* Thousand Oaks, CA: Sage.

Kellogg, W. K. (2004). *Logic model development guide.* Battle Creek, MI: W. K. Kellogg Foundation.

LoBiondo-Wood, G., & Haber, J. (2010). *Nursing research: Methods and critical appraisal for evidence-based practice.* St. Louis, MO: Mosby Elsevier.

McLaughlin, J. A., & Jordan, G. B. (1999). Logic models: A tool for telling your program's performance story. *Evaluation and Program Planning, 22*(1), 65–72.

Rossi, P. H., Lipsey, M. W., & Freeman, H. E. (2004). *Evaluation: A systematic approach* (7th ed.). Thousand Oaks, CA: Sage.

Sanders, J. R., & The Joint Committee on Standards for Educational Evaluation. (1994). *The program evaluation standards* (2nd ed.). Thousand Oaks, CA: Sage Publications.

Stufflebeam, D. L., Foley, W. J., Gephart, W. J., Guba, E. G., Hammond, R. L., Merriman, H. O., & Provus, M. M. (1971). *Educational evaluation and decision making.* Itasca, IL: Peacoct.

Weiss, C. H. (1998). *Evaluations: Methods for studying programs and policies* (2nd ed.). Upper Saddle River, NJ: Prentice Hall.

Wholey, J. S., Hatry, H. P., & Newcomer, K. E. (Eds.). (2010). *Handbook of practical program evaluation* (3rd ed.). San Francisco, CA: Jossey-Bass.

Zhang, G., Zeller, N., Griffith, R., Metcalf, D., Williams, J., Shea, C., & Misulis, K. (2011). Using the context, input, process, and product evaluation model (CIPP) as a comprehensive framework to guide the planning, implementation, and assessment of service-learning programs. *Journal of Higher Education Outreach and Engagement, 15*(4), 57–84.

# CHAPTER NINE

# QUALITY IMPROVEMENT

Eileen R. Giardino

> *The truth is rarely pure and never simple.*
> —*Oscar Wilde*

Quality improvement (QI) in health care is a process of systematic and continuous actions, which cause measurable improvements in the health status of patient populations and health care services (Health Resources and Services Administration [HRSA], 2011). A QI initiative provides a formal approach to the analysis of performance in health care and then determines systematic efforts to improve the delivery of health care patient safety (PS). In essence, the QI process involves the development and implementation of a systematic approach to apply evidence-based standards to a given health care system for the purpose of improving determined outcomes (McCarthy, 2008).

The 1999 Institute of Medicine (IOM) report entitled *To Err Is Human* reported that the health care industry delivers inconsistent and unsafe care that harms people (Kohn, Corrigan, & Donaldson, 1999). A subsequent IOM report, *Crossing the Quality Chasm*, suggested that change in the delivery of health care was needed and identified six aims that health care should be: effective, safe, patient-centered, timely, efficient, and equitable (Institute of Medicine, 2001). *Crossing the Quality Chasm* (2001) found that gaps in the quality of care delivered in institutions and health care systems nationwide were evidenced by suboptimal outcome measures in health care institutions along with breeches in PS (Institute of Medicine, 2001). Outcome studies across health care institutions identified widespread problems with PS along with mediocre to poor outcomes in patient care parameters at all levels of health care delivery (Institute of Medicine, 2001; Reid, Compton, Grossman, & Fanjiang, 2005). The identification of inconsistent and unsafe care practices in all care delivery systems helped to shift the focus of health care delivery to the expectation that people should receive safe, high quality, and consistent care in all institutions, not just in one hospital (Leape et al., 2009). Health care delivery has shifted from individuals providing the care that they think is best to systems that focus on the goals of delivering quality health care, decreasing premature deaths associated with preventable harm, and decreasing expenses that preventable adverse events cause (Leape et al., 2009; U.S. Department of Health and Human Services, 2000).

The doctor of nursing practice (DNP) graduate has a strong role in the areas of QI and safety, as the DNP should be a champion for identifying and developing processes to improve care at all levels of health care delivery. DNP Essential II, entitled "Organizational and Systems Leadership for Quality Improvement and Systems Thinking," outlines the role of the DNP in quality and safety within all health care organizations. DNP Essentials state that DNP graduates are leaders within systems and organizations to improve health care systems and patient outcomes. It is the responsibility of the DNP to understand what QI is and know how to guide and direct the improvement of outcomes in systems (American Association of Colleges of Nursing, 2006).

This chapter describes what QI is within a health care system, where QI initiatives fall along the research continuum, and how models of care are used to enhance quality and safety to improve PS and health care outcomes.

## QI IN HEALTH CARE

There is a history of mistakes in health care that have resulted in harm or death. Errors range from giving the patient an incorrect medication dosage to performing the wrong surgery on the wrong body part. The IOM's report published in 2000, *To Err Is Human,* revealed that between 44,000 and 98,000 Americans die each year as a result of medical errors (Botwinick, Bisognano, & Haraden, 2006; Kohn, Corrigan, & Donaldson, 2000). The report drew attention to overwhelming quality and safety problems in all areas of health care delivery. The cost of errors that resulted in injury was estimated to be between 17 and 29 billion dollars, with over 50% of these costs related to medical errors. The IOM report identified a widespread problem throughout all areas of health care delivery and recommended the need for improvement in the delivery of care to decrease medical errors, make health care outcomes more consistent across institutions, and decrease the rising cost of health care (Kohn et al., 2000).

Since the 2000 IOM report, the goal to decrease the rising costs of health care while improving patient outcomes and institutional safety and efficiency has not yet been met. A 2008 report showed that medical errors cost the US $19.5 billion annually with approximately $17 billion associated directly with costs (Andel, Davidow, Hollander, & Moreno, 2012; Van Den Bos et al., 2011). A later study estimated the number of premature deaths associated with preventable harm to patients to be more than 400,000 per year (James, 2013).

Past and current costs of medical errors is another indication of poor consistency in the delivery of quality care in U.S. hospitals that result in high mortality rates and injuries that result in longer hospital stays, increased medical costs, and preventable disability (Brennan et al., 1991; Carter, Zhu, Xiang, & Porell, 2014). Conversely, quality care focuses on providing the right care at the right time, every time, and ensures that fewer people are harmed or injured by incorrect procedures, incorrect medications, and incorrect treatment plans (Andel et al., 2012). It is less expensive, more efficient, and less wasteful to provide safe and quality health care all the time than to provide care that engenders higher costs from errors and improper medical treatment plans. Therefore, it is incumbent that health care leaders and clinicians understand what quality care involves, and how to develop protocols and programs that focus on quality and PS to improve patient outcomes.

The focus of many DNP student projects is on small scale QI and safety initiatives within health care practices and organizations. Such projects enable the DNP student to learn principles of QI, how to develop and implement QI projects in an organizational setting, and then how to measure whether desired outcomes have been achieved through the protocols and processes of the QI program. More importantly, students learn the theory, principles, and methods of QI and develop skill in developing QI initiatives (see Exhibit 9.1 for examples of DNP student-developed QI initiatives).

| EXHIBIT 9.1 | |
|---|---|
| **Examples of DNP Student QI Projects** | |
| Justina Megwa, DNP, MSN, RN, FNP-BC | Integration of Palliative Care Into Primary Care Practice |
| Christine Nguyen-Moen, DNP, RN, FNP-BC | A Comprehensive Family-Based Group Appointment for Addressing Overweight Hispanic Children |
| Sherly Sebastian, DNP, MSN, RN, ANP-C | Web Based Education and Support Tool for Brain Tumor Patients and Their Families |
| Mary Lou Warren, DNP, MSN, RN, CNS-CC | The Development, Implementation, and Evaluation of an Early Mobilization Program for Critically Ill Adult Oncology Patients |
| Scott A. Zela, DNP, MSN, ANP-BC, GNP-BC | Implementation of a Hepatocellular Carcinoma Surveillance Monitoring System for At-Risk Patients in a Private Hepatology Clinic |
| L. Denise Johnson-Vaught, DNP, MSN, RN, ACNP-BC, ENP | Optimizing Patient Flow in the Emergency Department |
| Vianey Quintana Casarez, DNP, MSN, CRNA | Integrating Cost Methodology in Health Care at a Proton Radiotherapy Center |
| Lesley Boyko, DNP, MSN, CRNA | Quality Care and Process Improvement Project Implemented in Endoscopy |
| Johnny Dang, DNP, MSN, CRNA | Cost Effective Methodologies in Health Care: Bridging the Gap Between Efficiency and Quality of Care in the Bronchoscopy Suite |
| Dorothy Andrew, DNP, MSN, RN, CCM, NE-BC | Improving the Transition of Care From Hospital to Home, a Pilot Program |
| Maureen S. Beck, DNP, MSN, RN, GNP-BC | Implementation of a Comprehensive Clinical Practice Guideline for Osteoporosis Screening in Primary Care |
| Rosslyn Blake, DNP, MSN, RN, GNP-BC, FNP-BC | Reducing Medication Errors Through Workflow Redesign |

*(continued)*

**EXHIBIT 9.1**

**Examples of DNP Student QI Projects (*continued*)**

| | |
|---|---|
| Kimberly Curtin, DNP, MS, RN, APRN, ACNS-BC | Implementation of the Care and Communication Bundle in an Oncology Intensive Care Unit |
| Puneet Freibott, DNP, MSN, RN, CCRN, NE-BC | Optimizing Emergency Department Throughput—Using Best Practices to Improve Patient Flow |
| Kerrie Guerrero, DNP, MSN, MBA, RN, NE-BC | Improving the Transition of Care From Hospital to Home: Using a Transition Coach |
| Marcia K. Gamez, DNP, MSN, RNFA, CNS | Education for the Prevention of Ankle Injuries in Young Persons Participating in Sports Activities |

## QUALITY IN THE U.S. HEALTH CARE SYSTEM

Quality is a direct link to an organization's care delivery systems and their ability to deliver service to patients and populations (HRSA, 2011; Massoud, 2001). The U.S. health care system as a whole has trailed behind other nations and industries in demanding better outcomes for patient care and initiating safety efforts to prevent errors that result in morbidity and death (Schimpff, 2012). The airline industry is an exemplar of an industry that could not afford to allow tragic accidents to occur, and has focused on providing safety systems since World War II. While the airlines have pioneered QI and safety initiatives to avoid preventable accidents (Reid et al., 2005; Shojania, Duncan, McDonald, Wachter, & Markowitz, 2001), the health care industry has not met the challenge of providing safe and quality care all the time in the same way that the airline industry has done.

In health care, QI initiatives focus primarily on the outcome performance of patient-care delivery and attempt to implement evidence-based best practices to improve outcomes. The measure of success or failure of a QI initiative is if the outcomes achieved through the QI protocol were improved over the baseline outcomes that were measured prior to implementing the best practice protocol.

The Institute for Healthcare Improvement (IHI) identified questions to guide QI work (IHI-How to Improve, 2015; Langley et al., 2009). Those questions are:

- What does the system want to accomplish?
- What is the evidence needed to show that an improvement has occurred?
- What changes are necessary to make that will cause improvement and positive change in the system?

It is important to understand what types of activities are considered to be QI initiatives to improve performance and outcomes. The following are functions considered in the realm of QI (O'Kane, 2009):

- Designing processes of care—best process translated into a standard of care, treatment protocol, or practice guideline.
- Monitoring to detect conformance with standards of care.
- Detecting negative outcomes through surveillance, both predictable and unexpected (e.g., monitoring of infection rates and surgical outcomes, examining sentinel events).
- Reporting about performance at the unit, group, or individual level.
- Measuring and improving patient-centered aspects of care.

All of these activities address a need to understand and then improve deficits in performance and ways to improve outcomes (O'Kane, 2009).

## THE IOM: SIX AIMS TO IMPROVE DELIVERY OF HEALTH CARE

In response to the identification of gross errors within the health care system, the IOM identified aims to improve health care in the report *Crossing the Quality Chasm* (Institute of Medicine, 2001). The report included a strategy and framework to improve the overall delivery of health care and, in turn, improve the quality and safety of health care delivery (Ortiz & Clancy, 2003). Each aim describes an aspect of health care delivery that addresses quality, safety, and effectiveness of the care from provider to patient.

The six IOM aims are to provide safe, effective, patient-centered, timely, efficient, and equitable care (Institute of Medicine, 2001). The following is an overview of what each aim means:

1. *Safe*: Avoiding injuries to patients from care that is intended to help them
2. *Effective*: Providing services based on scientific knowledge to all who could benefit, and refraining from providing services to those unlikely to benefit (avoiding underuse and overuse)
3. *Patient-centered*: Providing care that is respectful of and responsive to individual patient preferences, needs, and values and ensuring that patient values guide clinical decisions
4. *Timely*: Reducing waits and sometimes harmful delays for both those who receive and give care
5. *Efficient*: Avoiding waste, such as waste of equipment, supplies, ideas, and energy
6. *Equitable*: Providing care that does not differ in quality because of personal characteristics such as gender, ethnicity, geographic location, and socioeconomic status

## QI VERSUS RESEARCH INITIATIVES

The question arises as to where QI initiatives fall along the research continuum. Does a QI initiative fall within the category of research, and as such is subject to the guidelines and consideration of research projects within an institution? Does a QI initiative need to seek institutional review board (IRB) approval to protect the safety and rights of those individuals affected by the QI protocol? To answer these questions, it helps to compare the activities of QI initiatives to research initiatives that seek to describe, explain, predict, and control observed phenomenon, and in turn uncover new knowledge in health care.

There are distinctions between QI and research methodologies. For example, a research project may focus on determining whether drug A or drug B is the best treatment for a disease condition, while a QI initiative may focus on first identifying care processes that need improvement and then setting in place processes based on already determined evidence for the purpose of improving patient care outcomes. QI initiatives are structured to yield improvements in care outcomes through the use of best practices in the clinical setting (James, 2007).

A QI initiative identifies intended outcomes, initiates a best practice protocol, and then measures outcomes to determine if the measures have indeed improved clinical outcomes over what the usual or baseline practice was in the clinical setting. A QI project is not structured to compare two competing protocols, as might be done in a research study. Research projects often involve random assignment of patients to competing treatments, while QI implements an already established best practice protocol to achieve outcomes over baseline measures. Research initiatives may put a patient (subject) at risk by using unproven therapies for the purpose of generating new knowledge, while QI initiatives use already proven best practice protocols to improve care outcomes (McCarthy, 2008; see Table 9.1).

**TABLE 9.1  Intermountain Healthcare: Characteristics of QI Versus Research**

| QI Activities | Research Activities |
|---|---|
| Focus on performance of local patient-care delivery protocols, to apply evidence-based practice to improve outcomes | Focus on an experimental design or unproven therapies (not evidence-based treatment) to generate new knowledge in the field |
| Attempt to implement established best practices based on existing evidence (including randomized controlled trials, observational studies, and consensus-expert opinion) | Randomly assign patients to competing treatments, potentially conflicting with an ethical commitment to preserve each patient's well-being |
| Involve "open-loop systems" where implementation protocols are modified based on patient need (so that it does not conflict with the clinician's primary ethical commitment to the patient's well-being) | Follow a strict, unchangeable research protocol that may impose additional testing burdens that may cause risk to patients, while not providing an alternative benefit to patients |
| Are usually funded from an initiating organization and implemented as part of the normal operating procedures | May be funded by external grants or awards with primary or secondary goals of knowledge generation, such that the research investigator may have potential conflicts of interest that could place patients' interests secondary to some other goal |

Adapted from McCarthy (2008).

## Institutional Review Board Oversight of QI Initiatives

The role of the IRB for protection of human subjects is to ensure that ethical standards are in place to protect the welfare and rights of humans participating in research initiatives. To that end, the IRB reviews research protocols and materials such as investigator brochures and informed consent documents to make certain that all parts of the research protocol are in accordance with ethical standards to protect the human subjects. Research in which the intervention could in some way harm study participants requires the oversight of an IRB to ensure that participant safety and privacy are upheld throughout the research process (American Psychological Association, 2015; FDA, 2014).

The need for IRB review of a QI initiative depends on a number of factors. In research study initiatives, IRB oversight looks at factors such as the potential for patient risk, testing new or nonstandard care, intent to publish, and confidentiality requirements (Weiserbs, Lyutic, & Weinberg, 2009). An IRB may not require its oversight to protect the participants of a QI initiative, as most QI initiatives involve the implementation of a protocol established from evidence-based and best-practice recommendations and there is no experimentation involved.

Institutions often use QI initiatives to improve compliance with national PS benchmarks, and therefore may require that its IRB be notified of the QI initiative. Usually an IRB exempts QI initiatives from IRB oversight when participant data are deidentified, or gives the QI initiative an expedited review status if the initiative tests a hypothesis, includes data with personal identifiers, or anticipates publication. Some institutions have instituted an IRB-QI subcommittee to fast-track QI proposals (Weiserbs et al., 2009).

Depending on the details of the quality initiative and the specific institution, it may be necessary or advisable to submit a QI project to the institution's IRB for review. In regards to student DNP projects in the academic setting where students carry out QI initiatives in other organizations, it is wise to submit all DNP QI projects to the university IRB for review. In most cases, QI initiatives receive expedited review when the protocol does not involve direct patient involvement with treatment changes or direct patient care. QI initiatives may need IRB approval when the protocol could potentially expose patients to risks and burdens, when questions are raised regarding possible ethical conflict, and when the results of the QI initiative may be published (Lynn, 2004; Shirey et al., 2011; see Table 9.2).

The Veterans Health Administration's National Ethics Committee recommends a systematic approach to ensure ethical conduct in QI initiatives. The committee suggests that the level of scrutiny should correspond to the level of potential ethical concern. A QI project that has minimal burdens or risks that do not go beyond any risks already inherent in the clinical situation may only need brief review discussions with quality management staff. Projects that have greater potential ethical or safety risks may require a formal review by a group such as an ethics committee or multisite review committee (Holm et al., 2007; National Ethics Committee of the Veterans Health Administration, 2002).

The most consistent way for a QI team to be certain of appropriate oversight for QI initiatives is to view every initiative in a framework of risk for conflict of interest (James, 2007). It is best to submit a QI initiative to the IRB for review if there is any question or concern as to whether a process of informed consent might be needed, or if there are any questions regarding the nature of the QI protocol

**TABLE 9.2  QI Initiatives That Warrant IRB Overview**

| Situation Concern | Process | Outcome |
|---|---|---|
| Risks to patient privacy | Publish summary QI results outside the organization (analogous to situation when physician publishes a case-series report on patients' clinical experience) | Ethical review (typically by a privacy board) is applied at that point in time to ensure the protection of patient confidentiality (not to approve the activity itself) |
| Risks to patient health: Randomly assign patients to different QI interventions to determine which evidence-based care is most effective (distinguished from nonrandomized pilot test comparing the experience of different organizational subunits) | Request IRB review of project | Dependent on project details, may qualify for "expedited" IRB review or for waiver of informed consent |

Adapted from James (2007).

(Holm et al., 2007). The IRB then determines whether an initiative requires oversight throughout its implementation.

## KNOWLEDGE GENERATED FROM QI PROJECTS

In order to describe the knowledge generated from QI initiatives, it is helpful to first understand the types of knowledge that encompass scholarly activities. Boyer developed a model of scholarship that broadened the focus of scholarly activity to include activities that expand beyond traditional research projects (Boyer, 1990). Boyer's four areas of scholarship are the scholarships of discovery, integration, application, and teaching and learning. QI initiatives often apply the knowledge and findings gained from research to develop processes or protocols that are then put in place to improve health care outcomes. Therefore, the knowledge that QI generates is in the realms of application and integration of knowledge (Boyer, 1990; see Table 9.3).

### The IHI and the Triple Aim

The IHI is a leader in health care improvement worldwide and a resource to help laypeople and professionals understand how to implement QI and safety initiatives in health care settings. The mission of IHI is to provide guidance to individuals and organizations who want to improve best practices and seek out innovative models of care. The IHI shares approaches to QI through a comprehensive website that includes white papers, reports, and information on the innovative ideas of leaders in QI and safety (Stiefel & Nolan, 2012).

**TABLE 9.3  Categories and Focus of Scholarship**

| Type of Scholarship | Focus of Scholarly Activity |
| --- | --- |
| Scholarship of discovery | Original research to advance knowledge |
| Scholarship of integration | Synthesizes information between disciplines, across topics within a discipline, or across time |
| Scholarship of application/Scholarship of engagement | Involves rigor and application of discipline-specific expertise with results shared with and/or evaluated by peers |
| Scholarship of teaching | Systematic study of teaching and learning processes. Teaching transmits, transforms, and extends knowledge |

Adapted from Boyer (1990).

The IHI developed the Triple Aim framework to describe an approach to optimizing health system performance. Triple Aim describes three dimensions that should be pursued simultaneously to ultimately improve the quality of health care, outcome measures, and cost of care. The three prongs of the Triple Aim are: improving the patient experience of care (including quality and satisfaction); improving the health of populations; and reducing the per capita cost of health care (Berwick, Nolan, & Whittington, 2008; Institute for Healthcare Improvement [IHI], 2015). The IHI Triple Aim advocates a focused approach to change based on the identification of target populations; defining what a system wants to accomplish and measure; development of a project that will affect change in the system; and the implementation of a change approach that is able to adapt to local needs and conditions (Institute for Healthcare Improvement [IHI], 2015).

## MODELS IN QI INITIATIVES

A model serves as a blueprint to guide the QI processes of problem identification, solution determination, evaluation of the implementation processes, and system evaluation while providing a standard format of how work flows that everyone can understand (Scoville & Little, 2014). Models guide people and systems to ensure that people get the right care, at the right time, by the right team, and in the right place, and outline best practice care and services for a person (Agency for Clinical Innovation, 2013). In QI, the improvement team uses the model to guide the approach and steps to change within the organization. This section introduces specific models that health care organizations can use to guide QI activities and shape quality program infrastructures to improve care and outcomes for patients and organizational systems (HRSA, 2011).

There are a number of models that guide change processes within organizations. Models include the FADE (Focus, Analyze, Develop, and Execute), QI

Model, IHI Model for Improvement, Plan-Do-Study-Act (PDSA), Lean Model for Performance Improvement, Six Sigma (DMAIC—Define, Measure, Analyze, Improve, and Control), Continuous Quality Improvement (CQI), and Total Quality Management (TQM), to name a few. Specific organizations tend to choose a model that they like and understand and continue with that framework. Conversely, it could be that one department in an organization likes to work with Model A while another department chooses Model B. Selecting the best and most appropriate model or framework may depend on the scale of the project, the scope, and the context of the outcomes that one wants to achieve (Scoville & Little, 2014).

A model is helpful in guiding a rigorous evaluation process for a QI/PS project. The model's diagram shows the process to follow as the steps of the plan unfold from identification of the problem, initiation of changes, and timing of evaluation processes to determination of how effective the change plan has been. Finally, models provide a pathway to take ongoing findings and use them to improve the system during the implementation process, to then make further changes that lead to the goal of improved outcomes.

## SPECIFIC MODELS USED IN QI INITIATIVES

### The Model for Improvement: PDSA

IHI describes the heart of their approach to QI as the Model for Improvement developed by Associates in Process Improvement. The Model for Improvement is an effective process that helps to guide purposeful action and enable learning from experience. It is a powerful tool for accelerating health care improvement, and many organizations have successfully used the improvement framework to improve health care processes and outcomes (IHI-Measures, 2015). The two essential steps of the model are: (a) the answering of three fundamental questions, and (b) testing changes through PDSA cycles (IHI-How to Improve, 2015).

The three fundamental questions essential for guiding improvement work are:

- What are we trying to accomplish?
- How will we know whether a change is an improvement?
- What changes can we make that will result in improvement?

The second step in the Model for Improvement is the PDSA cycle tool. The four cycles in the PDSA model are the development of a plan to test the change (Plan), carrying out the test (Do), observing and learning from the consequences (Study), and determining what modifications should be made to the test (Act). The PDSA cycle is a formula of change that helps accomplish desired outcomes and helps implementers determine if more change is needed to accomplish the desired outcomes or goals (Scoville & Little, 2014).

PDSA provides a blueprint for implementers to gain practical knowledge of the effects of the QI protocol and evaluate and revise the plan in an immediate and sequential process (Scoville & Little, 2014). PDSA cycles guide the development of changes, test interventions implemented to improve a system, and pilot changes in institution-specific situations, in order to gain confidence that changes will work and refine them as needed (Scoville & Little, 2014).

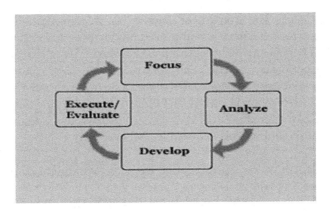

**Figure 9.1** The FADE model.
*Source:* Organizational Dynamics Institute (2014).

## FADE Model

The FADE model for use in QI initiatives involves the use of a cyclical process. The QI team uses a four-step process that repeats the steps again and again to evaluate how well the implementation processes are going and what the impact of the changes are in the system. The repeating process continues until the desired outcomes and goals are achieved. The FADE steps are (HRSA, 2011; Figure 9.1):

Focus: Define and verify the process to be improved
Analyze: Collect and analyze data to establish baselines, identify root causes, and point toward possible solutions
Develop: Based on the data, develop action plans for improvement, including implementation, communication, and measuring/monitoring
Execute: Implement the action plans, on a pilot basis as indicated; and Evaluate: Measure and monitor the system to ensure success.

## The Lean Thinking Model

The Lean model defines value by what a customer (and in health care, the patient) wants and maps how the value flows to the patient. The Lean approach to QI started in the manufacturing industry to streamline processes while right sizing an organization to produce a quality product in a safe, efficient, and outcomes oriented manner (Lean Enterprise Institute, 2015; Mi Dahlgaard-Park, Dahlgaard, & Mi Dahlgaard-Park, 2006). While the Lean approach guarantees the proficiency of a process through making the process time efficient and cost effective (HRSA, 2011), its focus is on eliminating waste, avoiding superfluous processes, and reducing production time and costs while preserving value with less work. Operations that fail to create value for the end customer are deemed "wasteful." The Japanese founders of Toyota listed the seven wastes as (a) transport, (b) inventory, (c) motion, (d) waiting, (e) overproduction, (f) overprocessing, and (g) defects (HRSA, 2011).

Leaders in health care have adapted Lean tools and principles to obtain higher quality outcomes at a lower cost to meet the needs of the organization (Lean Enterprise

Institute, 2014). The strength of Lean is fast implementation, immediate benefits regarding error reduction, and improved productivity and customer lead times while long-term benefits include improvements to customer satisfaction, staff morale, and financial performance. The Lean approach to QI works best in process-oriented industries that have clearly defined manufacturing or supply-chain elements such as the automotive, pharmaceutical, and industrial engineering industries.

The Lean approach to QI is a five-step process to guide the implementation of the model (Lean Enterprise Institute, 2014):

1. Identify value: Specify value from the standpoint of the end customer by product family.
2. Map the value stream: Identify all steps in the value stream for each product family, eliminating whenever possible those steps that do not create value.
3. Create flow: Make the value-creating steps occur in tight sequence so the product will flow smoothly toward the customer.
4. Establish pull: As flow is introduced, let customers pull value from the next upstream activity.
5. Seek perfection: Value is specified, value streams identified, wasted steps removed, and flow and pull introduced. The process goes on indefinitely and continues until the ideal process is achieved in which perfect value is created with no waste.

## Six Sigma

Six Sigma is a set of strategies and tools used to limit variability and defects in business processes, with the ultimate goal of process and performance improvement. The Six Sigma approach to improvement is a strategy focused on changing the culture of an organization that is in need of improving its processes that fall below desired outcomes (Benedetto, 2002). Motorola Corporation designed Six Sigma to decrease process variations, reduce cost, and eliminate defects in the manufacturing of their products. The term "Sigma" is the number of standard deviations a given process is from perfection. At the Six-Sigma level, a manufacturing process is virtually error free with approximately 3.4 defects per million opportunities (99.9996%; HRSA, 2011).

The Six Sigma approach is described as a "revolutionary" performance improvement method used when there is need for drastic changes and improvements in an organization. An organization that initiates the Six Sigma approach to QI understands that the process will be timely and expensive due to the need for radical changes within the organizational structure (Benedetto, 2002). Due to the large scale organizational changes necessary when Six Sigma is used as the change model, small QI initiatives do not warrant the use of the Six Sigma approach.

Six Sigma uses two models to frame improvement: (a) DMAIC, which is designed to examine existing processes, and (b) DMADV (define, measure, analyze, design, and verify), which is used to develop new processes.

## Lean Six Sigma

Six Sigma and Lean are often used in conjunction with one another in health care initiatives. While both Lean and Six Sigma address profit maximization,

Six Sigma focuses on the customer and end product, while Lean focuses on waste and production methods. In health care, the Lean and Six Sigma approach to QI can reduce variability and waste, and improve errors, processes, patient care, and patient satisfaction rates which, in turn, improve outcomes (Mozammel, Mapa, & Scachitti, 2011).

## The Evaluation of QI and Patient Safety Initiatives

Evaluation of QI initiatives provides data that shows to what extent a QI project achieved the desired outcomes. A well-organized QI initiative clearly outlines from beginning to end of the project what needs to be evaluated in the protocol, at what points in the QI protocol evaluation measures take place, specific evaluation tools used throughout the QI protocol, and statistical measures indicated for each part of the evaluation process (Hopkins Medicine, 2015). A QI project should systematically approach program evaluation and articulate what evaluation processes are used to assess if the desired outcomes are achieved (Mittman & Salen-Schatz, 2012). QI projects should articulate methods utilized to evaluate project processes, where and when those methods will be implemented within the quality initiative, and if desired outcomes were achieved (Hopkins Medicine, 2015).

Evaluation processes for QI and PS initiatives occur throughout the implementation of the change process to determine if intended outcomes resulted from the QI project protocols. A weak QI initiative results from poor conceptualization of evaluation methods to determine the efficacy of protocol processes and final outcomes. As such, QI project developers need to determine appropriate evaluation methods prior to the start of the QI initiative.

## Measurement in QI Initiatives

Since the development and implementation of evaluation measures is essential in a robust QI/safety initiative, then measurement is the part of testing that tells the team whether the changes they are making actually lead to improvement.

Measurement is a critical part of testing and implementing change in QI initiatives. Chosen measures tell a team whether the protocol introduced and changes made actually lead to improved outcomes (IHI-How to Improve, 2015). Measurement of quality processes helps determine in what direction the outcome measures have gone, what might have contributed to both intended and unintended results in the system, and what further changes might be necessary to achieve desired outcomes (IHI-How to Improve, 2015). There are three types of measures used in QI initiatives: outcome measures, process measures, and balancing measures. IHI recommends a balance between the three types of measures used in QI initiative. Table 9.4 defines each type of measure.

The types of measures and the process for measurement of outcomes may vary from research for the discovery of new knowledge to research for the application of knowledge, as in QI initiatives. Measurement for improvement should not be confused with measurement for research. This difference is outlined in Table 9.5.

**TABLE 9.4   Types of Measures**

| Type of Measure | Definition |
|---|---|
| Outcome measure | • The standard against which one assesses the end result of the intervention<br>• End result of a test used to objectively determine the baseline function of a patient at the beginning of treatment and then determine treatment efficacy by using the same test at the end of treatment |
| Process measure | • Determines whether the parts/steps in the system are performing as the protocol planned<br>• Process measures help determine if the initiative is on track with its efforts in place to improve the system |
| Balancing measure | • Help project implementers to view the system from a different direction or dimension in an effort to determine if changes made in one part of the system (through the initiation of a QI protocol) are causing problems in other parts of the system |

**TABLE 9.5   Comparison of Measurement for Quality Improvement Versus Research**

| | Measurement for Research | Measurement for Learning and Process Improvement |
|---|---|---|
| Purpose | To discover new knowledge | To bring new knowledge into daily practice |
| Tests | One large "blind" test | Many sequential, observable tests |
| Biases | Control for as many biases as possible | Stabilize the biases from test to test |
| Data | Gather as much data as possible, in case needed | Gather "just enough" data to learn and complete another cycle |
| Duration | Can take long periods of time to obtain results | "Small tests of significant changes" accelerates the rate of improvement |
| Variables | Controls as many variables as possible | Makes no attempt to control variables; accepts environment as is |

Adapted from IHI-How to Improve (2015).

## Dissemination of Findings of QI Initiatives

At the conclusion of a quality initiative, the results should be communicated to the stakeholders and organizations. There are a number of ways to disseminate findings including presentations to stakeholders, detailed reports, news releases, meetings with key people in the organization, and press conferences, to name a few.

It is imperative that the findings are shared with those who are then in charge of continuing the process within the institution (Unite for Sight, 2015).

## NATIONAL INITIATIVES FOR QI AND SAFETY IN HEALTH CARE

### The Patient-Centered Outcomes Research Institute

The Patient-Centered Outcomes Research Institute (PCORI) is an independent, nonprofit organization mandated by Congress in 2010 as part of the Patient Protection and Affordable Care Act to improve the relevance and quality of evidence in health care. The PCORI goal is to enable clinicians, lay people, and organizations to make informed health decisions based on evidence (PCORI, 2014). PCORI is a nongovernmental organization authorized to fund comparative clinical effectiveness research (CER) and support endeavors that improve methods used to conduct CER studies.

PCORI funds patient-centered outcomes research initiatives that address concerns most relevant to patient care and quality outcomes. PCORI funded initiatives strive to involve in the improvement process all stakeholders in health care services including caregivers, patients, clinicians, and researchers. The findings of PCORI-supported CER provide evidence-based information that addresses health care concerns and in turn helps health care providers determine which treatment options are best for individuals and populations (PCORI, 2014).

### Healthcare Effectiveness Data and Information Set

The Healthcare Effectiveness Data and Information Set (HEDIS) is a large data set that helps health insurance plans in America measure performance of hospitals and health care organizations on multiple dimensions of care and service. HEDIS measures a number of health issues such as asthma medication use, comprehensive diabetes care, and antidepressant medication management, to name a few. HEDIS measures help institutions determine their performance in specific areas and outcome measures so they can improve their quality of care and services and achieve outcomes that are standard with the national norms (NCQA, 2015a). Insurance health plans use HEDIS results to determine how well institutions perform on specific outcome measures individually and in comparison with other institutions (NCQA, 2015b).

The National Committee for Quality Assurance (NCQA) collects HEDIS data directly from Health Plan Organizations and Preferred Provider Organizations for multiple purposes via the Healthcare Organization Questionnaire and HEDIS non-survey data through the Interactive Data Submission System. NCQA maintains collected HEDIS in a central database with strict controls to protect confidentiality (Mainous & Talbert, 1998; NCQA, 2015b). A number of health plans use HEDIS data to make improvements in their quality of care and service while those who select health plans such as consultants and employers use HEDIS data to choose what seems to be the most effective health plan for the needs of an organization. Since HEDIS outcome measures effect a wide range of decisions that are based on the quality measures of specific health care institutions, the validity of HEDIS results is determined by rigorous audit of the measures by NCQA-designed process (NCQA, 2015b).

## SUMMARY

QI provides a systematic approach to improving the health status of patient populations through a process of problem identification followed by a determination of evidence-based approaches to reduce errors, improve systems, and, in turn, improve outcomes within health care organizations. This chapter provides insight into what QI is, how to understand what QI initiatives accomplish in health care, what kinds of processes are involved in QI initiatives, and how QI is an integral part of the goal to improve health care safety and efficiency.

## REFERENCES

Agency for Clinical Innovation. (2013). *Understanding the process to develop a model of Care: An ACI framework*. Agency for Clinical Innovation [On-line]. Retrieved from http://www.aci.health.nsw .gov.au/__data/assets/pdf_file/0009/181935/HS13-034_Framework-DevelopMoC_D7.pdf

American Association of Colleges of Nursing. (2006). *The essentials of doctoral education for advanced nursing practice*. American Association of Colleges of Nursing [On-line]. Retrieved from http:// www.aacn.nche.edu/publications/position/DNPEssentials.pdf

American Psychological Association. (2015). *Frequently asked questions about institutional review boards*. American Psychological Association [On-line]. Retrieved from http://www.apa.org/about/ gr/science/advocacy/2007/irbs.aspx

Andel, C., Davidow, S. L., Hollander, M., & Moreno, D. A. (2012). The economics of health care quality and medical errors. *Journal of Health Care Finance, 39*(1), 39.

Benedetto, A. R. (2002). Six Sigma: Not for the faint of heart. *Radiology Management, 25*, 40–53.

Berwick, D., Nolan, T., & Whittington, J. (2008). The Triple Aim: Care, health, and cost. *Health Affairs, 27*, 759–769.

Botwinick, L., Bisognano, M., & Haraden, C. (2006). *Leadership guide to patient safety*. IHI Innovation Series white paper. Retrieved from www.ihi.org/resources/Pages/IHIWhitePapers/Leadership-GuidetoPatientSafetyWhitePaper.aspx

Boyer, E. L. (1990). *Scholarship reconsidered: Priorities of the professoriate*. New York, NY: The Carnegie Foundation for the Advancement of Teaching.

Brennan, T. A., Hebert, L. E., Laird, N. M., Lawthers, A., Thorpe, K. E. Leape, L. L. . . . Hiatt, H. H. (1991). Hospital characteristics associated with adverse events and substandard care. *Journal of the American Medical Association, 265*, 3265–3269.

Carter, M. W., Zhu, M., Xiang, J., & Porell, F. W. (2014). Investigating the long-term consequences of adverse medical events among older adults. *Injury Prevention, 20*, 408–415.

FDA. (2014). *Institutional review boards frequently asked questions—Information sheet*. U.S. Food and Drug Administration. Retrieved from http://www.fda.gov/RegulatoryInformation/Guidances/ ucm126420.htm

Holm, M., Selvan, M., Smith, M., Markman, M., Theriault, R., Rodriguez, M., & Martin, S. (2007). Quality improvement or research: Defining and supervising QI at the University of Texas M. D. Anderson Cancer Center. In B. Jennings, M. Baily, M. Bottrell, & J. Lynn (Eds.), *Health care quality improvement: Ethical and regulatory issues* (pp. 144–168). New York, NY: Hastings Center.

Hopkins Medicine. (2015). *Evaluating quality improvement and patient safety projects*. Armstrong Institute for Patient Safety and Quality. Retrieved from http://www.hopkinsmedicine.org/ armstrong_institute/training_services/workshops/evaluating.html

Human Resources and Services Administration. (2011). *Quality improvement.* Rockville, MD: U.S. Department of Health and Human Services.

IHI-How to Improve. (2015). *How to improve: Improvement methods.* Institute for Healthcare Improvement. Retrieved from www.ihi.org/IHI/Topics/Improvement/ImprovementMethods/HowToImprove/

IHI-Measures. (2015). *Science of improvement: Establishing measures.* Institute for Healthcare Improvement. Retrieved from http://www.ihi.org/resources/Pages/HowtoImprove/ScienceofImprovementEstablishingMeasures.aspx

Institute for Healthcare Improvement. (2015). *The IHI Triple Aim.* Institute for Healthcare Improvement. Retrieved from http://www.ihi.org/engage/initiatives/tripleaim/pages/default.aspx

Institute of Medicine. (2001). *Crossing the quality chasm: A new health system for the 21st century.* Washington, DC: National Academies Press.

James, B. C. (2007). Quality-improvement policy at Intermountain Healthcare. In B. Jennings, M. A. Baily, M. Bottrell, & J. Lynn (Eds.), *Health care quality improvement: Ethical and regulatory issues* (pp. 169–176). Garrison, NY: The Hastings Center.

James, J. T. (2013). A new, evidence-based estimate of patient harms associated with hospital care. *Journal of Patient Safety, 9*(3), 122–128.

Kohn, L. T., Corrigan, J. M., & Donaldson, M. S. (1999). *To err is human: Building a safer health system.* Washington, DC: National Academy Press.

Kohn, L. T., Corrigan, J. M., & Donaldson, M. S. (2000). *To err is human: Building a safer health system. A report of the Committee on Quality of Health Care in America* (6th ed.). Washington, DC: Institute of Medicine.

Langley, G. J., Moen, R., Nolan, K. M., Nolan, T. W., Norman, C. L., & Provost, L. P. (2009). *The improvement guide: A practical approach to enhancing organizational performance.* San Francisco, CA: Jossey-Bass.

Lean Enterprise Institute. (2014). *A brief history of Lean.* Lean Enterprise Institute. Retrieved from http://www.lean.org/WhatsLean/History.cfm

Lean Enterprise Institute. (2015). *Principles of Lean.* Lean Enterprise Institute. Retrieved from http://www.lean.org/WhatsLean/Principles.cfm

Leape, L., Berwick, D., Clancy, C., Conway, J., Gluck, P., Guest, J., . . . Lucian Leape Institute at the National Patient Safety Foundation. (2009). Transforming healthcare: A safety imperative. *Quality and Safety in Health Care, 18,* 424–428.

Lynn, J. (2004). When does quality improvement count as research? Human subject protection and theories of knowledge. *Quality and Safety in Health Care, 13,* 67–70.

Mainous, A. G., & Talbert, J. (1998). Assessing quality of care via HEDIS 3.0: Is there a better way? *Archives of Family Medicine, 7,* 410.

Massoud, M. R. (2001). Advances in quality improvement: Principles and framework. *QA Brief, 9,* 13–17.

McCarthy, D. (2008). *Case study: Is it quality improvement or research? The experiences of Intermountain Healthcare and Children's Hospital Boston.* The Commonwealth Fund [On-line]. Retrieved from http://www.commonwealthfund.org/publications/newsletters/quality-matters/2008/july-august/case-study-is-it-quality-improvement-or-research-the-experiences-of-intermountain-healthcare

Mi Dahlgaard-Park, S., Dahlgaard, J. J., & Mi Dahlgaard-Park, S. (2006). Lean production, Six Sigma quality, TQM and company culture. *The TQM Magazine, 18,* 263–281.

Mittman, B., & Salen-Schatz, S. (2012). *Improving research and evaluation around continuous quality improvement in health care.* Princeton, New Jersey: Robert Wood Johnson Foundation.

Mozammel, A., Mapa, L. B., & Scachitti, S. (2011). *Application of Lean Six Sigma in healthcare—A graduate level directed project experience.* Calumet: American Society for Engineering Education.

National Ethics Committee of the Veterans Health Administration. (2002). *Recommendations for the ethical conduct of quality improvement.* Washington, DC: National Center for Ethics in Health Care, Veterans Health Administration, Department of Veterans Affairs.

NCQA. (2015a). *HEDIS and quality compass.* National Committee for Quality Assurance [On-line]. Retrieved from http://www.ncqa.org/HEDISQualityMeasurement/WhatisHEDIS.aspx

NCQA. (2015b). *Quality measurement products.* National Committee for Quality Assurance [On-line]. Retrieved from http://www.ncqa.org/HEDISQualityMeasurement/QualityMeasurementProducts.aspx

O'Kane, M. (2009). Do patients need to be protected from quality improvement? In B. Jennings, M. A. Baily, M. Bottrell, & J. Lynn (Eds.), *Health care quality improvement: Ethical and regulatory issues* (pp. 89–100). Garrison, NY: The Hastings Center.

Organizational Dynamics Institute. (2014). *The FADE model.* Retrieved from http://isepengage2013.yolasite.com/resources/Improvement%20model.pdf

Ortiz, E., & Clancy, C. M. (2003). Use of information technology to improve the quality of health care in the United States. *Health Services Research, 38,* xi–xxii.

PCORI. (2014). *Why PCORI was created.* Retrieved from http://www.pcori.org/about-us

Reid, P. P., Compton, W., Grossman, J. H., & Fanjiang, G. (2005). *Building a better delivery system: A new engineering/health care partnership.* Washington, DC: National Academies Press.

Schimpff, S. C. (2012). *The future of health-care delivery: Why it must change and how it will affect you.* Washington, DC: Potomac Books, Inc.

Scoville, R., & Little, K. (2014). *Comparing lean and quality improvement.* Cambridge, MA: Institute for Healthcare Improvement. IHI White Paper. August 18, 2015.

Shirey, M. R., Hauck, S. L., Embree, J. L., Kinner, T. J., Schaar, G. L., Phillips, L. A., . . . McCool, I. A. (2011). Showcasing differences between quality improvement, evidence-based practice, and research. *Journal of Continuing Education in Nursing, 4*(2), 57–68.

Shojania, K. G., Duncan, B. W., McDonald, K. M., Wachter, R. M., & Markowitz, A. J. (2001). *Making health care safer: A critical analysis of patient safety practices* (Rep. No. 43). Rockville, MD: Agency for Healthcare Research and Quality.

Stiefel, M., & Nolan, K. (2012). *A guide to measuring the Triple Aim: Population health, experience of care, and per capita cost.* Cambridge, MA: Institute for Healthcare Improvement.

Unite for Sight. (2015). *Dissemination and utility of evaluation findings.* Unite for Sight [On-line]. Retrieved from http://www.uniteforsight.org/evaluation-course/module7

U.S. Department of Health and Human Services. (2000). *The challenge and potential for assuring quality health care for the 21st century.* Washington, DC: Author.

Van Den Bos, J., Rustagi, K., Gray, T., Halford, M., Ziemkiewicz, E., & Shreve, J. (2011). The $17.1 billion problem: The annual cost of measurable medical errors. *Health Affairs, 30,* 596–603.

Weiserbs, K. F., Lyutic, L., & Weinberg, J. (2009). Should quality improvement projects require IRB approval? *Academic Medicine, 84*(2), 153.

# CHAPTER TEN

# EVALUATION OF PATIENT CARE BASED ON STANDARDS, GUIDELINES, AND PROTOCOLS

Ronda G. Hughes

> *Unless we are making progress in our nursing every year, every month,*
> *every week, take my word for it, we are going back.*
> —*Florence Nightingale*

Doctor of nursing practice (DNP) graduates are often called upon to evaluate individual and population health based on achievement of health outcomes that represent quality indicators of health and care. This chapter examines the evaluation of patient care based on accepted standards and guidelines. The Institute of Medicine Roundtable on Evidence-Based Medicine (2008) set a goal that "by 2020, ninety percent of clinical decisions should be supported by accurate, timely, and up-to-date clinical information that reflects the best available evidence." That is a lofty goal when it has been estimated that about 20% of clinical decisions are evidence based (McGlynn et al., 2003). Of the more than \$2 trillion annually invested in health care, less than 0.1% is devoted to evaluating the relative effectiveness of the various diagnostics, procedures, devices, pharmaceuticals, and other interventions in clinical practice. In order to appreciate what standards, guidelines, and protocols represent, a review of the background and development of each will be explored so that the advanced practice nurses (APNs) can critically review these entities before adoption or translation into practice.

The delivery and quality of health care services vary. Researchers continue to find variation associated with practice patterns, sociodemographics of populations, and geographic location. Health care leaders, managers, policy makers, and practitioners have been concerned about this variation and have been actively involved in various strategies to bring and drive health care toward high-quality consistency. Many of these efforts have involved developing, implementing, and enforcing standards, guidelines, and protocols as part of evidence-based practices (EBP).

## TYPES OF RESEARCH INFLUENCING PATIENT CARE

Research is evaluated through various mechanisms and can support or refute current or proposed standards, guidelines, and protocols. There are several major types of research that are used to influence patient care decisions.

Randomized controlled trials (RCTs), a form of a clinical trial or experiment type of research commonly used to test the safety and efficacy or effectiveness of health care services (e.g., a type of surgical procedure), are held by many to be the "gold standard." Considering the scope of depth of clinical and health care research and the cost of conducting an RCT, other forms of research can also be successfully used to inform practice. For example, descriptive research provides data and characteristics about a population or phenomenon, but does not describe what factors may have caused a situation. One example would be determining how many people within a specific population have been diagnosed and are being managed for diabetes.

There is also research that statistically assesses the relationship (or correlation) between two or more random variables. Determining a predictive relationship between the flu season and demand for visits or emergency department utilization serves to illustrate one example. Another type of research draws a sample from a larger population and makes a distinction between those with the risk factors and those without it. These two cohorts are followed over a period of time to determine the frequency and timing that the outcomes of interest occur. Additionally, qualitative research provides insight into the social processes, subcultures, experiences, and perceptions of individuals and populations that are generally not detectible through databases or other sources of information. Together, the different types of research can be used to inform the development, testing, and implementation of standards, guidelines, and protocols.

The information or research supporting practice and changes in how care is delivered varies. This information can range from a recommendation, a suggestion for practice that is not necessarily approved by expert groups, to a guideline that was the product of intensive research evidence and consensus among experts. The following section provides a brief discussion and definitions of a number of terms as a basis for discussion. These terms include *standards, standard of care, guidelines, protocols, recommendations, indicators, EBP,* and *best practices.*

## Indicators

Indicators are visible signs of whether or not an intervention or program is achieving the expected outcomes or progressing in the intended direction. An indicator is a measurable surrogate (e.g., number or percentage) that is considered representative of an outcome and can be tracked to determine if there is an increase or decrease or an improvement or deterioration in the outcome. Quality indicators are measures of health care quality that make use of readily available hospital administrative data.

## Standards

Standards are considered to be the expected level and type of care. They reflect a desired and achievable level of performance against which actual performance can be compared. Their main purpose is to promote, guide, and direct practice. According to the Healthcare Information and Management Systems Society (HIMSS), a standard is "a document established by consensus and approved by a recognized body, or is accepted as a de facto standard by the industry" (Healthcare Information and Management Systems Society [HIMSS], 2010, p. 113). Standards of care are developed over time or are the result of findings from clinical and health care research, and can vary by state or community (Emanuel, 1997).

In legal terms, a standard of care is used as the benchmark against what a clinician does in practice. If, for example, the U.S. Department of Health and Human Services (HHS) declares a treatment procedure as not safe and effective, then the practitioners who employ such a treatment procedure can be deemed as not meeting the professionally recognized standards of health care. Professionally recognized standards are applicable to practitioners providing care and are recognized by the professional peers of a clinician/clinical group. However, this does not mean that all other treatments meet the professionally recognized standards of care. In a malpractice lawsuit, the clinician's lawyers would want to prove that the clinician's actions were aligned with the standard of care. The plaintiff's lawyers would want to show how the clinician violated the accepted standard of care and was therefore negligent (Moffett & Moore, 2011).

All industries have some form of industry standards by which quality is judged. According to the American Nurses Association (ANA), a standard is an "authoritative statement enunciated and promulgated by the profession by which the quality of practice, service, or education can be judged" (ANA, 2010, p. 115). In another publication, the ANA says standards are authoritative statements by which the nursing profession describes the responsibilities for which its practitioners are accountable. Standards reflect the values and priorities of the profession and provide direction for professional nursing practice and a framework for the evaluation of this practice. Standards also define the nursing profession's accountability to the public and the outcomes for which registered nurses are responsible (ANA, 2010).

For nurses, there are nursing standards of care, promulgated by professional organizations. For example, the ANA promotes nursing excellence through standards, a code of ethics, and credentialing. The ANA standards describe the responsibilities for which its practitioners are accountable, reflect the values and priorities of the profession, and provide direction for professional nursing practice and a framework for the evaluation of this practice. These standards also define the nursing profession's accountability to the public and the outcomes for which registered nurses are responsible.

The ANA Standards of Professional Performance describe a competent level of behavior for professional nurses, including activities related to quality of care, performance appraisal, education, collegiality, ethics, collaboration, research, and resource utilization. These standards serve as guidelines for accountability, a method to assure patients receive high-quality care; specificity, so that the nurses know exactly what is necessary to provide nursing care; and measures that can be used to determine whether the care meets the standards. Of these standards, two, in particular, will be discussed for illustrative purposes.

First, the quality of practice is defined as the registered nurse systematically enhances the quality and effectiveness of nursing practice. The measurement criteria are (ANA, 2004):

1. Demonstrates quality by documenting the application of the nursing process in a responsible, accountable, and ethical manner
2. Uses quality improvement activities to initiate changes in nursing practice and the health care delivery system
3. Uses creativity and innovation to improve nursing care delivery

4. Incorporates new knowledge to initiate changes in nursing practice if desired outcomes are not achieved
5. Participates in quality improvement activities

Second, the research standard is defined as the nurse integrates research findings in practice. This is measured with the following criteria (ANA, 2004):

1. Utilizes best available evidence including research findings to guide practice decisions
2. Participates in research activities as appropriate to the nurse's education and position such as the following:
   a. Identifying clinical problems suitable for nursing research
   b. Participating in data collection
   c. Participating in a unit, organization, or community research committee
   d. Sharing research activities with others conducting research
   e. Critiquing research for application to practice
   f. Using research findings in the development of policies, procedures, and practice guidelines for patient care
   g. Incorporating research as a basis for learning

Nurses demonstrate the standards of care for professional nursing through the nursing process. This involves assessment, diagnosis, outcome identification, planning implementation, and evaluation. The nursing process is the foundation of clinical decision making and encompasses all significant action taken by nurses in providing care to all patients. Accountability for one's practice as a professional rests with the individual nurse. The standards of care in the *ANA Nursing: Scope and Standards of Practice* (2004) describe a competent level of nursing care. The levels of care are demonstrated through the nursing process. Standards of care are also important if a legal dispute arises over whether a nurse practiced appropriately in a particular case.

## Guidelines

Guidelines can be defined generically or specifically to clinical practice. A guideline is a description that clarifies what should be done, and how, to achieve given objectives (HIMSS, 2010, p. 55). Guidelines are developed to standardize care based on what should be considered the best available evidence and information. Most guidelines are based on research when possible. Clinical practice guidelines are a set of systematically developed statements, usually based on scientific evidence, to assist practitioners and patient decision making about appropriate health care for specific clinical circumstances (HIMSS, 2010, p. 21). Clinical practice guidelines are produced by government agencies, health care systems, professional organizations, and specialty centers.

There are many steps to develop guidelines, each of which can be vulnerable to bias or error; as a result, a practitioner may misinterpret the research evidence and its translation while developing a clinical practice guideline. There are various strategies to developing guidelines, but no universal standard mechanism to ensure that each published guideline was developed in the best way possible (Guyatt et al.,

2006). Generally, the process begins with identifying and refining the subject area of a possible guideline. Next, a group (optimally versus an individual) is created to engage stakeholders and identify and assess the evidence. Again, optimally, this group summarizes, categorizes, and critically evaluates available evidence. This evaluation of the evidence is then translated into a clinical practice guideline. The guideline should then be reviewed by experts in the field and key stakeholders. After a guideline is published, it should be updated frequently to reflect new research knowledge when available.

Acknowledging that clinical guidelines were becoming more of a part of clinical practice, Woolf, Grol, Hutchinson, Eccles, and Grimshaw (1999) discussed concerns with guidelines in terms of the benefits of encouraging the use of interventions proven to be successful and informing decision making, as well as the harms of misleading decision makers because the evidence informing the guideline was thin or misinterpreted or biases may have incorrectly influenced the recommendation(s) (Woolf et al., 1999). These and many other concerns have been raised about guidelines. In a recent report, the Institute of Medicine (IOM) set forth eight standards for clinical practice guidelines:

1. Establishing transparency
2. Managing conflict of interest
3. Overseeing guideline development group composition
4. Examining clinical practice guideline-systematic review intersection
5. Establishing evidence foundations for and rating strength
6. Addressing articulation or recommendations
7. Providing for external review
8. Updating (IOM, 2011a)

As such, APNs must be careful in implementing/adapting clinical guidelines in that for many topics/situations, there are a multitude of guidelines. These guidelines may not concur with each other and most likely were developed using different processes and different sources of evidence. To address these concerns, APNs must carefully consider each guideline and evaluate the best match to their practice and patient population.

## Protocols

A clinical protocol is a set of rules defining a standardized treatment program or behavior in specific circumstances (HIMSS, 2010, p. 21). A protocol is a detailed guide for approaching a clinical problem and is designed to address a specific practice situation. It is often agency specific; for example, a checklist for pressure ulcer prevention including assessment steps and timeline for turning and repositioning patients.

Protocols exist to reduce variation in care for a specific patient population. They are generally to be adhered to in practice, particularly when the recommended actions have been scientifically studied and experts in the field have considered and advised on their application. Clinical protocols are defined as standards of care that define specific care actions that should be given to a defined patient population. Many specify how, when, and by whom a specific action should be performed. Some clinical protocols present a comprehensive plan of care, such as perioperative and postoperative care for elderly patients receiving joint replacement surgery, whereas other protocols address just one aspect of care, such as prophylactic antibiotics before joint replacement surgery.

## Best Practices

A best practice describes a process or technique whose application results in improved patient and/or organizational outcomes. A best practice is something that an individual, group, or organization can apply to an action to perform significantly better than other individuals, groups, or organizations. From a nonscientific perspective, best practices can also be defined as the most efficient (least amount of effort) and effective (best results) way of accomplishing a task, based on repeatable procedures that have proven themselves over time for large numbers of people. A best practice is applicable to a particular condition or circumstance and may have to be modified or adapted for similar circumstances.

Various organizations, professional associations, and many others publish "best practices" to inform clinical decision making. Generally, best practices are accepted, informally standardized techniques, methods, or processes that have proven themselves over time to accomplish given tasks. These practices are commonly used, but are generally based on no specific formal methodology. It is assumed that if done right, using best practices will achieve a desired outcome across organizations that can be delivered more effectively and consistently.

A DNP searching for best practices for any given question will usually begin with a review of the literature so that research and other sources of evidence inform best practices. It rests upon the DNP to evaluate the literature to determine the basis and strength of a possible intervention based on the source, reliability, and quality of the information and the methods used to define the "best practice." Although meta-analysis is considered the highest level of research evidence, clinical questions in practice do not always have research of quantity and quality to provide this level of evidence. Therefore, the DNP must review what literature is available to make a judgment about what might potentially be a better or best practice in a given situation.

## Evidence-Based Practice

EBP is a problem-solving approach to clinical decision making within a health care organization that integrates the best available research evidence with the best available experiential (patient and practitioner) evidence. Both internal and external influences on practice, as well as critical thinking in the judicious application of evidence, are considered (Newhouse et al., 2007). EBP is based on research evidence about the effectiveness of interventions that are used to guide decision making about patient care. It relies on a ranking of the multiple research studies that critically differentiate the most to the least reliable research findings. This is important because individual research findings can be misleading for a variety of reasons, ranging from poor study design to small sample size that is not generalizable (Sackett, Strauss, Richardson, Roenberg, & Haynes, 2000).

Even when evidence is available, many research studies have identified significant gaps between actual practice and the best possible practice. Part of this gap has been because of the lack of research evidence to inform and standardize practice to achieve predictable outcomes. Another part of this gap reflects the view that EBP discounts individual clinical skills and patient preferences (Close & Cheater, 1999). Although in many instances there is no research evidence, the aim of EBP is to integrate current best evidence from research (when it is available) with clinical policy and practice. In doing so, clinical decision making can be based on evidence-informed tools of what works to improve performance, narrow the gap between practice and research, and improve patient outcomes (Bates et al., 2003).

To apply EBPs, APNs need to implement the best interventions and practices that are informed by the best evidence. From the perspective of quality and safety, EBP is considered the gold standard of care. EBP can "raise the bar" within a clinical practice and achieve more predictable patient outcomes.

## MAJOR INFLUENCES ON SHAPING AND EVALUATING HEALTH CARE

### Institute of Medicine (Now the Health and Medicine Division of the National Academies of Sciences, Engineering, and Medicine)

The IOM is a nonprofit, private organization whose purpose is to provide national advice on issues relating to biomedical science, medicine, and health to improve health care. It relies on a volunteer workforce of scientists and other experts, operating under a rigorous, formal peer-review system. The IOM strives to provide unbiased, evidence-based, and authoritative information and advice concerning health and science policy issues. With the release of *To Err Is Human* (Kohn et al., 1999), the IOM began a series of reports on improving quality and safety of health care. These reports have been instrumental in influencing national policy reimbursement policies.

In *Crossing the Quality Chasm: A New Health System for the 21st Century* (IOM, 2001), the IOM set forth six aims for health care improvement. These aims—safety, effective, timely, patient centered, efficient, and equitable—have become a standard throughout health care. In terms of other standards, the IOM also asserted that chronic diseases were best managed when using a "protocol or plan that provides an explicit statement of what needs to be done for patients, at what intervals, and by whom, and that considers the needs of all patients with specific clinical features and how their needs can be met" (IOM, 2001, p. 94).

The report, *Keeping Patients Safe: Transforming the Work Environment of Nurses* (IOM, 2004a), emphasized the evidence for nursing and set forth policy recommendations primarily regarding nurse staffing. The IOM focused their recommendations on improving patient safety through strategies that would improve the work environment for nurses. Among the many recommendations were adequate staffing, organizational support for ongoing learning and decision support, using mechanisms that promote interdisciplinary collaboration, and implementing a work design that promotes safety. While important for patients, practitioners, and organizations, the challenge is acting upon these recommendations in lieu of sufficient evidence for specific interventions that can optimize outcomes across organizations. The IOM also recommended changes in the minimum standards for registered and licensed nurse staffing in nursing homes, but only recommended them because of the lack of evidence for minimum standards in hospitals (IOM, 2004a).

In *Patient Safety: Achieving a New Standard for Care*, the IOM set forth recommendations to improve patient safety. One of the major recommendations was to better manage health information technology and data systems to enable patient safety as a standard across care delivery sites. The health information technology and data systems are needed to inform care decisions and support patient safety. To operationalize these recommendations, the IOM specified the need for common data standards for information sharing and utilization (IOM, 2004b).

The IOM has also addressed issues relating to evidence and how it should be used. In *Knowing What Works in Health Care: A Roadmap for the Nation* (2008), the IOM recommended government oversight of the production of information for comparative effectiveness and to set forth high priority topics for systematic reviews of clinical effectiveness. The IOM also recommended that methodologic standards and a common language for characterizing the strength of the evidence be developed for systematic reviews (IOM, 2008). Since these recommendations were made, an oversight committee has been developed and millions of dollars have been allocated by the federal government for comparative effectiveness research (CER) under the health care reform law passed in March 2010.

In *Finding What Works in Health Care: Standards for Systematic Reviews*, the IOM (2011b) responded to a directive from Congress to develop standards for conducting systematic reviews of the comparative effectiveness of medical and surgical interventions. These standards are intended to assure that systematic reviews will be objective, transparent, and scientifically valid. In this report, the IOM recommended standards for the entire systematic review process, making specific recommendations on finding and assessing individual studies, synthesizing the body of evidence, and reporting systematic reviews.

## The Joint Commission

Formerly called The Joint Commission on Accreditation of Healthcare Organizations, The Joint Commission is a private nonprofit organization that provides elective accreditation of over 19,000 health care organizations and programs in the United States. The Joint Commission seeks to improve health care by encouraging and evaluating health care organizations. Organizations can receive accreditation only when they demonstrate achievement of specific performance standards. Government recognizes The Joint Commission accreditation as a condition for Medicare and Medicaid reimbursement and licensure (The Joint Commission, 2008).

The Joint Commission's standards for acute care hospitals set the precedent for standards in other settings, and are even quoted in the judgments of some civil malpractice cases. When there are changes in The Joint Commission's standards, they are generally consistent with changes in federal policy and precedent-setting court cases as well as changes in national concerns (e.g., sentinel events) or major reports (e.g., the IOM report, *To Err Is Human*).

Consistent with its stated mission of "improving health care for the public," The Joint Commission has set forth standards, goals, and measures to promote improvements in patient safety. To receive accreditation, health care organizations need to achieve a series of standards that represent high-quality care. The Joint Commission's National Patient Safety Goal (NPSG) highlights problematic areas in health care and describes available evidence and expert-based solutions to these problems (The Joint Commission, 2011a), if they exist. The NPSGs have become a critical method by which The Joint Commission promotes and enforces major changes in patient safety. The Joint Commission also sets forth quality improvement measures, and works with the Centers for Medicare and Medicaid Services (CMS) to set forth common national hospital performance measures (The Joint Commission, 2011b).

In 1990, the JCAHO dropped their Managed Care Accreditation Program and turned their accredited managed care organizations over to the National Committee for Quality Assurance (NCQA). NCQA's first standards for managed care were published in 1991, and have been revised about every 2 years since then. The NCQA works with managed care organizations, health care purchasers, state regulators, and consumers to develop standards and performance measures (see http://www .ncqa.org/tabid/59/default.aspx for information on the Health Plan Employer Data Information Set) that are intended to evaluate the structure and functions of medical and quality management systems in managed care organizations.

## Centers for Medicare and Medicaid Services

As part of the U.S. Department of HHS, the CMS, previously known as the Health Care Financing Administration, administers the Medicare program and works in partnership with state governments to administer Medicaid, the State Children's Health Insurance Program (SCHIP), and health insurance portability standards. CMS is also responsible for the administrative simplification standards from the Health Insurance Portability and Accountability Act of 1996 (HIPAA), quality standards in long-term care facilities, and clinical laboratory quality standards under the Clinical Laboratory Improvement Amendments (see www.cms.gov). Throughout its programs and responsibilities, CMS exerts tremendous influence on practice standards by setting forth reimbursement policies for covered services and by developing, interpreting, implementing, and evaluating policies for professional standards review, related peer review, utilization review, and utilization control programs under Medicare and Medicaid. Hospitals must meet specific requirements and conditions established by CMS to receive reimbursement for providing services to Medicare and Medicaid beneficiaries. These conditions include patients' rights, quality assessment and performance improvement, and utilization review.

## Agency for Healthcare Research and Quality

Formerly the Agency for Health Care Policy and Research, the Agency for Healthcare Research and Quality (AHRQ) is also part of the HHS. The mission of the AHRQ is to improve the quality, safety, efficiency, and effectiveness of health care for all Americans. AHRQ's mission helps HHS achieve its strategic goals to improve the safety, quality, affordability, and accessibility of health care; ensure public health promotion and protection, disease prevention, and emergency preparedness; promote the economic and social well-being of individuals, families, and communities; and advance scientific and biomedical research and development related to health and human services. AHRQ facilitates the development of evidence through research grants and evidence-based research syntheses through its EBP centers (www.ahrq.gov/clinic/epc). Research funded by AHRQ helps people make more informed decisions and improve the quality of health care services. Quality and patient safety indicators are found or the AHRQ website (www.qualityindicators .ahrq.gov). AHRQ works with organizations, such as the National Quality Forum, to set forth evidence-based indicators of quality.

After AHRQ's "near death experience" from Congress in 1995 over its release of guidelines for back surgery and patrician politics, it turned the business of developing guidelines over to nongovernmental organizations including professional organizations. While not directly involved in guideline development, an important repository of guidelines is maintained by AHRQ, covering a variety of topics (www.guidelines.gov).

## HOW STANDARDS, GUIDELINES, AND PROTOCOLS ARE DEVELOPED

There are significant variations and several major forces in defining practice guidelines and protocols. Researchers apply various science-based methodologies to develop the research that can serve as the evidence. Experts and practitioners weigh in with their opinions based on personal experience and continue the tradition through education and reinforcement in practice settings. National health policy leaders and insurers influence minimal standards of care and what services will be reimbursed and where. The public influences what type of care is expected through public opinion, the new media, and publications. Patients and their families influence what care is provided through preferences and interactions with practitioners. When standards, guidelines, and protocols are developed, many forces come together. For example, clinical, administrative, and academic experts developed the standards of nursing practice (ANA, 2004).

### Process of Developing Standards, Guidelines, and Protocols

In many instances, practice guidelines are used to convey a synthesis of the strengths and weaknesses of the research and its practice implications, as well as provide a basis to improve care quality by reducing practice variations (Baker, 2001). It can take 5 years for published guidelines to be adopted into routine practice (Lomas, Sisk, & Stocking, 1993). Even when guidelines exist and are broadly accepted, they are often not used in practice.

The IOM has asserted that clinical guidelines should be used to guide health care decisions by practitioners and patients (Field & Lohr, 1990). Yet, the strength of the guideline and its applicability to practice is dependent upon appropriate interpretation of the research evidence that is developed using formal methods. These methods should include identification of the area or areas of practice where a guideline could be helpful, a synthesis of relevant research evidence, a review by a guideline development group, and an external review of the recommendations for the guidelines (Eccles & Grimshaw, 2004; Shekelle, Woolf, Eccles, & Grimshaw, 1999).

### Research Evidence

Research tests innovations in laboratories and in practice. The millions of dollars that many public and private organizations invest in research provide hope that health care services can be improved. The challenge is evidence developed through research has a tendency to "sit" in research journals and not be used in practice.

Unfortunately, there is often a disconnect between research efforts and clinical practice. To improve research being used in practice, the research evidence needs to be synthesized because only rarely should findings from one research project be implemented into practice. Conclusions from synthesized research can then be used to develop clinical practice recommendations and policy. It is then up to organizational leaders and practitioners to apply the recommendations and policy in the right setting, at the right time, and in the right manner. These steps help to form a link between research and practice.

## Synthesizing and Grading the Evidence

Findings from research are published primarily in peer-reviewed research journals. Various strategies have been developed to assess the quality of the research evidence. Practitioners can find research syntheses from groups, such as EBP centers (see www.ahrq.gov/clinic/epc) and the Cochrane Collaborative (see www.cochrane.org), the peer-reviewed literature, and from information services that systematically review and evaluate the literature for specified topics and questions (Agency for Healthcare Research and Quality [AHRQ], 2010).

There are several challenges for both those doing the reviews and those reading the findings. First, these reviews and critical evaluations of research findings are dependent upon the research that has been completed, which may have only some bearing on the questions at hand. Second, many of the systematic reviews and efforts to inform guidelines hold randomized controlled trials (RCTs) as the gold standard where the majority of the knowledge gaps in clinical practice cannot be adequately addressed by RCTs. And third, how the research is synthesized and evaluated is dependent upon the reviewers, the inclusion and exclusion criteria, and the criteria they use to evaluate the research (Timmermans & Berg, 2003).

Another mechanism to locate and utilize synthesized research findings by integrating it into practice is through health information technology, such as clinical decision support systems that are sometimes integrated into electronic medical records. Optimally, electronic decision support systems enhance clinical practice and decision making with real-time information, but they must keep current with changes in evidence and clinical practice (Bates et al., 2003).

In practice, with particular patients, practitioners can search various sources of evidence. To effectively search EBP resources, it is helpful to decide what details are important to the clinical question at hand so the right questions can be asked. According to Sackett et al. (2000), a well-built clinical question includes the following components:

- The patient's disorder or disease
- The intervention or finding under review
- A comparison intervention (if applicable—not always present)
- The outcome

The acronym PICOT, from these four components, has been used to assist in remembering the steps: **P**, patient/population or problem; **I**, intervention or issue of interest; **C**, comparison intervention or issue of interest; **O**, outcome(s) of interest; and **T**, time it takes for the intervention to achieve the outcome(s) (Stillwell, Fineout-Overhold, Melynk, & Williamson, 2010).

**TABLE 10.1 U.S. Preventive Services Task Force Evidence Grading System**

| | |
|---|---|
| **High** | The available evidence usually includes consistent results from well-designed, well-conducted studies in representative primary care populations. These studies assess the effects of the preventive service on health outcomes. This conclusion is therefore unlikely to be strongly affected by the results of future studies. |
| **Moderate** | The available evidence is sufficient to determine the effects of the preventive service on health outcomes, but confidence in the estimate is constrained by such factors as:<br><br>• The number, size, or quality of individual studies.<br>• Inconsistency of findings across individual studies.<br>• Limited generalizability of findings to routine primary care practice.<br>• Lack of coherence in the chain of evidence.<br><br>As more information becomes available, the magnitude or direction of the observed effect could change, and this change may be large enough to alter the conclusion. |
| **Low** | The available evidence is insufficient to assess effects on health outcomes. Evidence is insufficient because of:<br><br>• The limited number or size of studies.<br>• Important flaws in study design or methods.<br>• Inconsistency of findings across individual studies.<br>• Gaps in the chain of evidence.<br>• Findings not generalizable to routine primary care practice.<br>• Lack of information on important health outcomes.<br><br>More information may allow estimation of effects on health outcomes. |

*Source:* USPSTF (2014).

Several strategies have been developed to evaluate the quality of evidence and the strength of practice recommendations. The strategies have different approaches to evaluating the evidence and have strengths and limitations (Atkins et al., 2004), according to the criteria used to evaluate the evidence and the subjectivity of the reviewers using a specific strategy. The U.S. Preventive Services Task Force (USPSTF) developed a system (see Table 10.1) to stratify evidence by USPSTF (2014).

In evaluating the research evidence, the USPSTF makes recommendations for a clinical service based on a balance of risk versus benefit and the level of evidence on which the recommendation can be based. The USPSTF used the following levels to reflect the strength of the recommendation for clinical practice (USPSTF, 2014):

Grade and Definition:

- Grade A: The USPSTF recommends the service. There is high certainty that the net benefit is substantial. Offer or provide this service.
- Grade B: The USPSTF recommends the service. There is high certainty that the net benefit is moderate or there is moderate certainty that the net benefit is moderate to substantial.

- Grade C: The USPSTF recommends selectively offering or providing this service to individual patients based on professional judgment and patient preferences. There is at least moderate certainty that the net benefit is small.
- Grade D: The USPSTF recommends against the service. There is moderate or high certainty that the service has no net benefit or that the harms outweigh the benefits.
- Grade I: The USPSTF concludes that the current evidence is insufficient to assess the balance of benefits and harms of the service. Evidence is lacking, of poor quality, or conflicting, and the balance of benefits and harms cannot be determined.

Another system for rating the hierarchy of evidence is as follows (Melnyk & Fineout-Overholt, 2005):

- Level I: Evidence from a systematic review or meta-analysis of all relevant RCTs, or evidence-based clinical practice guidelines based on systematic reviews of RCTs
- Level II: Evidence obtained from at least one well-designed RCT
- Level III: Evidence obtained from well-designed controlled trials without randomization
- Level IV: Evidence from well-designed case-control and cohort studies
- Level V: Evidence from systematic reviews of descriptive and qualitative studies
- Level VI: Evidence from a single descriptive or qualitative study
- Level VII: Evidence from the opinion of authorities and/or reports of expert committees

These and many other tools can be used to evaluate the quality of a guideline and the evidence that informed the guideline. APNs evaluating guidelines and the evidence will need to select which tool to use. However, it is important to appreciate the differences in the evaluation tools for guidelines and evidence as well as the significance of a guideline in altering clinical practice and the possibility of not achieving the preferred outcome because of the challenges involved in changing clinical practice.

## Comparative Effectiveness

Innovations in pharmaceuticals and therapeutic interventions have resulted in a tremendous amount of treatment options for clinicians, patients, and insurers. As the state of the evidence evolves, little is known or widely understood about the relative effectiveness of these various options. Efforts to compare the effectiveness among these options for a specific condition can focus on the benefits and risks of each option, or the costs and the benefits of those options. In some instances, one of the options may prove to be more effective clinically or more cost effective for a broad range of patients. However, a key issue is determining which specific type(s) of patient(s) would benefit most from a specific option.

CER was defined by the IOM as "the generation and synthesis of evidence that compares the benefits and harms of alternative methods to prevent, diagnose, treat, and monitor a clinical condition or to improve the delivery of care. The purpose of CER is to assist consumers, practitioners, purchasers, and policy makers to make informed decisions that will improve health care at both the individual and population levels" (IOM, 2009, p. 29). The core question of CER is which treatment works best, for whom, and under what circumstances. Findings from CER can provide invaluable information for clinical and coverage-related decision making. While the importance of CER increases, there continues to be both technical and policy-related questions about how CER is conducted, disseminated, and utilized.

Over the past few years, the federal government has made a substantial investment in CER. The American Recovery and Reinvestment Act of 2009 provided $1.1 billion for CER, dividing that money between the Office of the Secretary in the U.S. Department of Health and Human Services, the National Institutes of Health, and the AHRQ. Then in March 2010, Congress passed the Affordable Care Act, which created the Patient-Centered Outcomes Research Institute, a nongovernmental body that will establish a nationwide agenda for the research, much of which will be funded by a tax imposed on health insurers. The purpose of this institute is to review evidence and produce new information on how diseases, disorders, and other health conditions can be treated to achieve the best clinical outcome for patients. One of the organizations providing leadership in the area of CER is the AHRQ.

## Revising Existing Standards, Guidelines, and Protocols

Standards, guidelines, and protocols developed more than 5 years ago, and in some instances less than 5 years ago, may be out-of-date given more recent research evidence published. As research evolves with new information, guidelines need to be updated; some may need to be updated as often as every 3 years to reflect changes in empirical knowledge. Additionally, because the availability of new research evidence does vary by topic, guidelines generally become outdated in 5.8 years (Shekelle et al., 2001).

## Changing Practice

To implement EBPs in many organizations, decision makers need to balance the strengths and limitations of all relevant research evidence with the practical realities of the practice environment and patient population. This includes consideration of the clinical usefulness, the limitations of the available evidence, and understanding of the differentiation that exists among the multiple EBPs for the same issue. From a practical standpoint, evidence-based guidelines have to be tailored to the organization and the unique subculture(s) within.

Practitioners who want to improve the quality, safety, effectiveness, and efficiency of health care services can apply research evidence and best practices. However, practitioners are challenged to find, assess, interpret, and apply the current best evidence. Evidence is increasingly accessible through publications and information services such as electronic databases, systematic reviews, and health care journals. However, there are challenges to the successful application of the best information to changing practice.

To provide guidance on which factors practitioners should consider when determining whether research findings from a study should inform practice changes, the following has been proposed (Cone & Lewis, 2003, p. 418):

Factors related to the study in question:

1. The study should be of the highest possible quality (e.g., important and testable clinical question, prospective, large enough, randomized, blinded, controlled, minimal sources of bias).
2. The study results should be the best information available.
3. The study results should be valid and plausible.
4. The benefits of the change should outweigh the risks of implementing the change.

Factors not related to the study in question:

1. The costs of changing (or not changing) practice must be assessed.
2. The similarity of your clinical setting to that of the study.
3. The similarity of your health care system to that of the study.
4. "Expert" opinion and regulation.

Researchers have found that guidelines have minimal impact on changing physician behavior (Hayward, 1997; Woolf, 1993), but this could be due to a "lack of awareness, lack of familiarity, lack of agreement, lack of self-efficacy, lack of outcome expectancy, the inertia of previous practice, and external barriers" (Cabana et al., 1999, p. 1463). There may be similar issues for nurses (Creedon, 2005; Lyerla, 2008), yet several studies have indicated that nurses are more compliant with guidelines than physicians (Erasmus et al., 2010). However, one of the most significant challenges for nurses using guidelines is that much of the nursing knowledge has not been translated into evidence-based guidelines. Also, research is needed to understand advance practice nurses' challenges and compliance with guidelines to determine opportunities for improvement.

## Determining Which Guidelines to Use in Practice

Before a guideline is adopted or translated into practice, clinicians and organizations should critically review the guideline. There are two approaches to evaluating guidelines for potential use in clinical practice. The Appraisal of Guidelines for Research and Evaluation (AGREE) collaboration developed an evaluation instrument with 23 criteria for appraising the process used to produce clinical practice guidelines (see Table 10.2). The instrument is organized using six domains:

1. Scope and purpose
2. Stakeholder involvement
3. Rigor of development
4. Clarity
5. Applicability
6. Editorial independence (The AGREE Collaboration, 2013)

---

**TABLE 10.2  AGREE II Instrument**

**Scope and Purpose**
1. The overall objective(s) of the guideline is (are) specifically described.
2. The health question(s) covered by the guideline is (are) specifically described.
3. The population (patients, public, etc.) to whom the guideline is meant to apply is specifically described.

**Stakeholder Involvement**
4. The guideline development group includes individuals from all the relevant professional groups.
5. The views and preferences of the target population (patients, public, etc.) have been sought.
6. The target users of the guideline are clearly defined.

**Rigor of Development**
7. Systematic methods were used to search for evidence.
8. The criteria for selecting the evidence are clearly described.
9. The strengths and limitations of the body of evidence are clearly described.
10. The methods used for formulating the recommendations are clearly described.
11. The health benefits, side effects, and risks have been considered in formulating the recommendations.
12. There is an explicit link between the recommendations and the supporting evidence.
13. The guideline has been externally reviewed by experts prior to its publication.
14. A procedure for updating the guideline is provided.

**Clarity and Presentation**
15. The recommendations are specific and unambiguous.
16. The different options for management of the condition or health issue are clearly presented.
17. Key recommendations are easily identifiable.

**Applicability**
18. The guideline describes facilitators and barriers to its application.
19. The guideline provides advice and/or tools on how the recommendations can be put into practice.
20. The potential resource implications of applying the recommendations have been considered.
21. The guideline presents monitoring and/or auditing criteria.

**Editorial Independence**
22. The views of the funding body have not influenced the content of the guideline.
23. Competing interests of guideline development group members have been recorded and addressed.

*Source*: www.agreetrust.org

---

The other approach uses the Grading of Recommendations Assessment, Development and Evaluation (GRADE) system, which grades both the evidence and strength of the recommendation, taking into account the design of the research studies, the quality of the studies, and the consistency of the findings. The purpose of GRADE is to guide clinicians about which studies are likely to be the most valid by taking into account more than just the quality of the research evidence. Using this system, recommendations are graded taking into account five factors:

1. Certainty regarding the benefits, risks, and inconvenience
2. The size of the benefit produced
3. The importance of the benefit produced
4. The precision of the benefit estimate
5. The cost

This system also grades the quality of the evidence and the strength of the recommendations according to the following factors:

1. Quality of evidence for each outcome
2. Relative importance of outcomes
3. Overall quality of the evidence
4. Balance of benefits and harms
5. Balance of net benefits and costs
6. Strength of the recommendation
7. Implementation and evaluation (Atkins et al., 2004)

## Getting Research Into Practice

After the research and evidence and/or guidelines have been identified and evaluated for application to practice, getting research-based evidence into practice requires applying evidence-based recommendations at the right time, in the right place, and in the right way. Yet, there are most likely several barriers to implementation, from the organizational level to the actual process of care. First, senior staff and management must be committed to change and enable that change through resource allocation and policies. Second, leaders and clinicians must be invested in making the necessary changes to implement evidence into practice. Third, it is often necessary to make changes in how care is organized and how it is delivered. Fourth, clinicians will need skill development and training to successfully utilize the evidence in practice. Fifth, it is important to ensure clinicians have the tools they need to successfully use the evidence in practice, such as computerized decision support tools. Finally, it is important to build alliances with key partners and share ownership in ensuring the success of implementation and continued utilization of the evidence in practice. If any of these organizational-level factors are not in place and functioning, efforts to implement the evidence/guideline into practice may be thwarted or initially successful then fail over time.

While evidence/guidelines standardize care across settings and practitioners, there are aspects that need to be tailored to the patient and his or her circumstances. Because the delivery of health care involves complex decisions, implementing evidence/guidelines will not necessarily meet individual patient needs (Clancy & Cronin, 2005). In practice, practitioners need to integrate the best evidence, clinical expertise, and patient preferences and values in making decisions (Sackett et al., 2000).

Given the importance of patient- and family-centered care, practitioners need to consider involving patients in the decision-making process. Practitioners need to be able to define each patient's unique circumstances, determine what is wrong with the patient, and assess how it is affecting the patient. Once the possible interventions and treatments are discussed with the patient, it may be adverse to recommended interventions and care management. Using a patient-centered care approach injects the patient's preferences, values, and rights into the process of deciding on which interventions to use and the appropriate management. While this is appropriate and encouraged by policy makers and decision makers, guidelines, standards, and protocols are generally written in such a way that assumes patient consent to the evidence. As such, it is important to integrate research evidence into clinical decision making and customize it to the patient's clinical circumstances and wishes to derive a meaningful decision about interventions and care management.

## Evaluating Your Practice Outcomes

As important as using evidence in practice is, it is also important to understand the impact of both nonevidence-based and evidence-based practices on care processes and outcomes. Many organizations and practitioners continue to make the mistake of implementing evidence-based or evidence-informed changes in care processes but fail to measure the impact on care process as well as patient and organizational outcomes. This is a significant failure because there is always a cost associated with changes in care processes and decision making, and thinking that implementing evidence/guidelines will result in better outcomes cannot be proven unless appropriately measured and assessed. At a basic level, outcomes should be assessed before and after a change is made.

## SUMMARY

Patient and organizational outcomes can be improved and consistency in care across settings and practitioners achieved by applying evidence and clinical standards, guidelines, and protocols to practice. There are many influences on what evidence is available and how it may be used in practice. Practitioners and patients need to be actively involved in using the best evidence to inform decision making and improve outcomes.

## REFERENCES

Agency for Healthcare Research and Quality. (October 2010). *Evidence-based practice centers overview*. Retrieved from http://www.ahrq.gov/clinic/epc

American Nurses Association. (2004). *Nursing: Scope and standards of practice*. Washington, DC: Author.

American Nurses Association. (2010). *Standards*. Retrieved from www.nursingworld.org/MainMenu Categories/ThePracticeofProfessionalNursing/NursingStandards.aspx

Atkins, D., Eccles, M., Flottorp, S., Guyatt, G. H., Henry, D., Hill, S., . . . GRADE Working Group. (2004). Systems for grading the quality of evidence and the strength of recommendations I: Critical appraisal of existing approaches. The GRADE Working Group. *BMC Health Services Research, 4*, 38. Retrieved from http://www.biomedcentral.com/1472-6963/4/38

Baker, R. (2001). Is it time to review the idea of compliance with guidelines? *British Journal of General Practice, 51*, 7.

Bates, D. W., Kuperman, G. J., Wang S., Gandhi, T., Kittler, A., Volk, L., . . . Middleton, B. (2003). *Journal of the American Medical Informatics Association, 10*(6), 523–530.

Brouwers, M., Kho, M. E., Browman, G. P., Cluzeau, F., Feder, G., Fervers, B., &... Zitelsberger, L. (2010). AGREE II: Advancing guideline development, reporting and evaluation in healthcare. *CMAJ, 182*(18), E839-E842; doi: 10.1503/cmaj.090449

Cabana, M. D., Rand, C. S., Powe, N. R., Wu, A. W., Wilson, M. H., Abboud, P. A., & Rubin, H. R. (1999). Why don't physicians follow clinical practice guidelines? A framework for improvement. *JAMA, 282*(15), 1458–1467.

Clancy, C., & Cronin, K. (2005). Evidence-based decision making: Global evidence, local decisions. *Health Affairs, 24*(1), 151–162.

Closs, S. J., & Cheater, F. M. (1999). Evidence for nursing practice: A clarification of the issues. *Journal of Advanced Nursing, 30*(1), 10–17.

Cone, D. C., & Lewis, R. J. (2003). Should this study change my practice? *Academic Emergency Medicine, 10*(5), 417–422.

Creedon, S. A. (2005). Healthcare workers' hand decontamination practices: Compliance with recommended guidelines. *Journal of Advanced Nursing, 51*(3), 208–216.

Eccles, M. P., & Grimshaw, J. M. (2004). Selecting, presenting and delivering clinical guidelines: Are there any "magic bullets"? *Medical Journal of Australia, 180*(Suppl. 6), S52–S54.

Emanuel, L. L. (1997). Professional standards in health care: Calling all parties to account. *Health Affairs, 16*(1), 52–54.

Erasmus, V., Daha, T. J., & Brug H. (2010). Systematic review of studies on compliance with hand hygiene guidelines in hospital care. *Infection Control and Hospital Epidemiology, 31*(3), 283–294.

Field, M. J., & Lohr, K. N. (Eds). (1990). *Clinical practice guidelines: Directions for a new program.* Washington, DC: National Academy Press.

Guyatt, G., Vist, G., Falck-Ytter, Y., Kunz, R., Magrini, N., & Schünemann, H. (2006). An emerging consensus on grading recommendations? *ACP Journal Club, 144*(1), A8–A9.

Hayward, R. S. A. (1997). Clinical practice guidelines on trial. *Candian Medical Association Journal, 156*, 1725–1727.

Healthcare information and Management Society. (2010). *HIMSS dictionary of healthcare information technology terms, acronyms and organizations.* Chicago, IL: Author.

Institute of Medicine. (2001). *Crossing the quality chasm: A new health system for the 21st century.* Washington, DC: National Academies Press.

Institute of Medicine. (2004a). *Keeping patients safe: Transforming the work environment of nurses.* Washington, DC: National Academies Press.

Institute of Medicine. (2004b). *Patient safety: Achieving a new standard for care.* Washington, DC: National Academies Press.

Institute of Medicine. (2008). *Knowing what works in health care: A roadmap for the nation.* Washington, DC: National Academies Press.

Institute of Medicine. (2009). *Initial national priorities for comparative effectiveness research.* Washington, DC: National Academies Press.

Institute of Medicine. (2011a). *Clinical practice guidelines we can trust.* Washington, DC: National Academies Press.

Institute of Medicine. (2011b). *Finding what works in health care: Standards for systematic reviews.* Washington, DC: National Academies Press.

Kohn, L. T., Corrigan, J. M., & Donaldson, M. S. (Eds.). (1999). *To err is human: Building a safer health system.* Washington, D. C.: National Academic Press.

Lomas, J., Sisk, J. E., & Stocking, B. (1993). From evidence to practice in the United States, the United Kingdom, and Canada. *Milbank Q, 71*(3), 405–410.

Lyerla, F. (2008). Design and implementation of a nursing clinical decision support system to promote guideline adherence. *Computers Informatics Nursing, 26*(4), 227–233.

McGlynn, E. A., Asch, S., Adams, J., Keesey, J., Hicks, J., Decristofaro, A., & Kerr, E. (2003). The quality of health care delivered to adults in the United States. *New England Journal of Medicine, 348*(26), 2635–2645.

Melnyk, B. M., & Fineout-Overholt, E. (2005). *Evidence-based practice in nursing & healthcare. A guide to best practice*. Philadelphia, PA: Lippincott Williams & Wilkins.

Moffett, P., & Moore, G. (2011). The standard of care: Legal history and definitions. *Western Journal of Emergency Medicine, 12*(1), 109–112.

Newhouse, R. P., Dearholt, S., Poe, S., Pugh, L. C., & White, K. M. (2007). Organizational change strategies for evidence-based practice. *Journal of Nursing Administration, 37*(12), 552–557.

Sackett, D., Strauss, S., Richardson, W., Roenberg, W., & Haynes, R. (2000). *Evidence based medicine: How to practice and teach EBM*. New York, NY: Churchill Livingstone.

Shekelle, P. G., Ortiz, E., Rhodes, S., Morton, S. C., Eccles, M. P., Grimshaw, J. M., & Woolf, S. H. (2001). Validity of the agency for healthcare research and quality clinical practice guidelines: How quickly do guidelines become outdated? *JAMA, 286*(12), 1461–1467.

Shekelle, P. G., Woolf, S. H., Eccles, M., & Grimshaw, J. (1999). Developing guidelines. *BMJ, 318*, 593–596.

Stillwell, S. B., Fineout-Overhold, E., Melynk, B. M., & Williamson, K. M. (2010). Evidence-based practice, step by step: Asking the clinical question: A key step in evidence-based practice. *American Journal of Nursing, 110*(3), 58–61.

The AGREE Collaboration. (2013). *Appraisal of guidelines for research & evaluation (AGREE) instrument*. Retrieved from http://www.agreecollaboration.org/pdf/agreeinstrumentfinal.pdf

The Joint Commission. (2008). *About The Joint Commission*. Retrieved from http://www.jointcommission.org/about_us/about_the_joint_commission_main.aspx

The Joint Commission. (2011a). *National patient safety goals*. Retrieved from http://www.jointcommission.org/standards_information/npsgs.aspx

The Joint Commission. (2011b). *Specifications manual for national hospital inpatient quality measures*. Retrieved from http://www.jointcommission.org/specifications_manual_for_national_hospital_inpatient_quality_measures

Timmermans, S., & Berg, M. (2003). *The gold standard: The challenge of evidence-based medicine and standardization in health care*. Philadelphia, PA: Temple University Press.

U.S. Preventive Services Task Force. (May 2008). Grade definitions. Retrieved from http://www.uspreventiveservicestaskforce.org/uspstf/grades.htm

U.S. Preventive Services Task Force. (2014). *Grade definitions*. Retrieved from http://www.uspreventiveservicestaskforce.org/Page/Name/grade-definitions#grade-definitions-after-july-2012

Woolf, S. H. (1993). Practice guidelines: A new reality in medicine, III: Impact on patient care. *Archives of Internal Medicine, 153*, 2646–2655.

Woolf, S. H., Grol, R., Hutchinson, A., Eccles, M., & Grimshaw, J. (1999). Potential benefits, limitations, and harms of clinical guidelines. *BMJ, 318*(7182), 527–530.

# CHAPTER ELEVEN

# HEALTH CARE TEAMS

Joanne V. Hickey

> *None of us is as smart as all of us . . . . We all know that cooperation and collaboration grow more important every day. A shrinking world in which technological and political complexity increase at an accelerated rate offers fewer and fewer arenas in which individual action suffices.*
> —*Warren Bennis*

The current literature overwhelmingly exalts the value of teams—in particular, interdisciplinary and interprofessional health care teams—as the primary structural method to achieve better teamwork and improved patient/population outcomes. As one delves into the literature to find and examine the supporting evidence for such a claim, the results are mixed. What one finds are mostly descriptions, observations, case studies, and expert opinion reports, but fewer well-designed investigations of health care teams and the impact of teamwork on patient and population outcomes. A recent review of the literature suggests a shifting to more literature demonstrating the relationship of team training and teamwork on patient and population outcomes. Weaver, Dy, and Rosen (2014) conducted a 2000 to 2012 review of team training in acute care settings. Thirteen studies reported a statistically significant change in teamwork behaviors, processes, or emergent states, and 10 studies reported significant improvement in clinical care processes or patient outcomes. The investigators concluded that overall, moderate to high-quality evidence suggests team training can positively impact health care team processes and patient outcomes. The evidence also suggests that bundled team training interventions and implementation strategies that embed effective teamwork as a foundation for other improvement efforts may offer the greatest impact on patient outcomes. In the same vein, the Institute of Medicine (IOM) commissioned the Committee on Measuring the Impact of Interprofessional Education on Collaborative Practice and Patient Outcomes. The report examined the evidence that linked interprofessional education (IPE) to patient and health system outcomes. The committee provided general guidelines about approaches to strengthen the evidence in the future, especially about a conceptual model to guide research and expanded research methodologies to achieve the goals. They note that as contemporary health care has become more outcomes oriented, so have the questions about the impact and effectiveness of IPE and practice (Institute of Medicine [IOM], 2015). The committee noted that research is shifting from a focus on student learning about IPE to issues of patient safety, patient and provider satisfaction, quality of care, health promotion, population health, and cost of care, although methodological issues to conduct this complex research are still lagging (IOM, 2015; Moore, Green, & Gallis, 2009; Walsh, Reeves, & Maloney, 2014).

The work of teams is complex, and the magnitude of complexity increases with greater numbers of team members, the focus of the work, and contextual environmental factors. Teams are dynamic with complex internal and external interactions. Internal interactions occur within the team and include member-to-member and member-to-team interactions. External factors include interactions with the patient/family, other teams, and the organization; elements of the organization; oversight committees; and the overall health care delivery system.

Teams are ever changing as they undergo multiple transitions in their work and goals responding to the needs of patients, organizations, and the health care system requiring adaptability. A one-time snapshot of a team does little to capture the immense complexity and dynamics of the team, which suggests the need to study teams over time, thus creating multiple snapshots. In addition, current research methodologies are generally ineffective at enlightening investigators about the complex interactive processes and outcomes of teams. Most studies provide insight about a few variables of interest by reporting relationships among selected variables, but do not address causality or outcomes. The state of the science on health care teams is "messy," although it provides some direction for evaluation of teams.

The purpose of this chapter is to provide the reader with background information about health care teams, including the theoretical/conceptual basis, types, development, functions, and outcomes of teams as well as core competencies for interprofessional collaborative practice. This information serves as a basis for better understanding teams, foci for evaluation, and frameworks for evaluating teams.

## TEAMS

Teams have many definitions. Traditional definitions of teams conceptualize and define a team as identifiable groups of two or more individuals working interdependently toward a shared goal that requires the coordinated effort and resources to achieve mutually desired outcomes (Salas, Dickinson, Converse, & Tannenbaum, 1992; Salas & Frush, 2013). Another traditional definition of a team is "a small number of consistent people committed to a relevant shared purpose, with common performance goals, complementary and overlapping skills, and a common approach to their work" (Lorimer & Manion, 1996). Teams view themselves and are viewed by others as a distinct social entity working within a larger entity (Cohen & Bailey, 1997). Hackman (2002) describes teams and entities within defined boundaries of stable teams and notes that well-designed teams are those with clear goals, thought-out tasks that are conducive to teamwork, team members with the right skills and experiences for the task, adequate resources, and access to coaching and support. Teams in health care have been defined as "the interaction or relationship of two or more health care professionals who work interdependently to provide care for patients" (Lemieux-Charles & McGuire, 2006). Teams can be classified as *traditional teams,* defined as those teams whose members interact through traditional meetings and consultation, and *nontraditional teams*, whose structure, methods, and work is very fluid. Electronic teams are examples of nontraditional teams; their members interact mainly through communication processes augmented by electronic technology such as the Internet. Web-based tools using multifunctional software applications enable teamwork to occur at any time and anywhere (Wiecha & Pollard, 2004). The electronic medical record has created both opportunities and challenges for teams.

## TEAMWORK

The concept of teamwork has also evolved over time. *Teamwork* refers to the actual behaviors (e.g., exchange of information), cognitions (e.g., shared mental models), and attitudes (e.g., cohesion) that make interdependent performance possible (Salas, Rosen, Burke, & Goodwin, 2008). According to Xyrichis and Ream (2008), teamwork is "a dynamic process involving two or more health care professionals with complementary backgrounds and skills, sharing common health goals, and exercising concerted physical and mental effort in assessing, planning, or evaluating patient care." Teamwork occurs by using a number of strategies such as interdependent collaboration, open communications, shared decision making, and generated value-added patient, organizational, and staff outcomes (Xyrichis & Ream, 2008). Team-based care is defined "as an approach to health care whereby a group of people work together to accomplish a common goal, solve a problem, or achieve a specified result" (IOM, 2015). However, many teams in health care do not meet the definition of clearly identifiable individuals and stability of a team who work consistently together.

Stable teams are becoming less common in health care. The concept of teaming has been added to the nomenclature of teamwork in a knowledge economy. *Teaming* is defined as the activity of working together. Unlike the traditional concept of a team, teaming is an active process rather than a static entity. It is a way of collaboratively working that brings people together to generate new ideas, find answers, and solve problems. Teaming is further described as: blending of ways of relating to people; listening to other points of view; coordinating action; and making shared decisions. It is a dynamic process of working that provides the necessary coordination and collaboration without the luxury (or rigidity) of stable team structure. In health care, many teams come together for a circumscribed purpose, accomplish the task, and disband until the need arises again for their special expertise. There is an ebb and flow to the teamwork. The work may take minutes or occur over a short circumscribed time. Teaming has been described as teamwork on the fly, involving coordination and collaboration without the benefit of stable team structures. For example, many operations within hospitals and clinics require flexible staffing and make stable team composition rare (Edmondson, 2012).

Different competencies and leadership styles are required to work in these teams. Critical is the ability to act in the moment because there is no time to build a foundation of familiarity with others through sharing of personal history and prior experience nor experiential work. The new competencies included sharing crucial knowledge quickly and being able to quickly learn by asking questions clearly and frequently. This is particularly important because teaming is the engine of organizational learning and involves bringing people together to generate new ideas and make decisions, often about complex problems. Teaming is integral to any enterprise, but it is critical when any of the following conditions exist: work requires people to juggle multiple objectives with minimal oversight; need to shift from one situation to another while maintaining high levels of communication and tight coordination; need to integrate perspectives from different disciplines; collaboration required across dispersed locations; preplanned coordination is impossible or unrealistic due to rapid changing nature of the work; and complex information must be processed, synthesized, and used quickly (Edmondson, 2012). Weinberg, Cooney-Miner, Perloff, Babington, and Avgar (2011) describes *collaborative capacity* as the likelihood that providers, no matter how brief their exchange, will collaborate as if they were members of a conventional team even in the absence of a formal team structure. They recommend a "shift in emphasis from teams with their requirements for clear group boundaries and stable membership over time to collaborative capacity, which emphasized the ability of providers to engage in teamwork—sharing interdependent tasks with norms of respectful and helpful interaction and engaging in joint collaborative decision making" (Weinberg et al., 2011). For the evaluator, understanding team structure and processes are important in evaluating outcomes.

## CLASSIFICATION OF TEAMS

In health care, the teams of greatest interest are the teams classified as multidisciplinary, interdisciplinary, interprofessional, and transdisciplinary. Table 11.1 includes terms used in describing these teams. Choi and Pak (2006) addressed the development and clarity of terminology in a comprehensive review of terminology and suggested that these terms reflect a continuum of development. Although there continues to be some confusion about the definitions of terms, the following definitions are provided as a basis for discussion.

**TABLE 11.1  Definitions Related to Health Care Teams**

| Term | Definition |
|---|---|
| Collaboration | An active and ongoing partnership, often involving people from diverse backgrounds who work together to solve problems or provide services (IOM, 2015, p. xi).<br>Cooperatively working together, sharing responsibility for solving problems and making decisions to formulate and carry out plans for patient care (Baggs & Schmitt, 1988, p. 145; Baggs et al., 1999).<br>A complex process through which relationships are developed among health care professionals so that they effectively interact and work together for the mutual goal of safe and quality patient care (Freshman, Rubino, & Chassiakos, 2010, p. 110). |

*(continued)*

**TABLE 11.1   Definitions Related to Health Care Teams (*continued*)**

| Term | Definition |
|---|---|
| Interdisciplinary collaboration | An interpersonal process that facilitates the achievement of goals that cannot be reached when individual professionals act individually. |
| Interprofessional collaboration | A type of interprofessional work involving various health and social care professionals who come together regularly to solve problems or provide services (IOM, 2015, p. xi). |
| Interprofessional teamwork | A type of work involving different health or social care professionals who share a team identity and work together closely in an integrated and interdependent manner to solve problems and deliver services (IOM, 2015, p. xi). |
| Leadership | The ability to coordinate the activities of team members and teams by managing the resources available to team members and facilitating team performance by communicating plans, providing information about team performance through debriefs, and providing support to team members when needed (Agency for Healthcare Research and Quality [AHRQ], 2012). |
| Team effectiveness | The degree to which team goals and objectives are successfully met. |
| Team mental models | The shared and organized understanding and mental representation of knowledge or beliefs relevant to key elements of the team's task environment (Klimoski & Mohammed, 1994). |
| Team processes | Interdependent acts of members that convert inputs into outputs through cognitive, verbal, and behavioral activities directed toward organizing task work to achieve collective goals. Task work involves what the team is doing, and reflects skill and member competence. By contrast, teamwork describes how they do it, and relies on higher level behaviors, such as the ability to direct, align, communicate, negotiate, and monitor task work (Marks, Mathieu, & Zaccaro, 2001). |
| Value | Value has different meanings in different contexts. Value in health care is expressed as the physical health and sense of well-being achieved related to the cost (Institute of Medicine Roundtable on Evidence-Based Medicine, 2008). |

*Multidisciplinary* refers to a team where members of different disciplines/ professions work separately, each with its own treatment goals (Korner, Wirtz, Bengel, & Goritz, 2015). Although they contribute to the care of a patient, they often do so without knowledge of the overall specific goals or what other team members are doing. Although written documentation of care is available from each provider, it is a "silo" approach to care, with each provider "doing her or his own thing." Coordination, continuity of care, and a comprehensive approach to the achievement of common goals are lacking.

*Interdisciplinary* describes a deeper level of collaboration in which processes such as development of a plan of care or evaluation occur jointly, with professionals of different disciplines pooling their knowledge in an independent fashion. When the term *interdisciplinary* is attached to the term *practice*, then *interdisciplinary practice* refers to people with distinct disciplinary education and training working together for a common purpose through different but complementary contributions to patient-focused care (Leathard, 1994). In current practice, an interdisciplinary model of practice and care is considered best practice although interprofessional practice is rapidly replacing interdisciplinary practice. The interdisciplinary model is used across the continuum of care, including intensive care units (ICUs), long-term care facilities, geriatric acute and chronic care units, transitional care units, and community-based clinics.

*Transdisciplinary* is a specific form of interdisciplinary work in which boundaries between and beyond disciplines are transcended and knowledge and perspectives from different scientific disciplines, as well as nonscientific sources, are integrated. Transdisciplinary is the newest term in the disciplinarity nomenclature and is undergoing the process of consensus building around a definition. The prefix "trans" means to go across something. By going across, beyond, and over disciplinary boundaries, a process emerges to assemble the disciplines in new ways and to recombine disciplinary knowledge and information for the creation of new knowledge (Choi & Pak, 2006). There is interest in transdisciplinary teams because of the complexity of current problems and the belief that only transdisciplinary thinking and problem solving can adequately address these challenges. For example, transdisciplinary teams of molecular scientists, biological engineers, geneticists, ethicists, and others are needed to solve such complex questions related to stem cell and personal health issues (Massachusetts Institute of Technology, 2011).

*Interprofessional* describes the interactions among individual professionals who may represent a particular discipline or branch of knowledge, but who additionally bring their unique educational background, experiences, values, roles, and identities to the process of working across health care professions to cooperate, collaborate, communicate, and integrate care in teams to ensure that care is continuous and reliable. Each professional may possess some shared or overlapping knowledge, skills, abilities, competencies, and roles with other professionals with whom he or she collaborates (Ash & Miller, 2014; IOM, 2003). The term *interprofessional* excludes anyone who is not classified as a "professional" and thus excludes potential providers of information and knowledge to the work at hand, including the patient, family members, and community health workers (CHWs); this limitation is counterintuitive to patient-centered care.

The World Health Organization (WHO) defines *interprofessional collaborative practice* as "when multiple health workers from different professional backgrounds work together with patients, families, carers, and communities to deliver the highest quality of care" (WHO, 2010). The Interprofessional Education Collaborative Expert Panel (IECEP) defines *interprofessional teamwork* as the level of "cooperation, coordination, and collaboration characterizing the relationships between professions in delivering patient-centered care (Interprofessional Education Collaborative Expert Panel [IECEP], 2011, p. 8). *Interprofessional team-base care* is defined as "care delivered by intentionally created, usually relatively small work groups in health care, who are recognized by others as well as by themselves as having a collective identity and shared responsibility for a patient or group of patients, e.g., rapid response team, palliative care team, primary care team, or operating room team" (IECEP, 2011, p. 8).

The pursuit of multiple discipline work and teamwork is important for several reasons, including the following (Choi & Pak, 2006):

- To resolve real-world problems
- To resolve complex problems
- To provide different perspectives about a problem
- To create a comprehensive prospective theory-based hypothesis for research
- To develop consensus around clinical definitions and guidelines for complex diseases and conditions
- To provide comprehensive services such as health care and health education

In current practice, health care teams are responsible for managing the complex care of patients in a variety of settings. Care coordination and transitions in care to a variety of settings require teams to work together to achieve expected outcomes. Health care teams are now also beginning to work with CHWs to improve the quality of care and decrease costs.

## CHWs and Teams

CHWs are individuals from the community who provide care and services in a variety of settings, such as the client's home, provider officers, hospitals, social service agencies, schools, and in the community at large. The term CHW refers to many different job titles and roles, such as lay health worker, patient navigator, peer advisor, community health advocate, promotora, as well as others (Institute for Clinical and Economic Review [ICER], 2013). The CHW received a minimal amount of training (e.g., 2–6 weeks) and is a member of the community at large who has an appreciation and respect for the ethnic, linguistic, cultural, or experiential connections of the population that he or she serves (Brooks et al., 2014). They work as members of the health care team to increase the cultural competence by helping them to understand the beliefs and values of the individual that impact on the acceptance and adherence to health care. As trusted members of the same community from which the patient comes, CHWs assist the patient in achieving health care goals from preventive through treatment stages. For example, they assist the patient in understanding treatment options; take the patient to appointments, as needed; and run errands, such as getting a needed prescription at the local pharmacy. Their work contributes greatly to delivering patient-centered care. The CHW program is supported by the Affordable Care Act. A growing body of evidence suggests that the implementation of a CHW program produces meaningful and measurable results (Brooks et al., 2014). With the growing number of aged and persons with chronic diseases in the United States, the focus on chronic disease management and home care is expected to continue to grow along with the need for CHWs to decrease readmission and emergency department visits, increase patient adherence, improve health and wellness, and reduce cost. Members of the interprofessional team must learn how to incorporate CHWs into the team and work effectively with them to achieve optimal outcomes for patients and communities.

## INTERPROFESSIONAL TEAM EDUCATION

Interest in team-based education for U.S. health professionals is not new. At the first IOM conference entitled Interrelationships of Educational Programs for Health Professionals, 120 leaders from allied health, dentistry, medicine, nursing, and pharmacy considered key questions about promoting IPE. A report produced was entitled *Educating for the Health Team* (IOM, 1972). Another report, *Health Professions Education: A Bridge to Quality* (IOM, 2003), underscored the need for all health professionals to be competent in working in teams.

A 2013 Cochrane (Reeves, Perrier, Goldman, Freeth, & Zwarenstein, 2013) report updated a previous systematic review of the literature on IPE. The update identified nine new studies, which were added to the six studies from the 2008 review for a total of 15 studies that met inclusion criteria (eight randomized controlled trials, five controlled before-and-after studies, and two interrupted time-series studies). All of the studies measured the effectiveness of IPE. Although these studies reported some positive outcomes, the small number of studies and the heterogeneity of interventions and outcome measures precluded making any generalizable inferences about the key element of IPE effectiveness. To improve the quality of evidence for IPE education and patient outcomes or health care process outcomes, three gaps will need to be filled: studies that assess the effectiveness of IPE interventions compared with separate, professional specific interventions; studies that include qualitative strands examining processes relating to the IPE; and cost-benefit analysis.

### Core Competencies for Interprofessional Collaborative Practice

As a response to the continued call for IPE from the IOM and multiple other sources, the IECEP was formed to set standards. The Core Competencies for Interprofessional Collaborative Practice is the work of the IECEP (2011), which represents six national professional education associations (nursing, osteopathic medicine, pharmacy, dentistry, medicine, and public health). The report provides key definitions and principles that guide the identification of core interprofessional competencies and eight reasons why it is important to agree on a core set of competencies across the professions. The interprofessional collaborative practice competency domains include the following:

- Competency domain 1: Values/ethics (VE) for interprofessional practice
- Competency domain 2: Roles and responsibilities (RR)
- Competency domain 3: Interprofessional communication
- Competency domain 4: Teams and teamwork (TT)

Table 11.2 includes a general competency statement for each domain followed by the specific competencies (IECEP, 2011, pp. 16–25). These domains and competencies are useful for the doctor of nursing practice (DNP) nurse to consider in evaluating team functionality and team performance.

---

**TABLE 11.2  Interprofessional Collaborative Practice Competency Domain, Competency Statements, and Specific Competencies for Each Domain**

**Competency Domain 1: Values/Ethics for Interprofessional Practice**
General Competency Statement-VE. Work with individuals of other professions to maintain a climate of mutual respect and shared values
*Specific VE Competencies:*
  VE1. Place the interests of patients and populations at the center of interprofessional health care delivery
  VE2. Respect the dignity and privacy of patients while maintaining confidentiality in the delivery of team-based care
  VE3. Embrace the cultural diversity and individual differences that characterize patients, populations, and the health care team
  VE4. Respect the unique cultures, values, roles/responsibilities, and expertise of other health professions
  VE5. Work in cooperation with those who receive care, those who provide care, and others who contribute to or support the delivery of prevention and health services
  VE6. Develop a trusting relationship with patients, families, and other team members (CIHC, 2010)
  VE7. Demonstrate high standards of ethical conduct and quality of care in one's contributions to team-based care
  VE8. Manage ethical dilemmas specific to interprofessional patient-/population-centered care situations
  VE9. Act with honesty and integrity in relationships with patients, families, and other team members
  VE10. Maintain competence in one's own profession appropriate to scope of practice

**Competency Domain 2: Roles and Responsibilities**
General Competency Statement-RR. Use the knowledge of one's own role and those of other professions to appropriately assess and address the health care needs of the patients and populations served
*Specific RR Competencies:*
  RR1. Communicate one's RR clearly to patients, families, and other professionals
  RR2. Recognize one's limitations in skills, knowledge, and abilities
  RR3. Engage diverse health care professionals who complement one's own professional expertise, as well as associated resources, to develop strategies to meet specific patient care needs
  RR4. Explain the RR of other care providers and how the team works together to provide care
  RR5. Use the full scope of knowledge, skills, and abilities of available health professionals and health care workers to provide care that is safe, timely, efficient, effective, and equitable
  RR6. Communicate with team members to clarify each member's responsibility in executing components of a treatment plan or public health intervention
  RR7. Forge interdependent relationships with other professions to improve care and advance learning
  RR8. Engage in continuous professional and interprofessional development to enhance team performance
  RR9. Use unique and complementary abilities of all members of the team to optimize patient care

*(continued)*

**TABLE 11.2 Interprofessional Collaborative Practice Competency Domain, Competency Statements, and Specific Competencies for Each Domain (*continued*)**

**Competency Domain 3: Interprofessional Communication**

General Competency Statement-CC. Communicate with patients, families, communities, and other health professionals in a responsive and responsible manner that supports a team approach to the maintenance of health and the treatment of disease

*Specific Interprofessional Communication Competencies:*

CC1. Choose effective communication tools and techniques, including information systems and communication technologies, to facilitate discussions and interactions that enhance team function

CC2. Organize and communicate information with patients, families, and health care team members in a form that is understandable, avoiding discipline-specific terminology when possible

CC3. Express one's knowledge and opinions to team members involved in patient care with confidence, clarity, and respect, working to ensure common understanding of information and treatment and care decisions

CC4. Listen actively, and encourage ideas and opinions of other team members

CC5. Give timely, sensitive, instructive feedback to others about their performance on the team, responding respectfully as a team member to feedback from others

CC6. Use respectful language appropriate for a given difficult situation, crucial conversation, or interprofessional conflict

CC7. Recognize how one's own uniqueness, including experience level, expertise, culture, power, and hierarchy within the health care team, contributes to effective communication, conflict resolution, and positive interprofessional working relationships (University of Toronto, 2008)

CC8. Communicate consistently the importance of teamwork in patient-centered and community-focused care

**Competency Domain 4: Teams and Teamwork**

General Competency Statement-TT. Apply relationship-building values and the principles of team dynamics to perform effectively in different team roles to plan and deliver patient-population-centered care that is safe, timely, efficient, effective, and equitable

*Specific Team and Teamwork Competencies:*

TT1. Describe the process of team development and the roles and practices of effective teams

TT2. Develop consensus on the ethical principles to guide all aspects of patient care and teamwork

TT3. Engage other health professionals—appropriate to the specific care situation—in shared patient-centered problem solving

TT4. Integrate the knowledge and experience of other professions—appropriate to the specific care situation—to inform care decisions, while respecting patient and community values and priorities/preferences for care

TT5. Apply leadership practices that support collaborative practice and team effectiveness

TT6. Engage self and others to constructively manage disagreements about values, roles, goals, and actions that arise among health care professionals and with patients and families

TT7. Share accountability with other professions, patients, and communities for outcomes relevant to prevention and health care

TT8. Reflect on individual and team performance for individual, as well as team, performance improvement

TT9. Use process improvement strategies to increase the effectiveness of interprofessional teamwork and team-based care

TT10. Use available evidence to inform effective teamwork and team-based practices

TT11. Perform effectively on teams and in different team roles in a variety of settings

## Team Strategies and Tools to Enhance Performance and Patient Safety (TeamSTEPPS)

The Agency for Healthcare Research and Quality (AHRQ) in collaboration with the Department of Defense (DoD) have developed a team training curriculum called TeamSTEPPS® designed to educate health professionals in teamwork and patient safety (2016). It is an evidence-based system designed to improve communication and teamwork skills among health care professionals, scientifically rooted in more than 20 years of research and learning from the application of teamwork principles. TeamSTEPPS provides a source of ready-to-use multimedia materials and a training curriculum to successfully integrate teamwork principles into all areas of an organization and health care system. Validated instruments, slides, an evidence-based detailed curriculum, and many more resources are provided. More information is available at their website: www.teamstepps.ahrq.gov/.

## DEVELOPMENT OF TEAMS

Team development is usually regarded as an informal process by which group members attempt to create effective social structures and work processes on their own (Kozlowski & Ilgen, 2006). A number of team developmental process models are available, but perhaps the most commonly cited model is that of Tuckman (1965). The model initially included the four stages of forming, storming, norming, and performing; a fifth stage, adjourning, was later added (Tuckman & Jensen, 1977). These are the stages that small groups are likely to go through as they come together and begin to function (Smith, 2005). The *forming stage* is described as a time of orientation through testing. The testing helps to identify boundaries of both interpersonal and task behaviors. Interpersonal work is around the establishment of dependency relationships with leaders, other group members, or preexisting standards. In the *storming stage*, there is conflict and polarization around interpersonal issues with concomitant emotional response around tasks. These behaviors serve as resistance to group influence and task requirements. In the *norming stage*, resistance is overcome because of the development of in-group feelings and cohesiveness, evolution of new standards, and adoption of new roles. Personal opinions are expressed. The *performing stage* is characterized by effective interpersonal structures to accomplish the work; roles become flexible and functional, and group energy is channeled into getting the work done. Structural issues have been resolved and an effective structure supports group work. Finally, in the *adjourning stage*, the focus is on dissolution or termination of roles, the completion of tasks, and reduction of dependency. Particularly if unplanned, the process of adjourning can be stressful with a component of mourning related to individual losses.

The following factors facilitate teams to progress through the stages of team development as a high-performance team (Ash & Miller, 2014):

- Shared purpose, goals, and commitment of team members
- Mutual trust and respect among team members
- Recognition and value of the unique role or skills that each member brings
- High performance in level of skills, ability, and practice

- Clear understanding of RR and accountability of each team member to meet the goals
- A work culture and environment that supports team and collaborative processes
- Collective cognitive responsibility and shared decision making

The Tuckman (1965) model of the development sequence of small groups is a linear model that has stood the test of time, although some have challenged the linearity in favor of models that reflect the fluctuations of groups. There does appear to be general support that small groups tend to follow a fairly predictable developmental path (Smith, 2005). From the perspective of evaluation, the Tuckman model can provide insight into the group process and achievement of outcomes. The developmental stage of the group is one variable in understanding and evaluating groups. Although this model may be useful to understand the development of a traditional stable team, it is unclear how it applies to the nontraditional teams commonly seen in current practice.

## THEORETICAL PERSPECTIVES OF TEAMS

Most of the literature about teams is opinion/expert commentary, descriptive, and case studies. The literature about teams in general, and health teams specifically, is voluminous. Teams can be viewed from multiple perspectives. Since the 1950s, the social, organizational, and business/management sciences have investigated teams from a variety of discipline-specific perspectives, resulting in an overwhelming number of frameworks to view teams. A number of theories have been developed with a focus on teams, including how teams are organized, how they work, and how they achieve outcomes. One can evaluate teams based on group dynamics, effectiveness, efficiency, interpersonal communications, satisfaction, and outcomes. A brief discussion of the theoretical basis of teams is useful to better understand the multiple lenses that can be used to examine and evaluate teams.

### Sociological Influence

Team behavior through the conceptualization of group processes was strongly influenced by sociological studies of hierarchical differentiation (Ingersoll & Schmitt, 2004). The primary focus of research was on a group's social structure and its influence on team communications and problem solving (Feiger & Schmitt, 1979). Another example of a sociological view is the theory of Groupthink (Janis, 1982), defined as a condition in which highly cohesive groups in "hot" decision situations display excessive levels of concurrence seeking that suppresses critical inquiry and result in faulty decision making. Farrell, Heinemann, and Schmitt (1986, 1988), and Farrell, Schmitt, and Heinemann (1988, 2001), proposed guidelines to counteract poor team decision-making processes with the following: (a) emphasize open, honest, and direct communications; (b) facilitate team development through orientation of new team members and team retreats; (c) focus on the team's mission statement, goals, policies, and procedures; (d) acknowledge effective individual and team work; and (e) identify team processes that lead to poor decision making with a focus on finding more effective decision making processes (Ingersoll & Schmitt, 2004).

## Organizational Influence

The organizational literature has focused on theories such as high-reliability organizations (HRO), organizational structure, organizational culture, team performance, and learning organizations. Team structure is the fundamental characteristic of teams, and structure includes size, membership, leadership, identification, and distribution. Weick and Roberts (1993) examined HROs that espoused to be nearly error free operations. They found that these HROs integrate highly developed mental models and processes that all members follow, which are a reflection of overlapping knowledge and performance standards. Another example of organizational theory is that of learning organizations. Senge (1990), in addressing systems thinking, notes that team learning is vital because teams, not individuals, are the fundamental learning unit in modern organizations. Unless a team can learn, the organization cannot learn. Excellence in any organization is not a specific arrival destination; rather, great organizations are always in a state of learning to become better or worse by expanding their capacity to create their futures. Still another area of interest is organizational culture and its influence on interprofessional teamwork, team effectiveness, and patient/organizational outcomes (Korner et al., 2015).

## Business/Management Influence

Microsystem theory and macrosystem theory are other paths of organizational investigation. A microsystem refers to the next coherent organizational level above individuals, typically a small team of people working together as one unit to get jobs done (Nelson, Batalden, Godfrey, & Lazar, 2011, pp. 2–4). In aviation, the microsystem is the flight crew and air traffic controllers. In health care, it is the health care team. Microsystem theory focuses on the front-line component of service delivery. Nelson et al. (2002) used a qualitative methodology to investigate high-performance clinical microsystems. The researchers identified characteristics across sites that led to excellent systemic outcomes. These characteristics include: leadership and the culture of the microsystems; macroorganizational support of the microsystem; a focus on patients and staff; interdependence of care teams; easy access to information and information technology; a focus on process improvement; and high-level performance patterns (Nelson et al., 2002).

As described in Chapter 1, a macrosystem refers to the overarching structure above the microsystem, such as the organization or the system. A macrosystem includes the policies, procedures, culture, and leadership that oversee the microsystems. Interactions between the microsystem and macrosystem affect performance and outcomes at both levels.

Finally, the generic input–process–output (IPO) model is used as a framework for studying teamwork effectiveness and outcomes. The IPO model describes the impact of input (e.g., organizational culture, team composition, communication patterns, task design) and the processes of teams (e.g., communication, coordination, collaboration, cooperation, leadership) on the team's outputs (team performance, cost effectiveness, quality of care, treatment outcomes, patient safety; Korner et al., 2015). The parsimony of the model allows for flexibility. Researchers can examine a few or several variables in a study. Because of the inherent complexity in understanding the multiple variables that influence team outcomes and effectiveness, researchers usually select a few variables of interest in the model to study.

## Theoretical Basis of Team Effectiveness

Effectiveness of teams refers to an evaluation of the results of performance by the team. The limited published integrative reviews provide some insights into the development of knowledge about health care teams. The research on effectiveness of interdisciplinary teams was reviewed (Schmitt, 2001; Schmitt, Farrell, & Heinemann, 1988) and concluded that teams improve functional outcomes, although there were also mixed findings. The studies reviewed did not examine greater use of resources, cost variables, or multidimensional factors of team relationships and their impact on care.

Schofield and Amodeo (1999) reviewed the education, psychology, sociology, and medical databases to identify reports about interdisciplinary teams. Of the 138 articles reviewed, 55 were descriptive, addressing some component of interdisciplinary teams; team processes or the influence of data on process or outcomes were not examined. Another 51 articles described interdisciplinary team processes, but did not provide supporting data. Although research based, another 21 articles examined a variety of variables and their effect on the team. Finally, another group of 11 articles was described as outcome based because research methods were used to assess the impact of an interdisciplinary team on selected outcomes other than team functioning. In summarizing the literature, Schofield and Amodeo (1999) noted the following: (a) although the literature endorses the team model and assumes the value of interdisciplinary teams, there is little evidence to evaluate team effectiveness or impact; and (b) the absence of well-conceived conceptual models of interdisciplinary teamwork or models to assess components of the interdisciplinary process makes it difficult to draw any reliable conclusions.

A major focus in health care is outcomes and what contributes to achievement of superior outcomes and team effectiveness. Collaboration has been identified as a key variable in teamwork that contributes to superior outcomes. Weaver, Feitosa, Salas, Seddon, and Vozenilek (2013) noted that teamwork is not synonymous with collaboration, although these terms are often used interchangeably. Teamwork is the broader concept and includes many elements such as collaboration and common goals and mental models. Collaboration continues to be a frequently addressed concept in the literature.

The need for greater interprofessional collaboration has been emphasized since the 1970s (IOM, 2010). A growing body of research has begun to highlight the potential for collaboration among teams composed of diverse individuals to generate successful solutions to complex, knowledge-driven problems (Paulus & Nijstad, 2003; Pisano & Verganti, 2008; Singh & Fleming, 2010; Wuchty, Jones, & Uzzi, 2007). Researchers have also emphasized the importance of building interprofessional teams and establishing collaborative cultures to identify and sustain continuous quality improvement of care (Kim, Barnato, Angus, Fleisher, & Kahn 2010; Knaus, Draper, Wagner, & Zimmerman, 1986; Pronovost et al., 2008). Interest in collaboration as a concept integral to interdisciplinary practice was explored. Ingersoll and Schmitt (2004) noted that this basic shift in conceptualization is important because it highlights the concept of collaboration in the delivery of care among diverse health professions.

Beginning in the late 1980s, Baggs and Schmitt (1988) investigated collaboration and interdisciplinary teams within health care organizations. *Collaboration* was defined as "cooperatively working together, sharing responsibility for solving problems and making decisions to formulate and carry out plans for patient care" (Baggs & Schmitt, 1988, p. 145). An aim of collaboration is to coordinate care and improve patient outcomes. Baggs and Schmitt (1997) focused much of their early work on physician–nurse collaboration in critical care settings. Concurrently, Knaus et al. (1986) developed the Acute Physiology and Chronic Health Evaluation (APACHE) score to predict mortality in ICU patients. They also observed that high levels of interdisciplinary practice and coordination contributed to better patient outcomes.

Using a nurse–physician questionnaire to evaluate perceptions of the multiple dimensions of the processes of care in ICUs, Shortell et al. (1992, 1994) noted that communication, leadership, coordination, and conflict management were related to better technical care, meeting of family needs, and decreased length of stay (LOS). In a national study, a total of 25 ICUs were investigated by Mitchell, Shannon, Cain, and Hegyvary (1996). Flow of information characteristic of interdisciplinary collaboration was associated with better staff perceptions of unit conflict management, collaboration, staff quality, and quality of care, but it was not associated with better clinical outcomes. Other evidence of the benefits of teamwork has emerged and includes increased learning and development of people and organizations, better utilization of resources and planning, minimization of unnecessary costs, improved job performance work quality, increased discussion among participants, networking, professional development, and positive effect on career (Choi & Pak, 2006).

Many other studies have examined interdisciplinary teams and collaboration in relationship to patient outcomes in a variety of settings, such as nursing homes, long-term care facilities, acute/critical care units, rehabilitation, and primary care, as well as with specific populations, such as geriatrics, the chronically ill, and others (Boaro, Fancott, Baker, Velji, & Andreoli, 2010; Boult et al., 2009; Famadas et al., 2008; Korner, 2010; Meier & Beresford, 2010; Neumann et al., 2010; Pezzin et al., 2011; Pyne et al., 2011; Reader, Fin, Mearns, & Cuthbertson, 2009; Rocco, Scher, Basberg, Yalamanchi, & Baker-Genaw, 2011). What is clear is that little is known empirically about interdisciplinary teams and collaboration, including team effectiveness and impact on health care delivery. Health care teams are complex dynamic entities working in complex dynamic environments. Marks, Mathieu, and Zaccaro (2001) noted that the framework of team processes and outcomes are multidimensional, and team behavior is constantly changing. The changing nature of a team and team member behavior is tempered by the developmental level of the team and the work of the team that transitions between existing goals and new goals, including evolving processes. As previously noted, a single snapshot of a team provides little information in understanding how teams work in the achievement of outcomes. Therefore, new models to investigate teams are needed if theoretical frameworks based on evidence are to be useful in health care delivery.

A Cochrane systematic review addressed interprofessional collaboration practice and health outcomes. The review suggests that practice-based interprofessional collaboration can improve health care processes and outcomes, but because of the limitations of the literature (e.g., small number of studies, sample sizes, problems with conceptualization and measurement of collaboration, and heterogeneity of interventions and settings), it was not possible to draw generalizable conclusions about the key elements of interprofessional collaboration and its effectiveness

(Zwarenstein, Goldman, & Reeves, 2009). More studies and methodological rigor were recommended to better understand interprofessional collaboration. No updates of this Cochrane systematic review are available.

Andretta (2010) conducted an observational study of teams using qualitative methods of observation and categorization to inform a model of team development strategies. The results suggested that health care teams may be more complicated than nonhealth care teams. Team models with associated competencies identified from other professions may not transfer completely to health care. Further, a single model to inform best practices for health care team development may not adequately address the specific performance challenges of each team type found in health care, thus requiring a variety of different strategies to optimize team performance.

Nurse researchers have tried to untangle the role and contributions of the nurse in teams and have found it to be methodologically challenging. The Magnet Recognition Program®, administered by the American Nurses Credentialing Center, is a credential for nursing excellence awarded to health care facilities. It is based on extensive self-review that demonstrates achievement of established criteria of nursing excellence that achieves outstanding patient outcomes. A health care organization that chooses to seek this credential begins the Magnet journey to create a sustainable culture and work environment that supports excellence in professional nursing practice. The initial qualitative research that was foundational to creating the Magnet program was conducted by McClure, Poulin, Sovie, and Wandelt (1983). Participant hospitals were nominated as places that were able to attract and retain professional nurses. The study included 41 hospitals representative of all the regions of the country. Among the characteristics identified as essential in these facilities were good interdisciplinary relationships, defined as interdisciplinary effort and shared decision making, along with a sense of mutual respect exhibited among all disciplines. Among the 14 forces of magnetism outlined in the current Magnet model, interdisciplinary relationships continued to be a force within the category of exemplary professional practice.

Using a structure–process–outcome framework to examine research supporting interdisciplinary relationships, Reid-Ponte, Creta, and Joy (2011) suggest that there is limited research evidence supporting the premise that effectively led, collaborative, interdisciplinary care teams improve patient care processes and outcomes (Boyle & Kochinda, 2004; Cowan et al., 2006; DeChairo-Marino, Jordon-Marsh, Traiger, & Saulo, 2001; Grumbach & Bodenheimer, 2004; Horbar, Plsek, Leahy, & Ford, 2004; Houldin, Naylor, & Haller, 2004). They go on to say that practice environment research supports the idea that the more mutually collaborative and respectful a team is perceived, the higher the quality of care they perceive is delivered (Aiken, Clarke, Cheung, Sloane, & Silber, 2004; Aiken, Clarke, & Sloane, 2002; Friese, Lake, Aiken, Silver, & Sochalski, 2008).

Lemieux-Charles and McGuire (2006) reviewed health care team effectiveness literature from 1985 to 2004 and distinguished among intervention studies that compared team with usual (nonteam) care, intervention studies that examine the impact of team redesign on team effectiveness, and field studies that explore relationships among team context, structure, processes, and outcomes. Using an Integrated Team Effectiveness Model (ITEM) to summarize research findings and to identify gaps in the literature, their analysis suggested that the type and diversity of clinical expertise involved in team decision making largely accounts for improvements in patient care and organizational effectiveness. Collaboration, conflict resolution, participation, and cohesion are most likely to influence staff satisfaction and perceived team effectiveness. The studies examined here underscore the importance of considering the contexts in which teams are embedded.

These examples offer a glimpse of some theoretical challenges from disciplines both outside and inside of health care to provide a foundation for viewing health care teams, as well as insight into the investigational paths pursued. Research is slowly evolving regarding teams and interdisciplinary practice teams and how they affect patient outcomes. Table 11.3 provides a list of variables related to health care teams that have been investigated. These variables have been extracted from studies cited in this chapter, and have been organized into arbitrary categories. Each category is mutually exclusive from the other categories, although variables from a number of categories may be examined during a particular evaluation. From a cursory review of the list, it is clear that there are multiple perspectives that can be used to examine and evaluate teams.

---

**TABLE 11.3   Perspectives for Evaluating Health Care Team**

**Group Process Perspective**
- Interactions of team members
- Accomplishment of tasks
- Engagement in team activities
- Engagement in team development activities
- Decision-making processes (e.g., shared, hierarchal)
- Competition between and among members
- Team norms

**Communications Perspective**
- Open, honest, and direct communications
- Constructive feedback
- Effective conflict resolution

**Cohesiveness Perspective**
- Commitment to mutual purpose
- Understanding and commitment to team mission, goals, policies, and procedures
- Orientation of new members
- Supporting of team members
- Shared team mental model

**Leadership Perspective**
- Hierarchal versus shared leadership
- Interchange of leadership and followership

**High-Performance Perspective**
- Shared vision
- Clear responsibilities
- Mutual respect
- Trust
- Cohesiveness
- Collaboration
- Collaborative capacity
- Cooperation
- Expectation of accountability of all members for outcomes
- Appreciation of expertise and contribution of each discipline
- Interdisciplinary working together
- Individual and team effectiveness
- Shared decision making
- Team members supportive of team decisions and each other
- Use common mental models
- Coordination of care

**Structural Perspective**
- Vertical versus horizontal
- Shared versus hierarchal authority
- Hierarchal leadership
- Transformational leadership
- Make-up of the team (e.g., disciplines represented) and how this contributes to outcomes

*(continued)*

**TABLE 11.3   Perspectives for Evaluating Health Care Team (*continued*)**

- Person with the most knowledge for particular project leads
- Leadership development opportunities available to all members
- Organizational support for team

**Individual Team Member Perspective**
- Values
- Attitudes
- Autonomy
- Motivation
- Personal and professional development
- Confidence building
- Self-monitoring
- Emotional intelligence

**Team Development Perspective**
- Crew resource management (CRM)
- Culture of learning
- Individual and group competency

**Satisfaction Perspective**
- Patient/family satisfaction with team
- Individual team members satisfied with team
- Others external to the team such as employer, administrator, or funder

**Patient Outcome Perspective**
- Length of stay (LOS)
- Mortality
- Morbidity/complications
- Functionality (e.g., social, intellectual, activities of daily living [ADLs], instrumental ADLs)
- Cost of care
- Service utilization

**Safety and Quality Perspective**
- Culture of blame versus quality improvement
- Root cause analysis

## BARRIERS TO TEAMS

In the health care arena, there are many barriers to establishing and maintaining high-performance teams. Some barriers cut across all practice areas while others are specific to particular areas of practice and environments. Barriers to interprofessional teamwork and collaboration include the following (Ash & Miller, 2014, p. 224):

- Gender, power, socialization, education, status, and cultural differences between professions
- Lack of a payment system and structures that reward interprofessional collaboration
- Misunderstanding about the scope of contributions of each profession
- Turf protection

Durbin (2006) notes that local customs may be the most difficult barrier to overcome. In addition, resistance comes from many sources such as hospital administration (concern about added cost), unit administrator (change in authority and control), bedside staff (must learn new ways of interacting with a team), and private physicians (altered authority gradient for patient management and decisions). Both technical competency and team competency are necessary to achieve high performance in interdisciplinary teams. Technical competency is based on professional training, education, and experience as well as licensure and certification. Team competency is based on education and the knowledge, skills, and attitude about interdisciplinary work. In addition, competency may be defined differently in each discipline.

## FAILURE OF TEAMS

Health care teams are often viewed through the lens of quality and safety. Understanding why and how teams fail is critical to understanding corrective interventions to support high-performance teams. Sassou and Reason (1999) reviewed adverse events in the nuclear, aviation, and shipping industries and found the most common cause of error was failure to communicate. The root causes of failure to communicate were authority gradient, excessive professional courtesy, overtrusting, projected confidence, inadequate resources, and poor task management, all of which resulted in a lack of ability to detect both individual and group error. Also noted was that there is a limit to how far any individual or process can be "perfected" and made "error-proof," and that a much higher degree of quality and safety can be achieved by using a team that spots for each. Strategies to keep teams and organizations functioning within industry-accepted safety standards have been developed and include crew resource management (CRM), also known as team cooperation training. CRM is used extensively by the military and aviation industry and encompasses a wide range of techniques to enhance communications, situational awareness, problem solving, decision making, teamwork, and making optimal use of all available resources (e.g., equipment, procedures, people) to promote and enhance efficiency of flight operations (AHRQ, 2016).

Blackmore and Persaud (2012) reviewed the literature and identified five critical domains important to optimize team functioning; a common team goal, the ability and willingness to work together to achieve team goals, decision making, communications, and relationships. Characteristics of behaviors for each domain were provided as well as a description of functional and dysfunctional teams. A brief discussion of how to improve team functioning was provided, including tables that summarized the information. The five domains and characteristic behaviors provide a useful framework for evaluating team function and effectiveness.

## MEASUREMENT INSTRUMENTS

Validated instruments to measure components of interprofessional practice have been developed. In 2013, the National Center for Interprofessional Practice and Education assembled and launched a web-based collection of existing IPE and collaborative practice (IPECP) measurement instruments (see www.nexusipe.org/measurement-instruments). The selection process for the initial 26 instruments included the following criteria:

- Measures one or more interprofessional outcomes (content)
- Defines a purpose (intended use)
- Provides subscale descriptions related to IPECP (content specificity)
- Has a verifiable record of use through peer-reviewed publications (acceptance)
- Provides evidence of attention to measurement properties of the tool (psychometrics)
- Provides documented uses in multiple settings (adaptability)
- Users have access to the instrument (availability)

In reviewing these instruments, one will find some specific to a population (pediatrics) or clinical practice (surgery). Other instruments are more generic to interprofessional practice. See Table 11.4 for examples of selected instruments. Measurement instruments for IPECP are available at www.nexusipe.org/measurement-instruments. The website also provides a helpful primer to guide individuals in the selection of valid instruments. See www.nexusipe.org/evaluating-ipecp.

**TABLE 11.4  Examples of Measurement Instruments for Interprofessional Teams**

| Name | Description | Number of Items and Subscale(s) | Use |
|---|---|---|---|
| The Attitudes Toward Health Care Teams (ATHCT) Scale | Developed as a pre- and postmeasure or longitudinal monitor of ATHCT among team members and/or trainees and their supervisors in clinically based team training programs | 20-item tool on a four-point scale that has two subscales:<br>● Quality of care/process (14 items) measures team members' perceptions of quality of care delivered by health care teams and quality of teamwork to accomplish this<br>● Physician centrality (six items) measures team members' attitudes toward physicians' authority in teams and their control over information about patients | To determine the effect of educational interventions for teams and evaluate practice-based team training programs for health care students and clinicians |
| Collaborative Practice Assessment Tools (CPAT) (Baggs, Ryan, Phelps, Richeson, & Johnson, 1992; Baggs et al., 1997) | Assesses levels of collaboration and is intended to assist clinical teams in identifying strengths and weaknesses in their collaborative practice | 57-item tool with a seven-point scale that assesses collaborative practice and has eight subscales:<br>● Mission, meaningful purpose, and goals<br>● General relationships<br>● Team leadership<br>● General role, responsibilities, and autonomy | To identify gaps in performance related to collaboration and suggests areas for focused educational interventions |

*(continued)*

**TABLE 11.4  Examples of Measurement Instruments for Interprofessional Teams (*continued*)**

| Name | Description | Number of Items and Subscale(s) | Use |
|---|---|---|---|
| | | • Communication and information exchange<br>• Community linkages and coordination of care<br>• Decision making and conflict management<br>• Patient involvement | |
| Index of Interdisciplinary Collaboration (IIC) Bronstein (2002, pp. 113–126) | Measures collaboration among professionals (originally social workers and other professionals) | 42-item five-point scale is a modified version of the 2002 IIC created to assess interprofessional collaboration in an organization. The tool has four subscales:<br>• Interdependence and flexibility<br>• Professional activities<br>• Collective ownership of goals<br>• Reflection on process | To assess these professional interactions with the goal of improved services to clients |
| Teamwork Perception Questionnaire (T-TPQ) TeamSTEPPS | Assesses health professionals' perceptions of interprofessional teamwork within an organization and group-level team skills and behavior | 35-item tool with a five-point scale; a self-report measure of teamwork within a unit or department; based on the core components of teamwork that comprise TeamSTEPPS:<br>• Team structure<br>• Leadership<br>• Communication<br>• Mutual support<br>• Situation monitoring | To assess TeamSTEPPS effectiveness and identify areas for education |

(*continued*)

**TABLE 11.4  Examples of Measurement Instruments for Interprofessional Teams (*continued*)**

| Name | Description | Number of Items and Subscale(s) | Use |
|---|---|---|---|
| Teamwork Attitudes Questionnaire (T-TAQ) TeamSTEPPS | Assesses an individual's impressions of team behavior as it relates to patient care in her or his work setting | 55 items graded on a five-point Likert scale from strongly agree to strongly disagree. The items are grouped according to the themes of:<br>• Team foundation<br>• Team functioning<br>• Team performance<br>• Team skills<br>• Team leadership<br>• Team climate and atmosphere<br>• Team identity | Help determine whether the TeamSTEPPS tools and strategies enhanced an individual participant's attitudes toward teamwork, increased knowledge about effective team practice, and improved team skills |
| Team Performance Observation Tool TeamSTEPPS | | 25-item Likert rating scale of 1 (very poor) to 5 (excellent). The observer is asked to rate a number of team attributes around the areas of:<br>• Team structure<br>• Leadership<br>• Situation monitoring<br>• Mutual support<br>• Communication | Help determine level of performance in five areas important for team performance. |
| Collaboration and Satisfaction About Care Decisions (CSACD) | Assesses quality of interaction in making care decisions and satisfaction with the decision-making process in the health setting | Nine-item tool on a seven-point scale and has two subscales:<br>• Collaboration<br>• Satisfaction | Assess quality of interaction in making care decisions and satisfaction with the decision-making process in the health setting |

(*continued*)

**TABLE 11.4  Examples of Measurement Instruments for Interprofessional Teams (*continued*)**

| Name | Description | Number of Items and Subscale(s) | Use |
|---|---|---|---|
| Health Care Team Vitality Instrument (HTVI) Upenieks, Lee, Flanagan, & Doebbeling (2009) | Developed and revised to assess team collaboration and patient safety, with a specific emphasis on team vitality | 10 items with a five-point scale to assess health care team functioning with the following subscales: <br>• Support structures <br>• Engagement <br>• Empowerment <br>• Patient care transition <br>• Communication | The revised 10-item HTVI is a useful tool for assessing effects of improvement projects or other innovations for frontline health care workers <br>This instrument is accessible through the Institute for Health Care Improvement website. Registration on the site is required, but free |
| Mayo High Performance Teamwork Scale (MHPTS) (Malec et al., 2007) | Provides a brief, reliable, practical measure of crew resource management (CRW) skills that can be used by participants in CRM training to reflect on and evaluate their performance as a team | 16-item three-point scale (0 = never or rarely; 1 = inconsistently; 2 = consistently) <br>The scale examines behaviors related to performance in a team such as: <br>• Effective listening and communications <br>• Accountability to team goals <br>• Mutual dependence on the organization and each other <br>• Demonstration of decision-making ability, personal and team leadership, understanding team disadvantages and liabilities, conflict management, and innovation that provided evidence of competency <br>• These concepts included in the scale were based on the work of Salas, Sims, and Klein (2004) | |

There may not be a validated instrument appropriate for the evaluation that you plan to conduct. In that case, you will need to collect that information through another source such as through the development of an evaluation protocol that asks questions about the area of interest. Even when a validated instrument is used, it becomes one component of an evaluation protocol for the collection of information.

## EVALUATION OF TEAMS

With this background information in mind, how is a DNP nurse going to evaluate a team? There is no easy answer or single approach to the evaluation. However, there are a number of questions about purpose and scope of the evaluation that, once answered, will help to focus the evaluation. A number of evaluation models have been discussed in previous chapters that provide the DNP nurse with frameworks to view the evaluation process. There are also practical frameworks that help the DNP nurse to identify the steps and activities in evaluating a team in a concrete way. In Chapter 1, Table 1.3 outlined the basic steps in evaluation, thus setting a generic framework for evaluation. The approach described in the following text, while congruent with the evaluation approach described in Chapter 1, is also concerned with the evaluation of team interactions.

Herman, Morris, and Fitz-Gibbon (1987) outline a general framework for evaluation that includes the major process categories: (a) setting the boundaries of the evaluation, (b) selecting appropriate evaluation methods, (c) collecting and analyzing information, and (d) reporting the findings. Under each major heading are a number of steps that guide the process (Table 11.5). This framework may be used to guide the process of evaluating a team by the DNP nurse. To map the evaluation process in a concise and efficient format, a logic model framework can also be used (Table 11.6). The information provided is applicable regardless if the DNP nurse is internal or external to the organization. The following text takes the reader through the steps of the evaluation.

---

**TABLE 11.5   Practical Framework for Evaluating Health Care Teams**

| Activities | Focus |
|---|---|
| *Set boundaries of the evaluation* | |
| • Determine the purpose(s) of the evaluation<br>• Learn all you can about the team<br>• Describe the team<br>• Focus the evaluation<br>• Negotiate your role<br>• Establish timeline for the evaluation | • What are the purposes of the evaluation? Who is requesting it and how will the report be used?<br>• Investigate the historical background of the team, why was it formed, has its purpose changed over time, where is it developmentally, what is the composition, to whom does it report, and so on?<br>• How would you succinctly describe the team? |

*(continued)*

**TABLE 11.5  Practical Framework for Evaluating Health Care Teams (*continued*)**

| Activities | Focus |
|---|---|
| | • Based on the purpose, intended use, and characteristics of the team, how will you narrow the focus of the evaluation? See Table 10.2 for examples of perspectives<br>• How will you participate in the evaluation? To whom are you responsible? Will you be given access to the people and information that you need to conduct the evaluation? |
| *Select appropriate evaluation methods* | |
| • Refine the description of the team<br>• Make sure you are asking the right questions<br>• Determine the course of action that will result from the data you supply<br>• Design a plan from evaluating the team<br>• Decide what to measure and observe<br>• Determine how to measure areas of interest<br>• Determine any associated costs with the evaluation<br>• Come to a final agreement about services and responsibilities | • Why does the team exist; to whom are they responsible (broad stakeholders)?<br>• Verify and clarify what you want to address in your final report to be sure you are collecting the most appropriate data<br>• Be very clear on how the information you provide will be used so that there is a good match between purposes and collected information<br>• Do you have an overall plan?<br>• What will you measure and observe? Have a written plan<br>• What will the evaluation cost?<br>• Are you clear about your role and responsibilities? |
| *Collect and analyze information* | |
| • Construct or purchase instruments<br>• Set deadlines for data collection<br>• Determine expectations for interpretation of the data<br>• Make sure that your data collection plan is implemented properly<br>• Analyze data with an eye on team improvement | • How will you collect the data? What resources are available to you?<br>• Do you have a written timeline for your work (e.g., Gantt chart)?<br>• Is your implementation plan complete? List all activities to be completed<br>• Address interrater reliability<br>• How can you use the data to make recommendations to enhance performance? |
| *Report your findings* | |
| • Determine the format for reporting your findings<br>• Meet with a team leader and/or staff to verify factual information<br>• Present the report<br>• Come to closure | • Determine how you will report your findings (informal, formal, memo, e-mail, etc.) and to whom<br>• Select methods to verify with the team leader or team members that your facts are correct<br>• Leave a record of the evaluation<br>• Determine how you will come to closure with the project |

*Source:* Herman et al. (1987).

**TABLE 11.6  A Logic Model**

| Inputs | Outputs | | Outcomes—Impact | | |
|---|---|---|---|---|---|
| | Activities | Participation | Short | Medium | Long (Impact) |
| Multidisciplinary team (MDs, NPs, RT, PharmD) Time devoted for rounds Combined EMR and paper (for writing orders and progress notes) Leadership who wants improved outcomes Strong organizational commitment to evidence-based practice (EBP) with resource support Data on LOS Available national data for similar academic medical centers | Conduct meeting to focus evaluation Meet to discuss work processes of patient management to move patients across continuum of care Observe conduct of rounds, flow of information, and interactions Meetings to discuss flow Observe work patterns related to transfer/ discharge Review protocols for admission and discharge from unit | Leadership Leadership of multidisciplinary team Members of each discipline in team Multidisciplinary team Nursing staff and support staff (transcriber of orders, other departments) Nursing staff Written policies, procedures, and protocols | Awareness of barriers Removal of barriers Education of multidisciplinary team New attitudes and awareness Knowledge about EBP and best practices Revision of process maps for transfer and discharge Facilitator to help improve group communications, trust, mutual respect, and common goals Revision of policies, procedures, and protocols | Leadership satisfied with changes Improved function of multidisciplinary team Average LOS met or LOS less than national average Integration of EBPs and best practices Policies, procedures, and protocols followed Better communications Cost savings from shorter LOS | High-performance multidisciplinary team Increased esteem of multidisciplinary team Increased satisfaction of team members, staff, and patients/ families Sustained cost savings from shorter LOS Better overall patient outcomes |

**Assumptions:** High-functioning interprofessional teams can provide comprehensive cost-effective care. LOS can be facilitated by input of all team members using protocols based on EBP to move patients in a timely manner from one level of care to the next.

**External Factors:** Reimbursement for care is tied to LOS; longer than average LOS are not reimbursed by some insurers and create a huge burden on the health care facility to absorb those costs. EBPs can decrease LOS, if followed.

**Evaluation:** Interdisciplinary Team on ICU A. **Situation:** Examine team effectiveness in meeting patient outcome benchmarks for LOS in an ICU. Current data show that the LOS is 2.5 days longer than national averages. Evaluate the team to determine why the team is not meeting national benchmarks.

## SETTING THE BOUNDARIES OF THE EVALUATION

In order to conduct a useful evaluation of team effectiveness, the DNP nurse (i.e., evaluator) must be able to set the boundaries of the evaluation so that it is a doable and useful project.

## Purpose

A clear understanding of the purposes of the evaluation is imperative. This information comes from the person or persons requesting the evaluation, such as a director, chief nurse or executive officer, a board, a committee, or another initiator. The purpose or purposes are varied and may include: the impact of the team on quality indicators of patient outcomes or cost savings; examination of team processes in relation to compliance with evidence-based practice guidelines and best practices; comprehensiveness of care; team group dynamics; leadership practices; and team member and patient satisfaction with care delivered. Another way to think about the evaluation is from the perspective of problems. What are the specific problems with the team that are to be addressed? This approach also helps to identify desired outcomes from the evaluation and sets the evaluation criteria to be used. Because information from an evaluation may be used for decision making, it is helpful to know who is going to receive the information and how the information will be used (e.g., team redesign, continued funding of the team, improvement in patient outcomes). All of this information helps to shape the evaluation process.

## Gaining Knowledge About the Team and Describing the Team

The DNP nurse may or may not have knowledge of the team and should take the time to conduct a comprehensive assessment of the team. Even if the evaluator thinks he or she knows the team, take a fresh unbiased look at the team from the eyes of an evaluator. Examples of areas to consider are: historical background of the team (e.g., When was it formed? For what purpose? Who started the team?); the setting in which the team functions and how it is tied to the organizational structure; focus of the team work; changes in the purpose of the team over time; team membership; longevity of each member on the team; the team's organizational structure; leadership; how work gets done; and developmental stage of the team. This information can be gathered through discussions, observation, and review of written materials. Once necessary information has been collected, the evaluator will be able to describe the team and categorize it according to type, developmental level, work patterns and processes, and outcomes.

## Focusing the Evaluation and Negotiating the Evaluator Role

Once the DNP nurse has collected the information and formulated a description of the team, the evaluator can begin to clarify the rationale and objectives for the evaluation and narrow the scope. This should lead to a brief written outline of purpose, rationale, objectives, and scope, which should be shared with the person or persons requesting the evaluation to verify and clarify a common focus of the evaluation. This is also a time to negotiate the evaluator role. Be clear about the expectations, responsibilities, deliverables, timeline, and the person to whom you will report findings. Verify access to information and people for the conduct of the work, and determine what the team members have been told about the evaluation and who provided that information. In addition, identify the contact person who will act as facilitator if issues occur in the conduct of the evaluation. Discuss what format the final report should take and who should receive it. Finally, the conditions under which the work will be done should be addressed. If the evaluator is an outside consultant, conditions of work and compensation are addressed through a contract. If the evaluator is internal to the organization, how will this work be calculated into his or her current workload? Is there anyone available to help or provide support for data gathering? These and other questions need to be addressed prospectively to avoid misunderstandings later.

## Selecting Appropriate Evaluation Methods

To move the evaluation process forward, a number of refinements, double checks, and design and measurement decisions need to be made.

## Refine Description of the Team and Reexamine the Approach

In selecting appropriate evaluation methods, the evaluator should further refine and double check the description of the team, the rationale for the team, and the goals/objectives of the evaluation. This may seem like redundancy, but as the evaluator continues to work and plan, there may be new information and subtle changes in direction that influence the approach, including what questions and observations need to be completed in order to get to the heart of the evaluation. The evaluator will also want to be clear on the outcomes on which to focus (e.g., processes, outcomes). A clear understanding of how the resultant information will be used is important so that there is a congruency between purposes and collected information.

## Design a Plan Including Measurement

The next step is to develop a detailed, step-by-step written plan of activities, data to be collected, methods of collection, timeline for collection, and sources of data. Knowledge of the organization/system and team will help make these determinations. The evaluator should decide what to measure and observe, and may wish to measure contextual characteristics, participant characteristics, processes, patient outcomes, or costs. The variables selected to investigate must be operationally defined to determine how they can best be measured. For example, to investigate team communication patterns, the evaluator first must define communication patterns. The definition might include verbal interactions among team members, verbal interactions of team members with bedside staff nurses, written documentation of the plan of care, or exchange of information at team conferences. How the concept is operationalized will drive options for measurement. For example, the definition given earlier regarding verbal interactions among team members could be investigated by observation of team members at work, by a questionnaire, or both. The evaluator must decide what method or methods of measurement are available and which will best meet the objectives of the evaluation. If there is any cost associated with measurement, such as purchase of instruments, these costs need to be included in a budget for approval by the sponsor of the evaluation.

The DNP nurse must recognize the state of the science of evaluation of teams. Interpretive difficulties arise when examining how team outcomes are conceptualized and measured. Like the construct team, the outcome is also multidimensional, and poorly conceptualized outcomes make comparisons across studies difficult. Team studies usually examine processes or outcomes of teams, but not the linkages between the two (Schmitt et al., 1988; Schofield & Amodeo, 1999). Understanding the state of the science in evaluation of health teams will help to maintain realistic expectations of what can be accomplished from an evaluation.

## Collecting and Analyzing Information

In this phase, the evaluator constructs or purchases instruments, creates an evaluation protocol, and sets timelines for data collection and for analyzing the data with an eye on team improvement, which will be communicated in the form of summary remarks, conclusions, and recommendations.

## Construct or Purchase Data Collection Instruments

Depending upon the purposes and objectives of the evaluation, the evaluator will create an investigator-developed data collection instrument, purchase validated instruments, or use a combination of both. If any instruments are purchased, be sure that the intended purpose of the instrument and the purpose of the evaluation are congruent. For example, the Collaboration Assessment Tool (Baggs et al., 1992, 1997) was designed to measure nurse–physician collaboration in making specific decisions about patient care; it will not be useful to provide a comprehensive view of a team's overall effectiveness. Another instrument, such as the TeamSTEPPS Team Assessment Questionnaire, is better suited to provide a comprehensive view. Regardless if the instruments are evaluator created or purchased, the DNP nurse must follow a timeline for data collection. If another person is assisting with data collection, the DNP nurse will need to orient that person to the instrument and data collection process to ensure interrater reliability.

## Data Analysis

Once data are collected and organized in a usable format, the data analysis is conducted. Quantitative data may be entered into a spreadsheet of statistical analysis programs such as the Statistical Package for Social Sciences (SPSS). Qualitative data may be analyzed using content analysis or other qualitative data analysis methods. The data analyzed should be related clearly to the objectives outlined for the evaluation. As the evaluator analyzes the data, he or she must keep an eye on opportunities for quality improvement of team effectiveness around the areas evaluated. Are there any national standards or benchmarks that may be useful to frame the data collected? The evaluator should think about recommendations that may assist the decision makers who will receive the report.

## REPORTING THE FINDINGS

Once data analysis is completed and findings are formulated, the evaluator may wish to meet with the team leader and/or team members to discuss and follow up on the findings if this has been approved by the initiator of the evaluation. Such a meeting is directed at transparency and provides the opportunity to correct any factual information that was incorrect.

The next step is preparation of the final report. The format of the report is something that is negotiated during an earlier step in the process. The report can be informal or formal. An informal report may take the form of an e-mail or a memo; a formal report may require a detailed written report with an executive summary. A formal report may also include a presentation to a board or a committee with a detailed review of the processes and outcomes of the evaluation project. Regardless if the report is informal or formal, the evaluator should provide a tangible record of the evaluation in the form of a written report or electronic file, as well as a copy for his or her personal records.

The question of communicating the results of the evaluation with the team that was evaluated needs to be addressed. That decision usually lies in the hands of the person or persons who requested the evaluation. That person or persons must decide what information they wish to share with the team and how the information will be communicated.

Come to closure with the person or persons who requested the evaluation, those who assisted with the conduct of the evaluation, and the participants in the evaluation. It is clear from the brief overview of the conduct of an evaluation that it is a complex process that requires many decisions to be made along the way by the evaluator. That is true if conducting an informal focused evaluation of a team or a formal comprehensive evaluation. The principles are the same regardless of approach and the information provided in the evaluation should lead to useful information for the decision makers.

## SUMMARY

This chapter proposed to provide an overview of the state of the science of teams in health care and what is known about their effectiveness. Through a review of the literature, definitions and a view of the complexity of health care and teams delivering care was presented. Core competencies for interprofessional collaborative practice were briefly discussed. A list of variables that have been used in evaluating teams was offered. It was made clear that there are theoretical/conceptual and methodological challenges in the evaluation of teams that prevent a clear link between processes and outcomes. However, from a practical perspective, teams still need to be evaluated. To assist with this process, a generic approach to evaluation of a team was discussed. In addition, resources such as measurement instruments and a logic model were presented to assist the DNP nurse in the evaluation process. Further development in team theory and methodology will advance the science to better understand how teams contribute to team effectiveness and health care outcomes with the precision and clarity desired.

# REFERENCES

Agency for Healthcare Research and Quality. (2012). *TeamSTEPPS Instructor Guide Glossary.* Retrieved from http://www.ahrq.gov/professionals/education/curriculum-tools/teamstepps/instructor/reference/glossary.html

Agency for Healthcare Research and Quality. (2016). *TeamSTEPPS.* Washington, DC: Author, U.S. Department of Health and Human Services. Retrieved from http://teamstepps.ahrq.gov/

Aiken, L., Clarke, S., Cheung, R., Sloane, D., & Silber, J. (2004). Relationship between patient mortality and nurses' level of education. *Journal of the American Medical Association, 291*(11), 1322–1323.

Aiken, L., Clarke, S., & Sloane, D. (2002). Hospital staffing, organizational and quality of care cross-national findings. *International Journal for Quality in Healthcare, 14*(1), 5–13.

Andretta, P. B. (2010). A typology for health care teams. *Health Care Management Review, 35*(4), 345–354.

Ash, L., & Miller, C. (2014). Interprofessional collaboration for improving patient and population health. In M. E. Zaccagnini & K. W. White (Eds.), *The doctor of nursing practice essentials: A new model for advanced practice nursing* (2nd ed., pp. 217–256). Boston, MA: Jones and Bartlett Publishers.

Baggs, J. G., Ryan, S. A., Phelps, C. E., Richeson, J. F., & Johnson, J. E. (1992). The association between interdisciplinary collaboration and patient outcomes in a medical intensive care unit. *Heart and Lung, 21*(1), 18–24.

Baggs, J. G., & Schmitt, M. H. (1988). Collaboration between nurses and physicians. *Image Journal of Nursing Scholarship, 20*, 145–149.

Baggs, J. G., & Schmitt, M. H. (1997). Nurses' and resident physicians' perception of the process of collaboration in a MICU. *Research in Nursing and Health, 20*, 71–80.

Baggs, J. G., Schmitt, M. H., Mushlin, A. I., Eldredge, D. H., Oakes, D., & Hutson, A. D. (1997). Nurse–physician collaboration and satisfaction with the decision making process in critical care units. *American Journal of Critical Care, 6*(5), 393–399.

Baggs, J. G., Schmitt, M. H., Mushlin, A. I., Mitchell, P. H., Eldredge, D. H., Oakes, D., & Hutson, A. D. (1999). Association between nurse–physician collaboration and patient outcomes in three intensive care units. *Critical Care Medicine, 27*(90), 1991–1998.

Blackmore, G., & Persaud, D. D. (2012). Diagnosing and improving functioning in interdisciplinary health care teams. *The Health Care Manager, 18*(3), 195–207.

Boaro, N., Fancott, C., Baker, R., Velji, K., & Andreoli, A. (2010). Using SBAR to improve communication in interprofessional rehabilitation teams. *Journal of Interprofessional Care, 24*(1), 111–114.

Boult, C., Green, A. F., Boult, L. B., Pacala, J. T., Synder, C., & Leff, B. (2009). Successful models of comprehensive care for older adults with chronic conditions: Evidence for the Institute of Medicine's "retooling for an aging American" report. *Journal of American Geriatric Society, 57*(12), 2328–2337.

Boyle, D. K., & Kochinda, C. (2004). Enhancing collaborative communication of nurse and physician leadership in two intensive care units. *Journal of Nursing Administration, 34*(2), 60–70.

Bronstein, L. R. (2002). Index of interdisciplinary collaboration. *Social Work Research, 26*(2), 113–123.

Brooks, B. A., Davis, S., Frank-Lightfoot, L., Kulbok. P. A., Poree, S., & Sgarlata, L. (2014). *Building a community health worker program: The key to better care, better outcomes, and lower costs.* Chicago, IL: CommunityHealth Workers.

Canadian Interprofessional Health Collaborative. (2010). *A national interprofessional competency framework.* Retrieved from http://www.cihc.ca/resources/publications

Choi, B. C. K., & Pak, A. W. P. (2006). Multidisciplinarity, interdisciplinarity, and transdisciplinarity in health research, services, education and policy: 1. Definitions, objectives, and evidence of effectiveness. *Clinical Investigation Medicine, 29*(6), 351–364.

Cohen, S. G., & Bailey, D. R. (1997). What makes teamwork: Group effectiveness research from the shop floor to the executive suite. *Journal of Management, 23*(4), 238–290.

Cowan, M. J., Shapiro, M., Hays, R. D., Afifi, A., Vazirani, S., Ward, C. R., & Ettner, S. L. (2006). The effect of a multidisciplinary hospitalist/physician and advanced practice nurse collaboration on hospital costs. *Journal of Nursing Administration, 36*(2), 79–85.

DeChairo-Marino, A. E., Jordon-Marsh, M., Traiger, G., & Saulo, M. (2001). Nurse/physician collaboration: Action research and the lessons learned. *Journal of Nursing Administration, 31*(5), 223–232.

Durbin, C. G. (2006). Team model: Advocating for the optimal method of care delivery in the intensive care unit. *Critical Care Medicine, 34*(Suppl. 3), S12–S17.

Edmondson, A. V. (2012). *Teaming: How organizations learn, innovate and compete in the knowledge economy.* San Francisco, CA: Jossey-Bass.

Famadas, J. C., Frick, K. D., Haydar, Z. R., Nicewander, D., Ballard, D., & Boult, C. (2008). The effects of interdisciplinary outpatient geriatrics on the use, costs, and quality of health services in the fee-for-service environment. *Aging Clinical Experimental Research, 20*(6), 556–561.

Farrell, M. P., Heinemann, G. D., & Schmitt, M. H. (1986). Informed roles, rituals and humor in interdisciplinary health teams: Their relation to stages of group development. *International Journal of Small Group Research, 2*(2), 143–162.

Farrell, M. P., Heinemann, G. D., & Schmitt, M. H. (1988). Informal roles, rituals, and humor in interdisciplinary health care teams: Their relation to stages of group development. *International Journal of Small Group Research, 2*(2), 143–162.

Farrell, M. P., Schmitt, M. H., & Heinemann, G. D. (1988). Organizational environments of interdisciplinary health care teams: Impact on team development and implications for consultation. *International Journal of Small Group Research, 4*(1), 31–54.

Farrell, M. P., Schmitt, M. H., & Heinemann, G. D. (2001). Informal roles and the stages of interdisciplinary team development. *Journal of Interprofessional Care, 15*, 281–293.

Feiger, S. M., & Schmitt, M. H. (1979). Collegiality in interdisciplinary health teams: Its measurement and its effects. *Social Science and Medicine, 13A*, 217–229.

Freshman, B., Rubino, L., & Chassiakos, Y. R. (2010). *Collaboration across the disciplines in health care.* Sudbury, MA: Jones and Bartlett Publishers.

Friese, C., Lake, E., Aiken, L., Silver, J., & Sochalski, J. (2008). Hospital nurse practice environments and outcomes for surgical oncology patients. *Health Services Research, 43*(4), 1145–1163.

Grumbach, K., & Bodenheimer, T. (2004). Can health care teams improve primary care practice? *Journal of the American Medical Association, 291*(10), 1246–1251.

Hackman, J. R. (2002). *Leading teams: Setting the stage for great performances.* Boston, MA: Harvard Business School Press.

Herman, J. L., Morris, L. L., & Fitz-Gibbon, C. T. (1987). *Evaluator's handbook.* Newbury Park, CA: Sage.

Horbar, J., Plsek, P., Leahy, K., & Ford, P. (2004). The Vermont Oxford network: Improving quality and safety through multidisciplinary collaboration. *NeoReviews, 5*(2), e42–e49.

Houldin, A. D., Naylor, M. D., & Haller, D. G. (2004). Physician–nurse collaboration in research in the 21st century. *Journal of Clinical Oncology, 22*(5), 774–776.

Ingersoll, G. L., & Schmitt, M. (2004). Interdisciplinary collaboration, team functioning, and patient safety. In Institute of Medicine, *Keeping patients safe: Transforming the work environment of nurses* (pp. 341–383). Washington, DC: National Academies Press.

Institute for Clinical and Economic Review. (2013). *An action guide on community health workers (CHWs): Guidance for organizations working with CHWs.* Boston, MA: The New England Comparative Effectiveness Public Advisory Council.

Institute of Medicine. (1972). *Educating for the health team.* Washington, DC: National Academy of Sciences.

Institute of Medicine. (2003). *Health professions education: A bridge to quality.* Washington, DC: National Academies Press.

Institute of Medicine. (2010). *The future of nursing: Leading change, advancing health.* Washington, DC: The National Academies Press.

Institute of Medicine. (2015). *Measuring the impact of interprofessional education on collaborative practice and patient outcomes.* Washington, DC: National Academy of Sciences.

Institute of Medicine Roundtable on Evidence-Based Medicine. (2008). *Learning healthcare system concepts.* Washington, DC: The National Academies Press.

Interprofessional Education Collaborative Expert Panel. (2011). *Core competencies for interprofessional collaborative practice: Report of an expert panel.* Washington, DC: Author.

Janis, I. L. (1982). *Groupthink* (2nd ed.). Boston, MA: Houghton Mifflin.

Kim, M. M., Barnato, A. E., Angus, D. C., Fleisher, L. A., & Kahn, J. M. (2010). The effect of multidisciplinary care teams on intensive care unit mortality. *Archives of Internal Medicine, 170*(4), 369–376.

Klimoski, R. J., & Mohammed, S. (1994). Team mental model: Construct or metaphor? *Journal of Management, 20*, 403–437.

Knaus, W. A., Draper, E. A., Wagner, D. P., & Zimmerman, J. E. (1986). An evaluation of outcome from intensive care in major medical centers. *Annals of Internal Medicine, 104*(3), 410–418.

Korner, M. (2010). Interprofessional teamwork in medical rehabilitation: A comparison of multidisciplinary and interdisciplinary team approach. *Clinical Rehabilitation, 24*(8), 745–755.

Korner, M., Wirtz, M. A., Bengel, J., & Goritz, A. S. (2015). Relationship or organizational culture, teamwork and job satisfaction in interprofessional teams. *BMC Health Services Research, 15*, 243. doi:10.1186/s12913-015-0888-y

Kozlowski, S. W. J., & Ilgen, D. R. (2006). Enhancing the effectiveness of work groups and teams. *Psychological Science in Public Interest, 7*(3), 77–124.

Leathard, A. (Ed.). (1994). *Going interprofessional: Working together for health and welfare.* London, UK: Routledge.

Lemieux-Charles, L., & McGuire, W. L. (2006). What do we know about health care team effectiveness? A review of the literature. *Medical Care Research and Review, 63*(3), 263–300.

Lorimer, W., & Manion, J. (1996). Team-based organizations: Leading the essential transformation. *PFCA Review, 15*, 9.

Malec, J. F., Torsher, L. C., Dunn, W. F., Wiegmann, D. A., Arnold, J. J., Brown, D. A., & Phatak, V. (2007). The Mayo high performance teamwork scale: Reliability and validity for evaluating key crew resource management skills. *Simulation Healthcare, 2*(1), 4–10.

Marks, M. A., Mathieu, J. E., & Zaccaro, S. J. (2001). A temporally based framework and taxonomy of team processes. *Academy of Management Review, 26*, 356–376.

Massachusetts Institute of Technology. (2011). *The third revolution: The convergence of the life sciences, physical sciences, and engineering.* Washington, DC: Author.

McClure, M. L., Poulin, M. A., Sovie, M. D., & Wandelt, M. A. (1983). *Magnet hospitals: Attraction and retention of professional nurses.* Kansas City, MO: American Academy of Nursing.

Meier, D. E., & Beresford, L. (2010). Palliative care in long-term care: How can hospital teams interface? *Journal of Palliative Care, 13*(2), 556–561.

Mitchell, P. H., Shannon, S. E., Cain, K. C., & Hegyvary, S. T. (1996). Critical care outcomes: Linking structures, processes, and organizational and clinical outcomes. *American Journal of Critical Care, 5,* 353–363.

Moore, D. E., Jr., Green, J. S., & Gallis, H. A. (2009). Achieving desired results and improved outcomes: Integrating planning and assessment throughout learning activities. *Journal of Continuing Education in the Health Professions, 29*(1), 1–15.

Nelson, E. C., Batalden, P. B., Godfrey, M. M., & Lazar, J. S. (Eds.). (2011). *Value by design: Developing clinical microsystems to achieve organizational excellence.* San Francisco, CA: Jossey-Bass.

Nelson, E. C., Batalden, P. B., Huber, T. P., Mohr, J. J., Godfrey, M. M., Headrick, L. A., & Wasson, J. H. (2002). Microsystems in health care: Part 1. Learning from high-performing front-line clinical units. *Joint Commission Journal on Quality Improvement, 25,* 654–668.

Neumann, V., Gutenbrunner, C., Fialda-Moser, V., Christodoulou, N., Varela, E., Giustine, A., & Delarque, A. (2010). Interdisciplinary team working in physical and rehabilitation medicine. *Journal of Rehabilitation Medicine, 42*(1), 4–8.

Paulus, P. B., & Nijstad, B. A. (Eds.). (2003). *Group creativity: Innovation through collaboration.* New York: Oxford University Press.

Pezzin, L. E., Feldman, P. H., Mongoven, J. M., McDonald, M. V., Gerber, L. M., & Peng, T. R. (2011). *Journal of General Internal Medicine, 26*(3), 280–286.

Pisano, G. P., & Verganti, R. (2008). Which kind of collaboration is right for you? *Harvard Business Review, 86*(12), 78–86.

Pronovost, P. J., Berenholtz, S. M., Goeschel, C., Needman, D., Hyzy, R., Welsh, R., . . . Sexton, J. B. (2008). Improving patient safety in intensive care units in Michigan. *Journal of Critical Care, 23*(2), 207–221.

Pyne, J. M., Fortney, J. C., Curran, G. M., Tripathi, S., Atkinson, J. H., Kilbourne, A. M., . . . Gifford, A. L. (2011). Effectiveness of collaborative care for depression in human immunodeficiency virus clinics. *Archives of Internal Medicine, 171*(1), 23–31.

Reader, T. W., Fin, R., Mearns, K., & Cuthbertson, B. (2009). Developing a team performance framework for the intensive care unit. *Critical Care Medicine, 37*(5), 1787–1793.

Reid-Ponte, P., Creta, A., & Joy, C. (2011). Exemplary professional practice. In K. Drenkard, G. Wolf, & S. H. Morgan (Eds.), *Magnet: The next generation—Nurses making a difference* (pp. 68–69). Silver Spring, MD: American Nurses Credentialing Center.

Reeves, S., Perrier, L., Goldman, J., Freeth, D., & Zwarenstein, M. (2013). Interprofessional education: Effects on professional practice and health care outcomes. *Cochrane Databases Systematic Review, 3*(1), CD002213.

Rocco, N., Scher, K., Basberg, B., Yalamanchi, S., & Baker-Genaw, K. (2011). Patient-centered plan-of-care tool for improving clinical outcomes. *Quality Management in Health Care, 20*(2), 89–97.

Salas, E., Dickinson, T. L., Converse, S. A., & Tannenbaum, S. J. (1992). Toward an understanding of team performance and training. In R. W. Swezey & E. Salas (Eds.), *Teams: Their training and performance* (pp. 3–29). Norwald, NJ: Ablex.

Salas, E., & Frush, K. (2013). *Improving patient safety through teamwork and team training.* New York, NY: Oxford University Press.

Salas, E., Rosen, M. A., Burke, C. S., & Goodwin, G. F. (2008). The wisdom of collectives in organizations: An update of the teamwork competencies. In E. Salas, G. F. Goodwin, & C. S. Burke (Eds.), *Team effectiveness in complex organizations: Cross-disciplinary perspectives and approaches* (pp. 39–790). New York, NY: Psychology Press.

Salas, E., Sims, D. E., & Klein, C. (2004). Cooperation and teamwork at work. In C. D. Spielberger (Ed.), *Encyclopedia of applied psychology* (Vol. 1, pp. 497–505). San Diego, CA: Academic Press.

Sassou, K., & Reason, J. (1999). Team errors: Definition and taxonomy. *Reliability Engineering and Systems Safety, 65,* 1–9.

Schmitt, M. H. (2001). Collaboration improves the quality of care: Methodological challenges and evidence from U.S. health care research. *Journal of Interprofessional Care, 15,* 47–66.

Schmitt, M. H., Farrell, M. P., & Heinemann, G. D. (1988). Conceptual and methodological problems in studying the effects of interdisciplinary teams. *The Gerontologist, 40,* 343.

Schofield, R. F., & Amodeo, M. (1999). Interdisciplinary teams in health care and human services settings: Are they effective? *Health and Social Work, 24,* 210–219.

Senge, P. M. (1990). *The fifth discipline.* New York: Doubleday Currency.

Shortell, S. M., Zimmerman, J. E., Gillies, R. R., Duffy, J., Devers, K., Rousseau, D. M., & Knaus, W. A. (1992). Continuously improving patient care: Practical lessons and an assessment tool from the national ICU study. *Quality Review Bulletin, 18*(5), 150–155.

Shortell, S. M., Zimmerman, J. E., Rousseau, D. M., Gillies, R. R., Wagner, D. P., Draper, E. A., . . . Duffy, J. (1994). The performance of intensive care units: Does good management make a difference? *Medical Care, 32,* 508–525.

Singh, J., & Fleming, L. (2010). Lone inventors as sources of breakthroughs: Myth or reality? *Management Science, 56*(1), 41–56.

Smith, M. K. (2005). Bruce W. Tuckman—Forming, storming, norming and performing in group. *The encyclopedia of informal education.* Retrieved from www.infed.org/thinkers/tuckman.htm

Tuckman, B. W. (1965). Development sequence of small groups. *Psychological Bulletin, 63,* 384–399.

Tuckman, B. W., & Jensen, M. A. (1977). Stages of small group development revisited. *Group and Organizational Studies, 2,* 419–427.

Upenieks, V. V., Lee, E. A., Flanagan, M. E., & Doebbeling, B. N. (2009). Healthcare Team Vitality Instrument (HTVI): Developing a tool assessing healthcare team functioning. *Journal of Advanced Nursing, 66*(1), 168–176.

University of Toronto. (2008). *Advancing the interprofessional education curriculum 2009. Curriculum overview. Competency framework.* Toronto, Canada: University of Toronto, Office of Interprofessional Education.

Walsh, K., Reeves, S., & Maloney, S. (2014). Exploring issues of cost and value in professional and interprofessional education. *Journal of Interprofessional Care, 28*(6), 493–494.

Weaver, S. J., Dy, S. M., & Rosen, M. A. (2014). Team-training in healthcare: A narrative synthesis of the literature. *British Medical Journal of Quality and Safety, 23,* 359–372.

Weaver, S. J., Feitosa, J., Salas, E., Seddon, R., & Vozenilek, J. A. (2013). The theoretical drivers and models of team performance and effectiveness for patient safety. In E. Salas & K. Frush (Eds.), *Improving patient safety through teamwork and team training* (pp. 3–26). New York, NY: Oxford University Press.

Wiecha, J., & Pollard, T. (2004). The interdisciplinary eHealth Team: Chronic care for the future. *Journal of Medical Internet Research, 6,* e22. Retrieved from http://www.jmir.org/2004/3/e22

Weick, K. E., & Roberts, K. H. (1993). Collective mind in organizations: Heedful interrelating on flight decks. *Administrative Science Quarterly, 38,* 357–381.

Weinberg, D. B., Cooney-Miner, D., Perloff, J. N., Babington, L., & Avgar, A. C. (2011). Building collaborative capacity: Promoting interdisciplinary teamwork in the absence of formal teams. *Medical Care, 49*(8), 716–723.

Wuchty, S. B., Jones, F., & Uzzi, B. (2007). The increasing dominance of teams in production of knowledge. *Science, 316*(5827), 1036–1039.

World Health Organization. (2010). *Framework for action on interprofessional education & collaborative practice.* Geneva, Switzerland: Author. Retrieved from http://whqlibdoc.who.int/ hq/2010/WHO_HRH_HPN_10.3_eng.pdf

Xyrichis, A., & Ream, E. (2008). Teamwork: A concept analysis. *Journal of Advanced Nursing, 61*(2), 232–241.

Zwarenstein, M. J., Goldman, M. J., & Reeves, S. (2009). Interprofessional collaboration: Effects of practice-based interventions on professional practice and healthcare outcomes. *Cochrane Database of Systematic Reviews, 3*(3), CD000072.

# EVALUATION OF POPULATIONS AND HEALTH POLICY

# CHAPTER TWELVE

# EVALUATING POPULATIONS AND POPULATION HEALTH

Deanna E. Grimes and Nancy F. Weller

*The health of the people is really the foundation upon which all their*
*happiness and all their powers as a state depend.*
*—Benjamin Disraeli*

There was a time when the health of populations was considered to be the purview of public health agencies and public/community health workers, specifically nurses. Then, health care organizations and providers framed their responsibilities in terms of the populations served, such as workers in an industry, school children, residents of a long-term care facility, or enrollees in a managed care organization. Today, professional nurses recognize an expansion of their role from simply caring for individual patients in a clinic/hospital/nursing home to caring for a panel of patients seen regularly in those settings. Nurses recognize that their patients have health problems similar to those of the populations from which they come. In this time of promoting efficiency in health care, it is not always efficient to treat population health problems that could be prevented. Doctor of nursing practice (DNP) graduates increasingly find themselves working to change health and health care for the populations served.

The American Association of Colleges of Nursing (AACN) recognized the importance of focusing on the health of populations in their document *The Essentials of Doctoral Education for Advanced Nursing Practice*. The focus of Essential VII is clinical prevention and population health for improving the nation's health (AACN, 2006). The AACN (2006, p. 16) outlined its expectations of the doctoral nursing graduate as follows:

- Analyze epidemiological, biostatistical, environmental, and other appropriate scientific data related to individual, aggregate, and population health.
- Synthesize concepts, including psychosocial dimensions and cultural diversity, related to clinical prevention and population health in developing, implementing, and evaluating interventions to address health promotion/disease prevention efforts, improve health status/access

patterns, and/or address gaps in care of individuals, aggregates, or populations.

- Evaluate care delivery models and/or strategies using concepts related to community, environmental, and occupational health, as well as cultural and socioeconomic dimensions of health.

How can a DNP realize these expectations in practice? In the remainder of the chapter, we look at an example case in which a DNP is asked to assess a problem of increasing tuberculosis (TB) disease in a health care population. We examine the application of the Centers for Disease Control (CDC) guidelines for preventing transmission of *Mycobacterium tuberculosis* in health care settings (CDC, 2005) that are outlined in Exhibit 12.1. This presentation should highlight population-focused concepts/methods that may serve as a guide for the DNP in applying Essential VII requirements to practice.

DNPs are frequently faced with implementing patient- or population-focused guidelines, such as these updated TB guidelines, in a variety of different settings. What are the principles illustrated in this case that can be used by DNPs in any setting? The following questions will be the focus in the remainder of this chapter: (a) What is a population and what is the definition of population health? (b) What is meant by the terms *risk*, *risk factors*, and *populations at risk*? (c) What are the determinants of health that may contribute to risk? (d) How does one assess the distribution of a disease, such as TB, in a population? (e) How does one assess risk factors and populations at risk for TB? (f) What models may be used to analyze a health problem and disease in a population? and (g) How does one evaluate the impact of an intervention on the health problem?

---

**EXHIBIT 12.1**

**CDC Guidelines**

In 2005, the Centers for Disease Control and Prevention (CDC) published an update to their guidelines for preventing the transmission of *Mycobacterium tuberculosis* in health care settings (CDC, 2005). These new guidelines emphasized that health care organizations assess and categorize the risk for transmission of TB in their settings prior to implementing the guidelines. The guidelines cover valuable information directed to clinic/hospital administrators, clinicians, and TB control personnel on such topics as:

1. Health care workers who should be included in a TB surveillance program
2. Pathogenesis, epidemiology, and transmission of *M. tuberculosis*
3. Persons at highest risk for exposure to and infection with *M. tuberculosis*
4. Persons who are at high risk for progression to TB disease
5. Characteristics of a patient with TB disease that increases the risk for infectiousness
6. Environmental factors that increase the probability of transmission
7. Risk for health care-associated transmission of *M. tuberculosis*
8. TB risk assessment in populations, and so on.

## POPULATIONS AND POPULATION HEALTH

Population, as a general term, refers to a group of people who have a common characteristic, such as age, geography, political boundaries, race/ethnicity, religion, environmental exposures, occupation, education, sexual preference, and so on. According to the AACN, population health includes "aggregate, community, environmental/occupational, and cultural/socioeconomic dimensions of health. Aggregates are groups of individuals defined by a shared characteristic such as gender, diagnosis, or age" (AACN, 2006, p. 15).

In the field of health and health care, populations are identified by their health status or medical condition, such as persons with a disability or with a TB infection or active TB disease. They are also identified by their risk for certain conditions: smokers are at risk for lung cancer and persons with compromised immunity are at risk for active TB disease. For example, the 2005 CDC guidelines on TB referred to four different populations at risk for TB: (a) the geographic community (local, regional, state, and national) from which TB cases derived; (b) population groups that are at greatest risk for obtaining or transmitting TB, such as the homeless; (c) patients in a variety of health care settings, including clinics and nursing homes; and (d) the many categories of health care workers (HCWs) exposed to TB at their places of employment.

How do you, as a DNP, define the population you serve? How would you define population health relative to your population? With respect to the TB case study, who is the population served by the nursing administrator of a hospital? Who is the population served by the nurse in an outpatient clinic? Who is the population served by the triage nurse in the emergency department?

## RISK, RISK FACTORS, POPULATIONS AT RISK

Risk and assessment of risk are major foci of the CDC guidelines on TB. The guidelines identified risk associated with the transmission of TB, risk factors in certain groups that increase the risk of transmitting TB, populations at risk for acquiring TB infection, and populations at risk for acquiring TB disease.

Risk is simply the probability that something will occur. With respect to health, risk is the increased probability that a disease, injury, disability, or death will occur to an individual or a population. The term is generally applied to the probability that something specific will occur, such as the risk of infection with *M. tuberculosis*. Risk factors are those characteristics of an individual and/or a population that increase their risk for disease, illness, disability, or death. Living in proximity to a person with active TB is a risk factor for acquiring *M. tuberculosis*. The term *populations at risk* refers to all those persons who have a similar type of risk, such as health care workers (HCWs) with continuing exposure to patients with active TB infection. Individuals who are immune compromised are a population at risk for TB infection that can progress to active TB disease.

## DETERMINANTS OF HEALTH

Apart from risk and risk factors, why are some people healthy and others not? What are the conditions that contribute to disparities in health among individuals and populations? These conditions are commonly called the determinants of health. Determinants of health are the array of personal, social, economic, and environmental factors that impact the health status of populations. These determinants have been defined more formally as the "combined effects of individual and community physical and social environments and the policies and interventions used to promote health, prevent disease, and ensure access to quality healthcare" (U.S. Department of Health and Human Services [USDHHS], 2002, p. 7; Wilkinson & Marmot, 2003; World Health Organization & Commission on Social Determinants of Health, 2008). A model for the determinants of health can be seen in Figure 12.1.

Since the term *determinants of health* was coined, the number and types or categories of determinants have varied. Originally, there were four general determinants (human biology, health system, environment, and lifestyle) included in the Lalonde Report (Glouberman & Miller, 2003). The determinants of health depicted in the *Healthy People 2010* (Figure 12.1) and the *Healthy People 2020* documents include (a) social environment, (b) physical environment, (c) policies and interventions, (d) health services or access to quality health care, (e) individual behavior or lifestyle, (f) biology and genetics (USDHHS, 2001, 2009). These six categories of determinants are described in the following text.

### Social Environment

Social factors include relationships with family and friends, workplace colleagues, neighbors, and other community members. Social environment may also include access to resources in the community (public safety, parks, and recreational facilities), social institutions (law enforcement, school systems, governmental and social service agencies), and cultural features and practices. Social factors may directly or indirectly affect health, and their effects may accumulate across time and the life spans of individuals, and across generations of individuals and families. The social

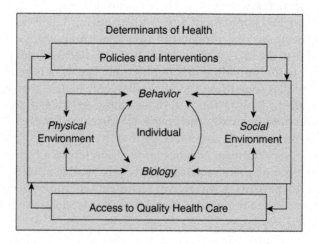

**Figure 12.1** The Healthy People model for determinants of health.
*Source:* U.S. Department of Health and Human Services (n.d.).

environment may lead to undesirable cycles between these social factors and health. Although genes and access to good health care are important overall, social factors may play a larger role than either genetics or health services because they interact with both. Fortunately, many of these social factors may be influenced by policies and programs designed and targeted to remediate their harmful effects. Many models of the social determinants of health, both early and especially later versions of these expanding models, include the following social factors: early life experience, education, income, housing, community, race/ethnicity, occupation/work, and the economy (USDHHS, 2009).

With respect to the case study on TB, the social environment may impact the spread of disease. Economic conditions may force some persons to live in crowded conditions, increasing the risk of transmission of the pathogen. Immigrant families, especially those within 5 years of arrival from geographic areas with a high incidence of TB disease, may be infected without awareness. They may live together in one apartment or in close proximity in congested urban neighborhoods and may be at greater risk for transmission of TB. Those isolated from resources because of language barriers may not have access to health care, particularly screening for TB infection. Residents and employees of congregate settings that are high risk (e.g., correctional facilities, long-term care facilities, and homeless shelters) may also be at greater risk due to their social environment.

## Physical Environment

Physical conditions in the environment in which people live, recreate, and work impact health, functioning, and quality of life. Examples of the physical determinants of health include: housing, homes, and neighborhoods; exposure to toxins and physical hazards (accumulated trash and debris); physical barriers to those with disabilities (lack of wheelchair ramps); natural environment (plants, weather, and air quality); man-made environment (buildings); occupational settings; educational institutions; and recreational areas (USDHHS, 2009). Poor quality housing may expose residents to undesirable conditions and contribute to poorer health. Inferior and substandard housing may lead to infectious diseases, injuries, and exposure to lead and other household toxins. In the case of TB, close contacts may expose others to TB disease. Close contacts are persons who share the same air space in a household or other enclosed environment for a prolonged period (days or weeks, not minutes or hours) with a person with pulmonary TB disease (USDHHS, CDC, 2010).

## Policies and Interventions

Governmental policies at the local, state, and federal levels may profoundly affect individual and population health. Individual- and population-level behavior change may occur with changes in government regulations. Cuts in programs, such as Medicaid, for dependent and low-income families due to changes in political structure at the state and federal level may greatly alter the resources of struggling, working-class families. In the case of TB, changing the restrictions on immigration between and among nations with a high incidence of TB may alter the numbers of high-risk TB cases coming into the United States. Most state public health agencies currently cover the cost of treatment with anti-TB drugs and for directly observed therapy (DOT) programs. Changes in how treatment is financed could dramatically alter the health outcomes for those with TB and those with whom they come in contact.

## Health Services or Access to Quality Health Care

Lack of or limited access to quality health services may seriously erode population health. The failure to maintain health insurance policies due to poverty and/or unemployment or underemployment, for example, may lessen participation in preventive health care and delay needed medical treatment. In addition to those already mentioned, barriers to health services include high cost of care, limited language access, and immigration status. These barriers lead to unmet health needs, delays in receiving needed care, lack of preventive care, and unnecessary hospitalizations. Lack of access to quality health care serves to increase health disparities among racial/ethnic and socioeconomic groups, profoundly affecting the health of certain components of the population (USDHHS, 2009). Populations who are medically underserved and who have low income may be at greater risk for exposure to and infection with TB; the infants, school-age, and adolescent children of these medically underserved adults, especially those with compromised immune function such as HIV, may be at high risk for exposure and acquisition of disease.

## Individual Behaviors or Lifestyle

Individual behaviors and lifestyle choices may also impact health outcomes. These factors include an individual's responses to internal stimuli and external conditions and often interact with an individual's biology. Lifestyle factors include risk behaviors, such as alcohol, tobacco, and other kinds of substance abuse; unprotected sexual behaviors; sedentary lifestyle and lack of regular physical activity; poor diet; and poor safety practices, such as neglecting seat belt and child restraint use in motor vehicles. Persons who use tobacco, alcohol, or illegal drugs, including injection drugs and crack cocaine, might also be at increased risk for infection and TB disease. Many population health interventions target such individual behaviors, reducing the rates of chronic disease and injury acquired from risky behaviors.

## Biology and Genetics

Biological factors include the effects of an individual's genetic makeup, family history, and physical and mental health problems acquired over the course of the individual's lifetime. Genetic factors may affect certain population groups more than others. Older individuals are more likely to acquire cancers due to the physical effects of aging on cells. Examples of genetic and biological determinants of health include: age, gender, immune status, and certain inherited conditions (sickle cell anemia, hemophilia, and cystic fibrosis); the BRCA1 or BRCA2 gene which increases the risk of breast and ovarian cancer; and a family history of certain forms of heart disease (USDHHS, 2009). Those who are immune compromised in any manner, including those with HIV infection, have an increased risk for progression from latent TB infection to TB disease.

## ASSESSING THE DISTRIBUTION OF DISEASE IN A POPULATION

How would one apply the previous discussion of risk and determinants of health to implement the CDC 2005 TB prevention guidelines? The guidelines (CDC, 2005, Appendix B) ask the following:

- What is the incidence of TB in your community (county or region served by the health care setting), and how does it compare with the state and national average?
- What is the incidence of TB in your facility and specific settings, and how do those rates compare?
- Are patients with suspected or confirmed TB disease encountered in your setting (inpatient and outpatient)? If yes, how many are treated in your health care setting in 1 year?
- Currently, does your health care setting have a cluster of persons with confirmed TB disease that might be a result of ongoing transmission of *M. tuberculosis*?

A review of basic concepts and methods pertaining to these measures of morbidity may be helpful here. Distribution of disease refers to the occurrence of a disease, injury, disability, or death according to the extent of the problem in the population during a time period. The common questions are: What is the disease or other health problem? How much is occurring? To whom? When? If one is counting new events in nursing staff, such as new TB infection cases diagnosed by positive conversions of the TB skin test, the new infections are called incidence. Newly diagnosed active TB disease during a time period also is called incidence. A count of all of the staff demonstrating a positive TB skin test at one time, regardless of when they were infected, is called prevalence. All patients treated for active TB disease and attending a TB clinic over a time period are referred to as prevalent cases.

It is also important to relate cases, whether new or existing, to the population from which they were counted. This process involves relating the cases (the numerator) to the whole (the denominator) to calculate a proportion, percentage, or rate. Rates are the basic measures of disease, injury, disability, or death in a defined population over a specified period of time. Rates allow comparisons between populations, between geographic areas, and over periods of time. Incidence rates are calculated by the number of events occurring in a population during a specific time period, divided by the number of persons in the population at risk for those events, and multiplied by a base number (100, 1,000, 10,000, or 100,000) that will result in a whole number answer. For example, one might calculate the incidence rate of TB during 2011 in a country as:

$$\frac{\text{Number of new cases of TB in 2011}}{\text{Number of residents in the country in 2011}} \times 100,000 = \frac{\text{TB incidence per}}{100,000 \text{ population}}$$

Prevalence rates are calculated by the number of existing events in a population during a time period or at one time, divided by the number of persons in the population at risk for those events, multiplied by a base number (100, 1,000, 10,000, or 100,000) that will result in a whole number.

$$\frac{\text{Number of persons with TB hospitalized today}}{\text{Total number of patients in the hospital today}} \times 100 = \frac{\text{\% of hospitalized}}{\text{patients with TB}}$$

(Subtract the TB cases from this number)

The 2005 CDC guidelines for TB also specify that the incidence rates of new TB cases should be compared with a state or national distribution of the disease. The state or national distribution of TB is sometimes called a standard population, that is, one that encompasses the population being studied. The process of comparison is similar to comparing one's weight with a standard weight chart for one's height and age. State or national TB incidence rates serve as a standard for comparing the local or regional rates. Therefore, assessment of the distribution of TB could include comparison of incidence rates of TB in the local population during the past year with those of the state or nation during the same time period, as well as incidence over time, incidence in certain high-risk groups, and incidence in the health care facility or clinic.

In addition, it is important to assess the characteristics of the populations who have TB disease and who have TB infection. What are their demographic characteristics such as ages, genders, race, or ethnicity? Where do they live (urban, rural, or suburban areas)? What is the geography and climate of their locale? What are their living conditions (single-family dwellings, multiple-family households, congregate living facilities)? What do members of the population do for a living and where do they work? Do they have comorbidities, such as cancers or HIV, which may exacerbate their infection with TB?

Because TB disease is a reportable condition, data on the numbers and rates of TB disease in the local, regional, and state geographic areas are available from local and state health departments and from the CDC. The presence of TB disease in health care facilities may be monitored by laboratory data and patient records. TB infection, as determined by skin testing, is not reportable to local health departments.

## ASSESSING RISK FACTORS AND POPULATIONS AT RISK

Understanding the mechanisms whereby a disease or health problem exists in a population provides a roadmap for assessing risk factors for the condition in the population. With respect to an infectious disease, an examination of such factors as the nature and virulence of the pathogen, mode of transmission, natural history of the disease, susceptibility of the potential host, and environmental factors that may increase the probability of transmission are important to understand in terms of disease control and prevention.

As discussed earlier in this chapter, risk and assessment of risk are major foci of the CDC guidelines. DNPs are frequently responsible for the care of populations afflicted by infectious disease, for example, H1N1 influenza, which is also spread by droplet transmission. The principles inherent in these guidelines may be used by the DNP in caring for patient populations, by the hospital/clinic administrator responsible for the health of the staff, and by ancillary personnel who contact ill patients.

The guidelines identified risks associated with transmission of TB, risk factors in certain groups that increase the risk of transmitting TB, populations at risk for acquiring TB infection, and populations at risk for acquiring TB disease. These are discussed in the following text.

## Risk Associated With Transmission of *M. tuberculosis*

*M. tuberculosis* is carried in airborne particles (droplet nuclei) released when persons with pulmonary or laryngeal TB disease cough, sneeze, or shout. The particles are small enough that air currents may keep them airborne for prolonged periods, allowing the droplets to travel. *M. tuberculosis* is generally not transmitted by contact with surfaces that might be covered with TB particles.

## Risk Factors That Increase the Risk of Transmitting TB

The more airborne particles released when a person coughs, the more the risk of transmission. According to the CDC (2005), the following conditions in a person with TB increase their infectiousness:

- Cough
- Cavitation on chest radiograph
- Positive sputum smear result for acid-fast bacilli
- Respiratory tract disease with involvement of the larynx
- Respiratory tract disease with involvement of the lung or pleura
- Failure to cover the mouth and nose when coughing
- Incorrect, lack of, or short duration of anti-TB treatment
- Undergoing cough-inducing or aerosol-generating procedures.

## Populations at Risk for Acquiring TB Infection

Characteristics of persons exposed to *M. tuberculosis* that may increase their risk for infection are broad and sometimes ill defined. Being in close contact, that is, sharing the same air space for a prolonged period of time with a person with pulmonary TB disease is the major risk factor for infection. The risk of contacting someone with TB disease increases when TB is highly prevalent in the surrounding environment or in one's living quarters. So, living or working in close contact with infected persons increases the risk of acquiring the infections. The guidelines list the following as populations at risk: (a) foreign-born persons who have arrived in the United States within 5 years of moving from an area with a high incidence of TB; (b) residents and employees in congregate settings, such as homeless shelters and correctional facilities; (c) HCWs in general; (d) HCWs with unprotected exposure to a patient with TB disease; (e) low income and medically underserved populations; and (f) infants, children, and adolescents exposed to adults in high-risk categories.

The new guidelines have expanded the list of HCWs who regularly should undergo screening for TB infection to 42. HCWs refer to all paid and unpaid persons working in health care settings who have the potential for exposure to *M. tuberculosis* through air space shared with persons with infectious TB disease. All HCWs who have duties that involve face-to-face contact with patients with suspected or confirmed TB disease (including transport staff) should be included for screening. In addition, any employee should be screened who:

- Enters patient rooms or treatment rooms whether or not a patient is present
- Participates in aerosol-generating or aerosol-producing procedures
- Participates in suspected or confirmed *M. tuberculosis* specimen processing
- Installs, maintains, or replaces environmental controls in areas in which persons with TB disease are encountered (CDC, 2005).

## Populations at Risk for Acquiring TB Disease

Not every person infected with *M. tuberculosis* will progress to have active TB disease. A compromised or undeveloped immune system seems to contribute to the progression of infection to active disease. The highest risk is for persons with HIV infection. Other groups include infants and children less than 4 years and persons with chronic and/or immune-compromising conditions (silicosis; diabetes mellitus; chronic renal failure; leukemia; lymphoma; carcinoma of the head, neck, or lung; prolonged corticosteroid use; other immune-suppressive treatments; organ transplant; end-stage renal disease; and intestinal bypass surgery). In addition, persons with a history of untreated or inadequately treated TB disease and substance abusers are populations at risk for progressing from a new TB infection to active TB disease (CDC, 2005).

DNPs frequently encounter infectious diseases in their practices and patient populations. Inadequate infection control practices in the health care facility increase the risk for nosocomial (health care-acquired) infections, which constitute a major population health hazard to patients, their families, and to health care professionals. The authors encourage DNPs to access the CDC Guidelines for Preventing the Transmission of *M. tuberculosis* in health care settings for more information on recognizing the risks and preventing transmission of TB (CDC, 2005).

## ANALYZING A HEALTH PROBLEM IN A POPULATION

A population of patients, a geographic population, or a well population with similar characteristics (such as pregnant women or school children) may experience multiple health problems. Some are overt health status problems, such as diabetes, asthma, or TB. Others are risk factors for future health problems, such as smoking, poverty, or environmental hazards. Still others may be categorized as a lack of resources, which is the case for populations who are uninsured, homeless, or live in areas remote from health care facilities. And, some health problems do not fit into a neat category but still are expressed by patients and populations as a need—a need for help with an elderly parent, a need to have someone with whom to talk, or a need to have a place to go during a hurricane.

In order to analyze a problem, such as a high incidence of new TB infections, for possible intervention, one begins with a measure of the extent of a problem in a specific group or population during a specific time period. Such would be the case if a DNP assesses that 30% of the hospital's housekeeping staff converted to a positive TB skin test during the past year. Although health status problems, particularly those that lead to death or are reportable infectious diseases, are the easiest to quantify in a population, it also is possible to have measures of the extent of risk factors and lack of resources. For example, a DNP may have observed that 80% of the hospital's housekeeping staff do not wear respiratory protection when working in the rooms of patients in respiratory isolation.

To plan interventions for a problem in a population, it helps to know what is causing the problem in the population. Therefore, the next step in analyzing a health problem is to organize the evidence on determinants of the problem in the population. Some of that evidence is available from firsthand experience with the population; other evidence is available from published research and guidelines.

The authors of this chapter have used the Problem Analysis Model (Figure 12.2) to analyze complex problems in a population. The model is an adaptation of a health problem analysis worksheet that was published by the CDC, Public Health Practice Program Office, in 1991 and reprinted in Turnock (2009, p. 74). The arrows at the bottom of the model represent a timeline. The CDC defined a *determinant* as a "scientifically established factor that relates directly to the level of the health problem. A health problem may have any number of determinants identified for it." For example, inhalation of *M. tuberculosis* in aerosolized mucous droplets is a determinant of infection with *M. tuberculosis*. A direct contributing factor is a "scientifically established factor that directly affects the level of the determinant." For example, near proximity to a person with active pulmonary TB is a direct contributing factor. An indirect contributing factor is a "community-specific factor that affects the level of a direct contributing factor. There may be many indirect factors contributing to a direct factor and indirect factors may vary considerably from one community to another" (CDC, cited by Turnock, 2009, p. 75). An example is crowded living conditions or a crowded waiting room, which may be an indirect contributing factor that increases the risk for exposure to the *Mycobacterium*. Figure 12.3 provides an analysis of a specific problem: 30% increase in new TB infections (diagnosed by new skin test conversions) in HCWs in one hospital.

Note that it is easier to start the analysis with the problem and to work backward in time and from right to left across the figure. Note, too, that the direct and

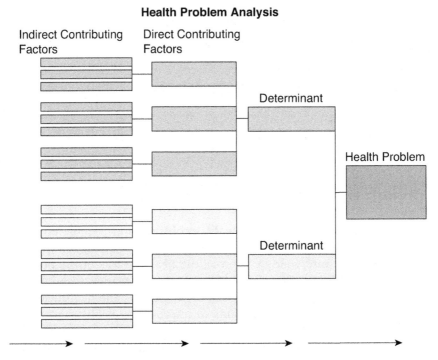

**Figure 12.2**   Problem Analysis Model.
Adapted from Turnock (2009).

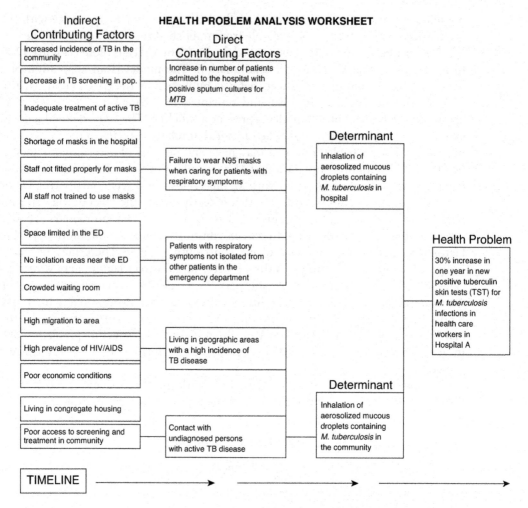

**Figure 12.3** Example of an analysis of tuberculosis infections in hospital staff.

indirect contributing factors provide places to intervene early to prevent the problem.

## EVALUATING POPULATION HEALTH OUTCOMES

Assessing and analyzing health problems in a population are not easy tasks. They are undertaken, however, to bring about change in the problem and, ultimately, to intervene to improve the health status of the population and of the individuals in the population. Multiple manuals, books, and web-based resources are available to assist organizations and health care providers to plan and implement new programs to improve the health status of the populations they serve (Exhibit 12.2). Figure 12.4 provides an overview of the process and emphasizes the ongoing and circular nature of the assessment, planning, implementation, and evaluation processes. The CDC guidelines provide ample examples of programs and interventions to prevent transmission of *M. tuberculosis* in health care facilities.

---

**EXHIBIT 12.2**

**Population Health and Program Planning Websites**

---

**Population Health Websites**

www.cdc.gov
www.commissiononhealth.org
www.healthypeople.gov
www.gapminder.org/
www.inequality.org/
www.thelaststraw.ca/
www.countyhealthrankings.org/
www.thecommunityguide.org/about/glossary.html
www.unnaturalcauses.org/
www.healthfinder.gov
www.ahrq.gov
www.who.int/hia/evidence/doh/en/
www.cdc.gov/nchhstp/socialdeterminants/docs/sdh-white-paper-2010.pdf
www.healthypeople.gov/2020/about/foundation-health-measures/determinants-of-health
www.populationhealthalliance.org
www.cdc.gov/nchhstp/socialdeterminants/definitions.html
www.iom.edu/~/media/Files/Report%20Files/2003/Unequal-Treatment-Confronting-Racial-and-
    Ethnic-Disparities-in-Health-Care/Disparitieshcproviders8pgFINAL.pdf
www.nytimes.com/interactive/2011/03/06/weekinreview/20110306-happiness.html?ref=weekinreview
www.iom.edu
www.who.org
www.cdc.gov/NCCDPHP/dph/
www.euro.who.int

**Program Planning Websites**

www.cdc.gov
www.wonder.cdc.gov/
www.wonder.cdc.gov/TB.html
www.thecommunityguide.org/index.html
www.health.gov/healthypeople/state/toolkit
www.cdc.gov/healthyplaces
www.healthypeople.gov/2010/
www.healthypeople.gov/2010/state/toolkit/default.htm
www.cdc.gov/CDCForYou/healthcare_providers.html
www.cdc.gov/CDCForYou/researchers.html
www.cdc.gov/healthcommunication/CDCynergy/editions.html
www.cdc.gov/eval/resources/index.htm
www.healthypeople.gov/2020/tools-and-resources/Program-Planning

---

Evaluating outcomes from a population-focused intervention is not difficult if the problem has been adequately assessed and analyzed. Evaluation officially begins when one assesses a problem according to its extent and distribution in the population. Knowing the answers to the following questions will provide guidance for the change that is desired:

- What is the extent of the problem and how is it distributed in the population?
- How does the extent compare with the extent and distribution of the problem in a standard population?

- Is the problem increasing or decreasing with time?
- Who has the problem and what are their demographic characteristics?

If one determines that the problem is greater than expected in some segments of the population, appropriate interventions then may be targeted to that population. The goal of the program would be a decrease in the extent of the problem in that population during the expected time period. Evaluation becomes straightforward: Was the stated goal achieved?

Of course, nothing ever is as easy as one would like. Let's look at the analysis of the problem of increasing TB infections in HCWs in Hospital A as seen in Figure 12.3. The authors of this chapter defined this problem as a 30% increase during the past year in new positive tuberculin skin tests (TSTs) for *M. tuberculosis* in HCWs in Hospital A. This statement is based on certain assumptions:

- Further evaluation of the problem finds that the majority of new infections are all in direct-care employees, specifically the nursing staff.
- The rate of positive TSTs last year is known and the number of new positive skin tests is known in the workers who were not infected last year. For example, if 10 of 1,000 employees tested positive last year, the prevalence of infection was 1%. A 30% increase this year would mean that 13 new infections occurred in the 990 employees who did not test positive last year.
- Let's also assume that these new positive TSTs are in employees who were employed at the hospital during the previous year and had negative TSTs during the screening 1 year ago. One could suspect, then, that the employees' risk for exposure to *M. tuberculosis* has increased and this exposure is more likely to have come from the hospital rather than the community.

Assuming that the analysis of the problem in Figure 12.3 is realistic and based on real information concerning the situation in Hospital A, the DNP or anyone responsible for employee health can develop intervention programs to improve infection control practices. Such programs could be to improve the availability, training, and fit of the N95 masks, or to add an isolation room in the emergency department. Once again, the CDC guidelines would help here. The primary question is: How should the DNP evaluate whether the interventions were successful? Clearly, the answer will be whether the prevalence of new infections in direct-care staff next year, as measured by positive TSTs in staff who were negative this year, has decreased. Ideally, the prevalence rate would be 0% or, at least, less than the previous 1%.

As anyone who has tried to bring about change in any population knows, the ideal does not always occur. What if there is not a decrease in new TB infections, as measured by TST conversions, in direct-care staff in Hospital A after 1 year of the improved infection control program? Or what if there is some decrease but not as much as expected? First, go back to the analysis of the problem. Is it possible that a major contributing factor was overlooked? For example, has there been such a rapid increase in infections in the community that staff may be exposed outside the hospital? Or is it possible that the number of patients admitted to the hospital with nonsymptomatic active TB disease that is undiagnosed has increased substantially? Have any other contributing factors been overlooked when planning the intervention?

**Program Development and Evaluation**

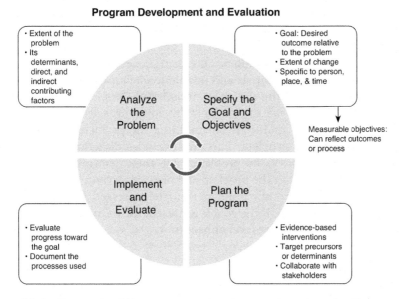

**Figure 12.4** Elements of the program development and evaluation process.
Developed by Deanna E. Grimes DrPH, RN.

Second, was the goal realistic? What is the average prevalence rate for new infections in other direct-care hospital staff working in the same region as Hospital A, in the state, and in the nation? Maybe the small decrease in new infections in Hospital A is comparable to the situation in other hospitals, and the original goal exceeded the standard at the time.

Third, were all of the infection control plans implemented as designed? For example, were new N95 masks ordered and made available on all patient care units in a timely manner? Were all staff fitted appropriately for the masks and trained to use them? Are staff members using the masks as they were trained to do? Was the isolation room in the emergency department available for use in a timely manner? Are patients with respiratory symptoms being triaged to the isolation area as soon as they arrive at the emergency area?

There are additional general factors, sometimes called intervening variables, to consider when desired outcomes in a population are not achieved within the desired time frame. Has something in the population changed, increasing their risk or making them more vulnerable? Have they aged or has their health status declined? For example, one might investigate whether the job of the direct-care staff has changed such that their potential exposure to M. tuberculosis has increased.

Also look at the environment for possible change that has increased the risk to staff. Has the ratio of patients to staff increased so much as to preclude staff using adequate infection control practices? Is it possible that patients, who have been inadequately treated for active TB disease and now have multidrug resistant tuberculosis (MDRTB), are being admitted to the hospital? Another possibility to consider is whether patients are sicker at admission because of changes in their insurance coverage, and, therefore, are expelling more bacteria in mucous droplets when they cough.

The new information learned from the evaluation can then influence further analysis of the problem and further planning, as depicted in Figure 12.4.

The process of improving the health of populations is not unlike that of improving the health of an individual patient. The process begins with an understanding of basic social, behavioral, biological, and physical environmental concepts influencing individuals and populations. One then proceeds to assess and diagnose health problems in both individuals and populations. Part of the diagnosis is to quantify a problem by comparing the characteristics of the problem with a standard. The next step is to analyze the problem by applying scientific evidence and direct observation of the conditions surrounding the problem to highlight the factors contributing to the problem. This step provides direction for the intervention to prevent progression of the problem. One then determines the outcome that is desired with respect to the problem and plans interventions to achieve that goal. If the goal is not reached, the problem is further assessed and analyzed and the planning circuit continued. If the goal is achieved, the individual patient or the population experiences a higher level of health.

## REFERENCES

American Association of Colleges of Nursing. (2006). *The essentials of doctoral education for advanced nursing practice*. Retrieved from www.aacn.nche.edu

Centers for Disease Control and Prevention. (2005). National Center for HIV, STD, and TB prevention. guidelines for preventing the transmission of *Mycobacterium tuberculosis* in health-care settings 2005. *Morbidity and Mortality Weekly Report, 54*(RR17), 1–144.

Glouberman, S., & Miller, J. (2003). Evolution of the determinants of health, health policy, and health information systems in Canada. *American Journal of Public Health, 93*, 388–392.

Turnock, B. J. (2009). *Public health: What it is and how it works* (4th ed.). Sudbury, MA: Jones and Bartlett Publishers.

U.S. Department of Health and Human Services. (2001). *Healthy People 2010: Understanding and improving health*. Retrieved from http://www.healthypeople.gov/

U.S. Department of Health and Human Services. (2002). *Healthy People 2010* (2nd ed.). Washington, DC: U.S. Government Printing Office.

U.S. Department of Health and Human Services. (2009). *Healthy People 2020*. Retrieved from http://www.healthypeople.gov/2020/about/DOHAbout.aspx

U.S. Department of Health and Human Services. (n.d.). *Healthy People 2010: A systematic approach*. Retrieved from http://www.healthypeople.gov/2010/Document/html/uih/uih_2.htm#deter

U.S. Department of Health and Human Services, Centers for Disease Control and Prevention. (2010). *Establishing a holistic framework to reduce inequities in HIV, viral hepatitis, STDs, and tuberculosis in the United States*. Atlanta, GA: Author. Retrieved from http://www.cdc.gov/socialdeterminants/docs/SDH-White-Paper-2010.pdf

Wilkinson, R., & Marmot, M. (2003). *The solid facts: Social determinants of health*. Copenhagen, Denmark: Center for Urban Health, World Health Organization. Retrieved from http://www.euro.who.int/__data/assets/pdf_file/0005/98438/e81384.pdf

World Health Organization & Commission on Social Determinants of Health. (2008). *Closing the gap in a generation: Health equity through action on the social determinants of health*. Final Report of the Commission on Social Determinants of Health. Geneva, Switzerland: World Health Organization.

# CHAPTER THIRTEEN

# TRANSLATING OUTCOMES FROM EVALUATION TO HEALTH POLICY

Deanna E. Grimes, Richard M. Grimes, and
Christine A. Brosnan

> *Knowing is not enough; we must apply. Willing is not enough;*
> *we must do.*
> —*Johann Wolfgang von Goethe*

Doctors of nursing practice (DNP) graduates may question the relevance of health policy to their patients' needs and to their ability to take care of their patients. One might also wonder why the American Association of Colleges of Nursing (AACN) specified Health Care Policy for Advocacy in Health Care as one of *The Essentials of Doctoral Education for Advanced Nursing Practice* (AACN, 2006). The purpose of this chapter is to address why and how DNPs can influence health policy. This chapter:

- Defines health policy
- Addresses the question of why nurses are involved in health policy
- Outlines guidelines for analyzing a health policy
- Summarizes the policy process
- Describes how nurses can influence health policy with outcome evaluation
- Describes the nursing roles of advocacy and leadership in the organizational, local, state, and national policy arenas

Two case studies with questions are provided to enable the reader to apply the principles of this chapter.

## WHAT IS HEALTH POLICY?

There are almost as many definitions of *health policy* as there are policies. A general definition of *policy* is the "authoritative guidelines that direct human behavior toward specific goals, in either the private or the public sector" (Hanley, 2002). Nurses are familiar with the myriad of policies within the private sector, such as organizational policies in the workplace dealing with staffing, chain of command, vacation time, evaluation, and salary. Nurses also live with countless public sector policies, such as the laws that determine licensure requirements, taxes, building codes, disposal of wastes, speed limits, and driving regulations. Some policy experts define *policy* only in terms of the public sector. Longest (2006, p. 7) defines *policy* as "authoritative decisions made in the legislative, executive, or judicial branches of government that are intended to direct or influence the actions, behaviors, or decisions of others." The term *authoritative* is key to most definitions of policy and suggests that there is a legal or administrative power or command behind the policy. When policies influence health, the determinants of health, or the use of the health care system, they can then be called health policies. Health policies can impact entire populations as well as selected individuals in the population. The authors of this chapter recognize that private sector as well as public sector policies influence health. As an example, hospital policies that control the quality and numbers of nurses on any shift can contribute to the health of patients as well as the health of the nursing staff.

The list of what constitutes health policy can be extremely long and varied. The list covers issues at the national level, such as health care reform, insurance for the currently uninsured, Medicare prescription drug policies, and policies regulating over-the-counter drugs and diet supplements. State health policies range from Medicaid policies to who is licensed to practice as an APN. Because states have the ultimate authority for the public's health and well-being, state policy also covers issues such as sanitation, the safety of the water supply, speed limits on the highways, and immunizations required to attend school, all of which impact health.

## WHY ARE NURSES INVOLVED IN HEALTH POLICY?

According to the AACN's *Essentials of Doctoral Education for Advanced Nursing Practice*, Health Care Policy for Advocacy in Health Care is Essential V (2006). The AACN (2006, p. 14) further specifies the expectations of the graduate of a DNP program with respect to policy and advocacy as follows:

- Critically analyze health policy proposals, health policies, and related issues from the perspective of consumers, nurses, other health professionals, and other stakeholders in policy and public forums.
- Demonstrate leadership in the development and implementation of institutional, local, state, federal, and/or international health policy.
- Influence policy makers through active participation on committees, boards, or task forces at the institutional, local, state, regional, national, and/or international levels to improve health care delivery and outcomes.
- Educate others, including policy makers at all levels, regarding nursing, health policy, and patient care outcomes.
- Advocate for the nursing profession within the policy and health care communities.
- Develop, evaluate, and provide leadership for health care policy that shapes health care financing, regulation and delivery.
- Advocate for social justice, equity, and ethical policies within all health care arenas.

Thus, one of the reasons DNPs are involved in health policy is that involvement is an expectation of the DNP role. Another equally important reason is that health policy has a downward influence on everything that happens and everything done in the health care system, including all aspects of nursing practice. Perhaps the most comprehensive depiction of the totality of the influence of health policy on health and health care can be seen in Figure 13.1 (Aday, Begley, Lairson, & Balkrishnan, 2004).

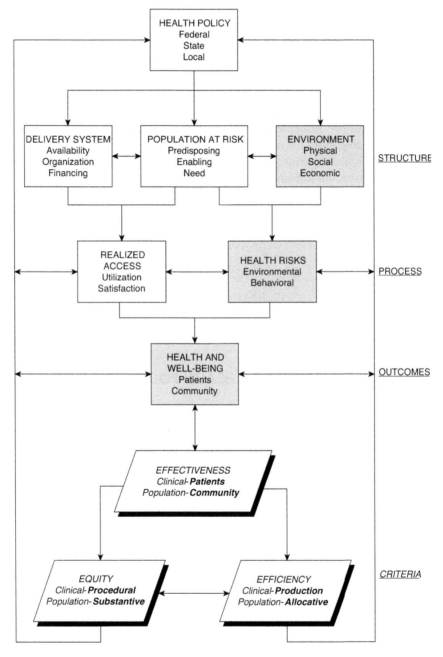

**Figure 13.1** Framework for applying health services research in evaluating health policy.

Source: Aday et al. (2004). Used with permission.

This model is discussed in Chapter 3 as a framework for evaluation. It is presented here because of its relevance to the influences of health policy. A quick review of definitions in the model in Figure 13.1:

- Structure refers to the composition of the health care system, the populations it serves, and the environment in which the system exists.
- Process is what providers do in the system and the health states of those who seek help from the system.
- Outcomes are what the system is trying to achieve.

The criteria are the standards whereby one can evaluate the outcomes from both a clinical or patient perspective and from a population perspective. One can expand the content in each of the boxes in the model to reflect the reality of one's nursing practice. For example, an APN providing primary care in a public health clinic in a medically underserved community has different available resources than one providing primary care in a private hospital outpatient clinic in a medical center. Additionally, patient needs are different in the different types of settings, and not all patients or communities achieve the same outcomes from their encounter with health care. Some are sicker at the onset or do not have the resources to follow a treatment or prevention plan and some never get to receive the primary care they need. This model is used as a reminder that health policy, whether federal, state, or local, impacts every aspect of the health care system and the health of the population served.

Nurses can monitor the impact of health policy on patient and population outcomes and, even more importantly, nurses can use that information to influence change in health policy. You can find more on this later in the chapter.

## GUIDELINES FOR ANALYZING A HEALTH POLICY

In order to use health policy to benefit patients, communities, and the nursing profession, and to influence the development of a new policy or a change in an existing health policy, it is useful to have a framework for understanding policies and the policy process. The policy process, according to Block (2008), is simply a way to solve problems. One may be trying to understand a new health policy in order to implement it or to analyze an existing health policy in order to change it. Policy analysis is the systematic study or appraisal of existing or proposed policies according to their background, purpose, content, and anticipated or actual effects (Hanley, 2002). The framework for policy analysis described by Stokey and Zeckhauser (1978) is a useful approach because it begins with the problem that the policy purports to solve. The five steps of their problem-focused analysis are:

- Establishing the context
- Laying out the alternatives
- Predicting the consequences
- Valuing the outcomes
- Making a choice

These steps are amplified here with questions to address for each step.

1. Establishing the context requires one to assess the circumstances surrounding the policy. One might ask some of the following questions: What is the underlying problem that the policy addresses and how is the problem defined? What are the background factors (e.g., history, emerging science, social, political, legal, ethical, and economic) leading to the problem? For example, the problem underlying the addition of Medicare drug coverage was defined by some as the high cost of drugs and by others as the inability of the elderly to pay for their drugs. The difference is subtle but real and leads to different solutions. If the costs of drugs are too high, then one would establish a policy to control costs. If elderly Americans do not have money for their drugs, then one would develop a policy to pay for the drugs. Another set of questions relating to context focuses on the major players in the environment. Who (e.g., governmental agency, community group, or private enterprise) is defining the problem? Who are the stakeholders in this policy; that is, who has something to gain or lose from the policy? The stakeholders may or may not have power, but they can and do have influence. Note that the focus is not just about the "political context" but rather about the entire environment surrounding a problem. Another important question might relate to the objectives of the policy; that is, what were the intended outcomes from the policy?

2. Laying out the alternatives relies on knowing how the problem was defined, as described in the preceding. Each definition of the problem may lead to alternative courses of action. And each stakeholder may have a different perspective on the "correct" course of action. Those who desire to influence the policy alternatives must provide additional information to expand the understanding of available choices for different courses of action.

3. Predicting the consequences of the alternative actions also relies on an understanding of how the problem was defined. The consequences of lowering the costs of drugs are certainly different from covering the costs of drugs with expanded insurance. One could explore different analytic approaches to predict the consequences, for example, economic versus efficacy, and the likelihood of each consequence.

4. Valuing the outcomes suggests that not everyone will view the outcomes of a policy through the same lens. Policy outcomes often are evaluated according to criteria similar to those used to define the problem (e.g., values of equity or justice, emphasis on liberty for the individual versus safety for society, ethical beliefs, economics, and benefits to whom).

5. Choose a policy. Evaluate whether the outcomes achieved or desired are the preferred outcomes. What is/was the preferred course of action? From which perspective? What can one conclude about the efficacy of the existent policy?

## THE POLICY PROCESS

Among the many published explanatory models of the public policy process, the one published by Longest (2006) stands out for its comprehensiveness and application for nursing (Figure 13.2). Longest describes three major phases, all of which can be impacted by nursing. The phases are policy formulation, policy implementation, and policy modification. The policy formulation phase is characterized by two separate sets of activities: agenda setting and development of legislation. If there is formal enactment of legislation, then one moves to policy implementation, which is composed of activities dealing with rulemaking and operations. Once a policy is put into operation, there is opportunity for a feedback loop to a policy modification phase where individuals, organizations, and governmental agencies can influence new phases of policy formulation and policy implementation.

Most of the information on the phases of the policy process is self-explanatory; however, the activities of agenda setting deserve further clarification and amplification, because this is the time in health policy formulation where nursing experience, expertise, and information from program evaluation are needed most. According to Longest (2006), agenda setting is comprised of problems, possible solutions, and political circumstances. When these conditions coalesce around an issue, a window of opportunity for change opens. This part of the model is based on the work of Kingdon in 1995, who conceptualized three streams of activities (e.g., a problem stream, a policy stream, and a political stream), all equally important. The problem stream defines the problem, the policy stream defines the policy goals of the stakeholders, and the political stream describes the political environment and power at the time (Hanley, 2002). Much of the content discussed in the previous section on policy analysis is relevant to agenda setting. The major questions are: What is the problem and how is it defined? How are various stakeholders defining the problem? What is the social, ethical, and scientific background of the problem? Who are the stakeholders in the context of the problem under question? What outcomes are desired by the stakeholders? Which alternative solutions are available and desired by the various stakeholders?

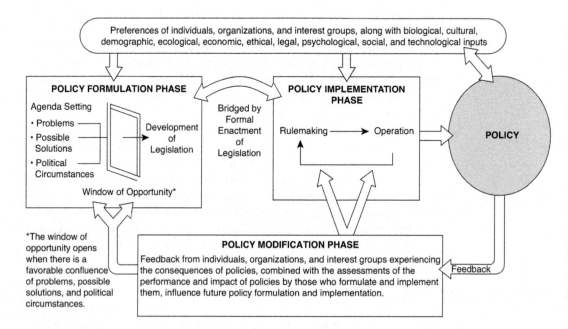

**Figure 13.2**   A model of the public policymaking process in the United States.
*Source:* Longest (2006). Used with permission.

## INFLUENCING HEALTH POLICY WITH OUTCOME EVALUATION

Sometimes the window of opportunity to provide good information to policy makers is very briefly open and, at other times, the window is partially open for long periods of time. An example of a narrow window was the time following the terrorist attacks on the United States on September 11, 2001, also known as 9–11. Health care professionals and organizations defined the problem as lack of education and training for disasters, particularly bioterrorism, for health care providers. The federal government defined the problem in terms of lack of preparedness and made grant money available for education and training of health professionals. Some state boards of nursing defined the problem similarly and determined that continuing education in bioterrorism should be a requirement for nursing licensure. In the year following 9–11, those who already had knowledge or experience in preventing infectious diseases were poised to receive funding to provide the training. Many nurses fit into that category.

Contrast that situation with the wide window around the human immunodeficiency virus (HIV) screening policies in the case study in this chapter (Exhibit 13.1). The window for changing the policies has been partially open since 1987. During the ensuing years, nurses have adapted their practices to implement the changing policies in general outpatient clinics, prenatal clinics, public health clinics, delivery rooms, emergency departments, HIV treatment centers, and schools of nursing. One hopes that nurses are evaluating and publishing outcomes for their patients and the populations they serve as the new screening procedures are implemented. Publishing or disseminating such information in other ways helps to establish one's credibility to influence future HIV screening and treatment policies. Because nurses are required to implement screening policies, nurses also should be serving on the government panels that devise the guidelines and on the committees within the health care organizations required to implement the guidelines. In Exhibit 13.2, one can see a window that has recently opened for the development of policies for long-term management of persons with HIV and/or other chronic conditions.

---

**EXHIBIT 13.1**

**Case Study: Changing Policy With Respect to Testing for HIV**

**Phase 1 in Testing**

The first cases of what was later to be called the acquired immunodeficiency syndrome (AIDS) were reported in 1981. By 1984, the causative agent, HIV, was discovered. Once the virus was known, it was possible to develop a test for antibodies to the virus. By 1985, very accurate tests were available that would determine if a person was HIV infected within a 6-month window after the infection occurred. By this time, all of the routes of transmission had been identified—sexual, blood transfusion, needle sharing, mother-to-child transmission, and needlestick injuries to health care workers. Associating needle sharing with illicit drug use and male-to-male sexual behaviors with this infection led to stigmatizing of anyone who had the HIV infection.

Once the test was available, public health authorities recommended that persons who considered themselves at risk for infection obtain HIV testing. Some segments of the health care community

*(continued)*

**EXHIBIT 13.1**

**Case Study: Changing Policy With Respect to Testing for HIV (*continued*)**

advocated that all patients be tested to prevent transmission from patients to health care workers. The HIV activist community questioned the value of testing in that there was no treatment for the infection or for its sequelae. In addition, the policy was seen as a mechanism by which any male who sought testing could potentially be identified as being gay. Therefore, community activists opposed any testing that would identify those being tested. As a result, the Centers for Disease Control and Prevention (CDC) issued guidelines that said that testing should be done only if the tested person was counseled about the meaning of the test before being tested and again when the result was reported. If the result was negative, posttest counseling also should include education on how to avoid future risk of becoming infected. If positive, counseling should include how to avoid transmission to others and when and where to seek medical care (Centers for Disease Control and Prevention, 1986, 1987). The CDC funded testing sites where names would not be taken during the testing process. The CDC also recommended that all testing be voluntary and that there be readily accessible sites where the test could be done anonymously. Many states passed laws requiring the expressed consent of the patient for testing. The laws usually had provisions for protecting the privacy of those who were found to be HIV infected. The exception to these guidelines and laws was screening for HIV of blood and tissue donations, which could be done without counseling or permission.

**Questions for Phase 1**

- How do the early CDC guidelines for testing fit the definition of a policy?
- How do the early testing guidelines fit the definition of a health policy?
- Are the guidelines an example of a public or a private health policy?
- What was the context for the guidelines in terms of the science and technology?
- Who were the stakeholders during this first stage of testing?
- How did each group of stakeholders define the problem?
- What were the values and beliefs that determined the CDC's approach to testing?
- In what way were nurses stakeholders in implementing these new recommendations?

**Phase 2 in Testing**

Eventually, epidemiologic and immunologic studies demonstrated that infection with HIV resulted in gradual destruction of the immune system, which typically occurred over 8 to 12 years. During most of this period, the infected person is asymptomatic. Toward the end of this asymptomatic period, infected adults may begin to experience opportunistic infections and cancers that meet the case definition for being classified as a case of AIDS. While AIDS was a reportable condition in all 50 states, HIV infection with patient names was not reportable in most states. This meant that tracking the growth and spread of the infection could only be done by analyzing AIDS cases, which reflected infections that had occurred 8 to 10 years earlier. Obviously, a much better system for tracking the epidemic would exist if persons with HIV infection but who had not progressed to AIDS would be reported to health departments.

Therefore, the CDC began encouraging state health departments to require reporting of HIV infections with patients' names. By 1988, 28 states required that HIV infections reported to the public health authorities include names. However, most of the states with large numbers of HIV-infected persons, including Florida, Texas, California, and New York, did not require reporting of HIV infection until 1999–2002. By 2003, 49 states and territories required such reporting. This slow accumulation of states requiring name-based reporting reflects the nature of the federal/state public health system in the United States. There is no national health authority that can require action by the states. Each state makes its own public health laws and regulations. The CDC can only provide evidence, suggest actions, and cajole state agencies to adopt its recommendations. In the case of name-based reporting, each state has had various levels of opposition and/or lethargy toward

(*continued*)

**EXHIBIT 13.1**

**Case Study: Changing Policy With Respect to Testing for HIV (*continued*)**

making HIV infection a reportable condition. In addition, requiring the reporting of HIV infection put an additional burden on state and local health departments. In most cases, additional funding was not made available to implement this new reporting requirement.

**Questions for Phase 2**

- What was the political and social context that determined whether states would require reporting of HIV infections by name?
- Who were the stakeholders in this situation?
- What optional policy alternatives might have been available to the CDC during the time period?
- In what way were nurses stakeholders in implementing these new recommendations?

**Phase 3 in Testing**

With minor modifications, the 1986–1987 recommendations with regard to HIV infection were the main way of conducting HIV testing for the next several years. The science of HIV infection, however, continued to advance. In 1994, there was evidence that treating HIV-infected women with zidovudine (also known as AZT) during pregnancy and delivery, as well as treating their infants, would reduce the rate of mother-to-child transmission by two-thirds. This introduced the issue of whether testing should become mandatory or remain voluntary. The CDC recommended routine HIV counseling and voluntary testing of all pregnant women. Women were to be informed about the importance of being tested. The CDC recommended, however, that women should give permission to be tested (Centers for Disease Control and Prevention, 1995). These recommendations were issued after a great deal of opposition against mandatory testing for HIV was expressed by activist groups.

By this time, the CDC had conducted studies on the risk of transmission from an HIV-infected person to health care workers following needlestick injuries. They learned that there were approximately 3 transmissions per 1,000 needlestick injuries. The rate of transmission was lowered to one-seventh this rate (approximately 4 per 10,000) when the health care worker started a course of zidovudine within 24 hours of the needlestick. The rate of transmission became even lower if the health care worker took a course of the multidrug therapies that had become available.

**Questions for Phase 3**

- How did advances in science change how the problem of testing was defined?
- Who were the stakeholders during this phase?
- What were the alternatives to the screening policy for pregnant women?
- What values seemed to underpin the policy to screen pregnant women?
- How did the data on outcomes influence policy for pregnant women and for health care workers?
- What kind of policy changes would be necessary for nurses working in inpatient obstetrical units to implement the CDC recommendations?
- What kind of policy changes would be necessary for nurses working in maternity clinics to implement the CDC recommendations?
- In what way were nurses stakeholders in implementing these new recommendations and evaluating the outcomes?

**Phase 4 in Testing**

By the beginning of the 21st century, there were two major changes in HIV/AIDS. Highly effective drug therapies became available. These suppressed the level of the virus and allowed the immune system to reconstitute itself. This converted HIV infection from a death sentence to a manageable, chronic disease. In addition, much of the stigma associated with HIV infection had gone away.

*(continued)*

**EXHIBIT 13.1**

**Case Study: Changing Policy With Respect to Testing for HIV (continued)**

Individuals who had HIV infection were more likely to be considered as persons with a chronic disease than as deviants. This changed the focus of AIDS activists from concerns about testing to advocating for access to anti-HIV medications.

In 2001, the CDC issued new guidelines for HIV testing and counseling. These recommendations included most of the previous guidelines but emphasized interactive HIV counseling that was directed toward the patient's personal risk behaviors rather than generic, didactic risk reduction education. Several studies had shown that this form of education was more effective in promoting positive behavior changes. The CDC also recommended that health care providers screen their patients for risk in order to make HIV testing more efficient. These guidelines also raised the possibility that early identification of HIV infection and treatment with highly active antiretroviral treatment (HAART) could lead to reduced transmission of the virus (Centers for Disease Control and Prevention, 2001). New scientific evidence had shown that HAART reduces the amount of circulating virus in blood, semen, and vaginal secretions. Experts believed that lower viral loads might result in lower rates of transmission.

**Questions for Phase 4**

- How did the definition of the problem of testing for HIV change during Phase 4?
- Who are the stakeholders during this phase?
- What criteria (individual benefit vs. societal benefit) should be used to evaluate outcomes from the policy to screen and treat in order to prevent transmission?
- What organizational policies would be necessary to allow nurses to implement the one-on-one, tailored counseling that CDC was recommending?
- In what way were nurses stakeholders in implementing these new recommendations and in evaluating the outcomes?

**Phase 5 in Testing**

In 2003, the CDC made several changes in its HIV testing guidelines following scientific advances and evaluations of the current HIV counseling and testing programs. By 2003, CDC-funded HIV test sites had provided approximately 2,000,000 tests and approximately 1% of these were newly discovered infections. However, of the newly discovered infections, 31% of those individuals did not receive their results. This was because the testing technology of that era required that confirmatory tests be done, and 1 to 2 weeks might pass between blood draw and when the test result was known and could be given to the individual. New tests using saliva had been developed that gave highly accurate results within 20 minutes. The test was relatively cheap, and no special equipment was required. Use of the test only required minimal training. Therefore, widespread use of this test was recommended for designated HIV testing sites and outreach programs to non-medical settings such as correctional facilities (Centers for Disease Control and Prevention, 2003).

Additionally, the CDC found that many health care providers were unwilling or uneasy in doing risk assessment and pretest counseling of their patients. Therefore, the CDC recommended that HIV testing be offered in settings serving populations with a high HIV prevalence. This could be done without ascertaining risk behaviors. These recommendations also removed the requirement for pretest counseling (Centers for Disease Control and Prevention, 2003).

**Questions for Phase 5**

- How did the definition of the problem for HIV testing change during Phase 5?
- Who were the stakeholders during this phase?
- Besides the change in the science of testing, what other values were determining changes in the screening policies?
- In what way were nurses stakeholders in implementing these new recommendations and in evaluating their outcomes?

(continued)

**EXHIBIT 13.1**

**Case Study: Changing Policy With Respect to Testing for HIV (continued)**

**Phase 6 in Testing**

The CDC further revised and expanded its guidelines in 2006. The agency recommended that all persons between the ages of 13 and 64 be offered HIV testing at each encounter with a health care provider. This recommendation was based on the knowledge that approximately 25% of HIV-positive people did not know that they were infected and were continuing to transmit the virus to others. Other research determined that routinely offering testing was more likely to be acceptable to patients than providers interviewing them to ascertain if they had engaged in risky behaviors. Experts believed that routine testing would no longer stigmatize those who agreed to be tested. Another major change in these guidelines was a recommendation that pregnant women should be tested according to an "opt out" protocol. Instead of asking women if they would like to be tested, they would be told that they are going to be tested unless they refused. This change was based on research that showed that pregnant women would be more likely to consent to HIV testing if presented with an "opt out" choice (Centers for Disease Control and Prevention, 2006).

The 2006 guidelines also emphasized that research now showed that patients with lower levels of circulating virus were less likely to transmit the virus. Reducing viral load was a major outcome of HAART so there was likely to be a prevention benefit if HIV-infected individuals were identified at an earlier stage and began receiving treatment. There was also evidence that individuals who knew that they were HIV infected were less likely to put others at risk. There was also evidence that persons who did not know their HIV status were 3.5 times more likely to transmit the virus to others (Centers for Disease Control and Prevention, 2006).

**Questions for Phase 6**

- How have program evaluation and outcome data influenced changes in screening policies during Phase 6?
- Has there been a shift in how the benefits to society are weighed against the benefits to individuals?
- Who are the stakeholders during this phase?
- What are the expected outcomes from the policy changes during Phase 6?
- What are your conclusions about the current screening policies?
- In what way were nurses stakeholders in implementing these new recommendations and in evaluating the outcomes?

**Questions for All Six Phases of the CDC Testing Recommendations**

- Do you think that the CDC's organizational emphasis on prevention of disease was the driving factor during all six phases of their recommendations on testing?
- Do you think that nurses would have made different recommendations if they had been directing the policies on testing between 1986 and 2006? What would they be?

In 2013, evidence indicated that patients who were treated early in the infection, when their CD4 cells were still ≥500, were less likely to transmit the virus (Centers for Disease Control and Prevention, 2013). In 2015, emerging evidence indicated that patients who are treated early in the infection and suppress their virus are only 5% as likely to transmit the virus. This has reinforced CDC's policy that all persons between 18 and 64 should be offered HIV testing. The policy should greatly improve HIV-infected persons' health and greatly reduce the incidence of HIV transmission.

You recognize that such testing will put a burden on your primary care practice and that of your colleagues. There is a window of opportunity here for you and other nurses to have input into either the development of the new policy or implementation of the policy.

- Who are the stakeholders now and what type of information do you want to provide to them?
- What additional information about the policy will you need to implement it?
- How would you evaluate whether the desired outcomes of the policy are met in your practice?

## EXHIBIT 13.2

### Case Study: Changing Policy in Response to the Paradigm of a Continuum of Care for HIV

The basic premise for encouraging HIV testing in the past was that individuals who were identified as HIV positive would seek care and receive proper treatment. However, two important papers challenged this thinking by pointing out that the most important issues in HIV care were occurring after testing and outside of the clinic (Gardner, McLees, Steiner, del Rio, & Burman, 2011; Giardano, Suarez-Almazor, & Grimes, 2005). These papers demonstrated that once individuals were found to be HIV positive they needed to be linked to care, retained in care, receive the proper treatment, and adhere to their treatment regimens. As shown in Figure 13.3, 70% of HIV-infected persons in the United States are not receiving the benefits of effective therapy. At each step in the testing, linking, retention, and care process, there is a drop-off in effectiveness.

Recognizing this, public health agencies have shifted their policies toward ensuring that persons who test positive are linked to care and that those who are in care are retained in care. This has led to the creation of a new health care worker called a service linkage worker (SLW). Some SLWs are tasked with assisting individuals who have recently tested positive to find competent HIV care. This has improved the linkage to HIV care. Other SLWs have the difficult task of finding those who have left care and facilitating those persons to return to care. This has proved to be a very difficult task because of the lag time between when a person is seen in a clinic and when the person later fails to keep an appointment (Udeagu, Webster, Bocour, Michel, & Shepard, 2013). Researchers are beginning to examine the reasons patients leave care and to develop interventions that facilitate retention in care. As of this writing there is little evidence that these questions have been resolved.

Doctors of nursing practice may wonder about the applicability of this case to their practice that may not involve HIV-infected patients. The issues for research and policy raised here about HIV may be applied to any chronic disease, such as hypertension, diabetes, and depression.

### Questions
● Are there similarities between the continuum of care illustrated in Figure 13.3 and the continuum of care for patients in your practice?
● Is there a "window of opportunity" for DNPs to advance the science for understanding the continuum for persons with chronic disease?

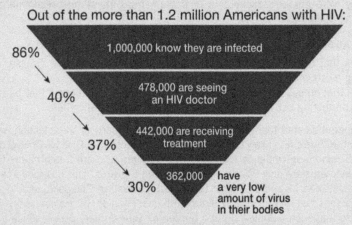

**Figure 13.3** Percentage of HIV-infected individuals engaged in selected stages of the continuum of HIV care, 2011.

*Source:* Centers for Disease Control and Prevention (2015). Used with permission.

*(continued)*

---

**EXHIBIT 13.2**

**Case Study: Changing Policy in Response to the Paradigm of a Continuum of Care for HIV (*continued*)**

- Given the widespread use of the electronic medical record, would it be possible to create a triangle like Figure 13.3 in your practice?
- Who would be the stakeholders in your practice to evaluate the continuum?
- Who would be the stakeholders to develop policies to improve outcomes at each stage of the continuum for your practice?
- What policies could be developed to improve testing for persons with chronic disease in the population you serve?
- What policies could be developed to improve early referral for diagnosis and treatment of persons with chronic disease in the population you serve?
- What policies could be developed in your health care setting to ensure that persons with a chronic disease are receiving treatment and are retained in care?
- How would you evaluate the outcomes from those policies and communicate the outcomes to stakeholders including other DNPs?

## ADVOCACY AND LEADERSHIP IN HEALTH POLICY

Nursing has a tradition of advocating for health policies that benefit patients. Florence Nightingale campaigned for effective care of hospitalized patients. Lillian Wald struggled to give poor women and children equal access to health care. Margaret Sanger fought to provide women with a choice about childbearing. These and many other nurses understood the connection between health policy and population health (Mullin, 2010; Mund, 2011; Nault & Sincox, 2014).

As the health care system became more complex, nursing leaders realized the need to provide nurses with sophisticated techniques to evaluate current policies and to develop innovative strategies for the future. The AACN's DNP Essentials (2006) specified seven policy activities for the DNP in Essential V, outlined at the beginning of this chapter. All of the Essentials addressed the expectation that DNPs will assume roles of leadership and advocacy in the health policy arena. Upon graduation, DNPs should have the knowledge and skills to advocate for effective, efficient, and equitable health care for individuals, groups, and populations.

The focus of advocacy depends not only on the DNP's education but also on professional practice, personal experience, and motivation. A nurse practitioner in Texas observes that individuals living below the federal poverty level and unable to afford health insurance do not qualify for Medicaid because their state opted out of the Medicaid expansion offered through the Affordable Care Act. A visiting nurse is concerned about the out-of-pocket costs incurred by an elderly patient with end-stage renal failure (Christopher, Duhl, Rosati, & Sheehan, 2015). The director of a continuing care retirement community discovers that hospitals are misplacing the advance directives of residents provided to the hospital during episodic admissions for acute care (Muller, 2015). A psychiatric nurse practitioner learns that a number of patients have been incarcerated instead of receiving appropriate treatment because psychiatric facilities in the area are overcrowded. In each of the situations, the work environment may trigger interest in a problem directly affected by health policies and laws. Regardless of clinical specialty, as members of the nursing profession, DNPs have an interest in the ongoing efforts to acquire an appropriate scope of practice and just reimbursement at the state and national levels (AACN, 2006; Mund, 2011).

Personal experience also plays a role in the choice of policies and issues most important to a nurse. Having a family member killed by a drunk driver, a parent in need of assistance with the activities of daily living, or a child with a serious congenital disease may prompt a DNP to assume an activist role with respect to those issues.

Motivation is arguably the strongest determinant of whether one will become an activist. A DNP must want to bring about change through the political process. Political activism is time-consuming, often frustrating, and frequently confrontational. Successful advocates maintain a commitment to a goal that enables them to take the negative aspects of advocacy in stride.

Concern about a professional or personal experience may lead a practitioner to find out more about an issue through reading health care policy journals, accessing the Internet, attending professional meetings, or discussing the problem with a mentor (Mullin, 2010). As the DNP learns more about a topic, the focus of advocacy sharpens. The DNP may be further motivated to contact politicians and lawmakers to discuss their perspectives on the issue. If a policy or law is already in place, the DNP examines it to determine if and how it can be improved.

"The goal of health policy . . . is to contribute to improving the health of individuals and communities" (Aday, Begley, Lairson, & Balkrishnan, 2004). Even after a thorough assessment in which the effectiveness and efficiency of a policy have been established, the DNP may be ambivalent about the direction advocacy should take because the perceived benefits to individual patients appear at odds with the perceived benefits to society (Mund, 2011). How does a practitioner decide on the most equitable course of action? Aday, Begley, Lairson, and Balkrishnan (2004) addressed this question using three paradigms that pertain to the just distribution of health care. The first paradigm is distributive justice. Adherents to this model have faith in individual autonomy and decision making. They believe that individuals are entitled to demand the health care that they need, regardless of the impact on the larger community. The second paradigm is social justice. Adherents to this model believe that society takes precedence over the individual. They believe that policies and laws should result in improved community health even though they result in a loss of benefits to some individuals. The third paradigm, deliberative justice, takes a centrist position. Adherents to this model argue that through public discussion, policy makers can reach a compromise between individual rights and the general good. Although these paradigms are expressed in political discussions, they have a philosophical foundation that reflects beliefs and values rather than facts. DNPs will become more successful advocates if they understand their own and their opponents' philosophical perspectives on justice in health care policy.

There is another issue to consider before becoming politically active. A natural tension exists between advocacy and evaluation. In fact, there are evaluators who believe that supporting a specific policy or law threatens the essential open-mindedness and impartiality of their role (Fitzpatrick, Sanders, & Worthen, 2004). A DNP who, as a result of education, experience, and motivation, chooses to become an activist should make an effort to maintain a certain detachment about the issues, to appreciate different viewpoints, and to reassess alternative options.

There are a number of approaches to political activism. One of the simplest is to join a professional organization (Hahn, 2009). There are numerous groups that provide support to nurses interested in advocacy. Professional organizations that are particularly relevant to the DNP include the American Association of Nurse Practitioners, the American Nurses Association, and AACN. Organizations such as the American Association of Nurse Anesthetists and the American College of Nurse Midwives provide a clinical focus. Professional organizations frequently have political action committees that offer a direct link to state and national legislators. These organizations present opportunities for mentoring, and facilitate collaboration with peers in developing successful strategies to evaluate and improve health care policy. Strategies may consist of meeting with legislators, preparing position statements and briefs, publishing in journals, giving interviews to the media, and organizing letter-writing campaigns (Betz, Smith, Melnyk, & Rickey, 2011; Mullin, 2010; Mund, 2011; Nault & Sincox, 2014).

Some DNPs may want to go a step further and assume a leadership role in advocacy. If that is the case, advanced education and experience are helpful. Universities, foundations, and professional associations offer advanced courses in leadership, health policy, and politics. Fellowships with agencies such as the Robert Wood Johnson Foundation provide a way to network with other health professionals who share common interests and to meet with policy makers at the local, state, and national levels (Mullin, 2010; Spross & Hanson, 2009). Ultimately, successful advocacy depends upon a long-term commitment of time, energy, and talent, a single-minded focus on an issue that is important to the DNP, and enthusiasm for the political process.

# REFERENCES

Aday, L. U., Begley, C. E., Lairson, D. R., & Balkrishnan, R. (2004). *Evaluating the healthcare system: Effectiveness, efficiency, and equity* (p. 14). Chicago, IL: Health Administration Press.

American Association of Colleges of Nursing. (2006). *The essentials of doctoral education for advanced practice nursing*. Retrieved from www.aacn.nche.edu

Betz, C. L., Smith, K. A., Melnyk, B. M., & Rickey, T. (2011). Disseminating evidence through publications, presentations, health policy briefs, and the media. In B. B. Melnyk & E. Fineout-Overholt (Eds.), *Evidence-based practice in nursing and healthcare* (2nd ed., pp. 355–393). Philadelphia, PA: Wolters Kluwer/Lippincott Williams & Wilkins.

Block, L. E. (2008). Health policy: What it is and how it works. In C. Harrington & C. L. Estes (Eds.), *Health policy: Crisis and reform in the U.S. health care delivery system* (5th ed., pp. 4–14). Sudbury, MA: Jones and Bartlett Publishers.

Centers for Disease Control and Prevention. (1986). Current trends: Additional recommendations to reduce sexual and drug abuse-related transmission of human T-lymphotropic virus type III/ lymphadenopathy-associated virus. *Morbidity and Mortality Weekly Report, 35*(10), 152–155.

Centers for Disease Control and Prevention. (1987). Perspectives in disease prevention and health promotion public health service guidelines for counseling and antibody testing to prevent HIV infection and AIDS. *Morbidity and Mortality Weekly Report, 36*(31), 509–515.

Centers for Disease Control and Prevention. (1995). U.S. public health service recommendations for human immunodeficiency virus counseling and voluntary testing for pregnant women. *Morbidity and Mortality Weekly Report, 44*(RR-7), 1–15.

Centers for Disease Control and Prevention. (2001). Revised guidelines for HIV counseling, testing, and referral. *Morbidity and Mortality Weekly Report, 50*(RR-19), 1–58.

Centers for Disease Control and Prevention. (2003). Advancing HIV prevention: New strategies for a changing epidemic—United States 2003. *Morbidity and Mortality Weekly Report, 52*(15), 329–332.

Centers for Disease Control and Prevention. (2006). Revised recommendations for HIV testing of adults, adolescents, and pregnant women in health-care settings. *Morbidity and Mortality Weekly Report, 55*(RR-14), 1–24.

Centers for Disease Control and Prevention. (2013). Prevention benefits of HIV treatment. Retrieved from http://www.cdc.gov/hiv/prevention/research/tap

Centers for Disease Control and Prevention. (2015). Today's HIV/AIDS Epidemic. Retrieved from http://www.cdc.gov/nchhstp/ux-test-2015/newsroom/hivfactsheets/epidemic/index.htm

Christopher, M. A., Duhl, J., Rosati, R. J., & Sheehan, K. M. (2015). Advocacy for vulnerable patients: How grassroots organizations can influence health care policy. *AJN, 115*(3), 66–69.

Fitzpatrick, J. L., Sanders, J. R., & Worthen, B. R. (2004). *Program evaluation. Alternative approaches and practical guidelines.* Boston, MA: Pearson Education.

Gardner, E. M., McLees, M. P., Steiner, J. F., del Rio, C., & Burman, W. J. (2011). The spectrum of engagement in HIV care and its relevance to test-and-treat strategies for prevention of HIV infection. *Clinical Infectious Diseases, 52*(6), 793–800.

Giardano, T. P., Suarez-Almazor, M. E., & Grimes, R. M. (2005). The population effectiveness of HAART: Are good drugs good enough? *Current HIV/AIDS Reports, 2*, 177–183.

Hahn, J. (2009, August, September, October). Power dynamics, health policy, and politics. *Virginia Nurses Today.* Retrieved from www.virginianurses.com

Hanley, B. E. (2002). Policy development and analysis. In D. J. Mason, J. K. Leavitt, & M. W. Chaffee (Eds.), *Policy and politics in nursing and health care* (pp. 55–69). St. Louis, MO: Saunders.

Longest, B. B. (2006). *Health policymaking in the United States* (4th ed.). Chicago, IL: Health Administration Press.

Muller, L. S. (2015). Advocacy: The key to dignified end of life. *Professional Case Management, 20*(3), 150–153.

Mullin, M. H. (2010). DNP involvement in healthcare policy and advocacy. In L. A. Chism (Ed.), *The doctor of nursing practice: A guidebook for role development and professional issues* (pp. 141–167). Sudbury, MA: Jones and Bartlett Publishers.

Mund, A. (2011). Healthcare policy for advocacy in health care. In M. E. Zaccagnini & K. W. White (Eds.), *The doctor of nursing practice essential. A new model for advanced practice nursing* (pp. 195–234). Sudbury, MA: Jones and Bartlett Publishers.

Nault, D. S., & Sincox, A. K. (2014, July). Nursing's voice in politics: The ongoing relationship between nurses and legislators. *Michigan Nurse, 87*(3), 17–19.

Spross, J. A., & Hanson, C. M. (2009). Clinical, professional, and systems leadership. In A. B. Hamric, J. A. Spross, & C. M. Hanson (Eds.), *Advanced practice nursing: An integrative approach* (pp. 249–282). St. Louis, MO: Saunders Elsevier.

Stokey, E., & Zeckhauser, R. (1978). *A primer for policy analysis.* New York, NY: W. W. Norton & Company.

Udeagu, C.-C. N., Webster, T. R., Bocour, A., Michel, P., & Shepard, C. W. (2013). Lost or just not following up: Public health effort to re-engage HIV-infected persons lost to follow-up into HIV medical care. *AIDS, 27*, 2271–2279.

# CHAPTER FOURTEEN

# FUTURE TRENDS AND CHALLENGES IN EVALUATION

Christine A. Brosnan and Joanne V. Hickey

*We shall not cease from exploration*
*And the end of all our exploring*
*Will be to arrive where we started*
*And know the place for the first time.*
—*T.S. Eliot*

The previous chapters have addressed the evaluation of health care from a number of different perspectives in which the doctor of nursing practice (DNP) graduates will undoubtedly share now and in the future. There is no way to predict with any degree of certainty how events in the health care sector will pan out. Some developments seem more likely than others. However, there is, and will continue to be, an increased demand for comprehensive, high-quality evaluation. The primary purpose of evaluation is to inform and support decision making based on relevant data that are collected, organized, and analyzed according to the high standards of evaluation.

Although there are many approaches for evaluation, the type and design of an evaluation are linked to its purpose. The complexity of health care delivery systems, organizations, and models of practice and care contribute to the complexity of decision making. Not only is complexity a hallmark of the current health care environment, but health care and all associated entities are undergoing extraordinary and unprecedented rapid changes that will add uncertainty to that complexity. More fundamental and rapid changes are expected in the future as the U.S. health enterprise struggles to align itself with the demands of a 21st century economy. The limited financial and human resources dedicated to health care, and the national imperative for quality and safety, will continue to be major drivers for informed and responsible decision makers.

## REFORMING HEALTH CARE

The Patient Protection and Affordable Care Act (P.L. 111–148) signed into law by President Barack Obama on March 23, 2010, addressed the challenge of providing quality health care for all Americans. The Affordable Care Act (ACA) was an attempt to overhaul the U.S. health care system. The ACA provides for systematic and robust methods of evaluation in order to ensure more effective, efficient, and equitable health care. A few examples of some of the changes scheduled to occur over a period of 8 years are discussed in the following text.

The ACA established the nonprofit Patient Centered Outcomes Research Institute and charged it with evaluating the *effectiveness* of health care interventions and programs. The ACA authorized changes to Medicare that included linking payment to quality outcomes, using short-term and long-term indicators in measuring outcomes of care, and developing and evaluating home care programs to keep high-risk patients out of hospitals. The law also directed the establishment of a national quality improvement strategy with the goal of improving the health care of individuals, groups, and populations (Kaiser Family Foundation, 2013).

There are a number of provisions in the ACA aimed at improving health care *efficiency*. The legislation encouraged a shift from uneven and patchy health care to a comprehensive and accountable system. Through structural and process changes, the new health care system offers incentives to provide seamless and holistic health care (Ebner, 2010). An example is the provision for Accountable Care Organizations. These organizations are composed of groups of health care professionals who collaborate in assessing patient needs, developing comprehensive and long-term plans of care, implementing the plans, and evaluating the effectiveness and efficiency of interventions and programs (Kocher & Sahni, 2010).

The ACA has the potential to increase health care access for about 32 million individuals who, prior to the law, could not afford care (Oberlander, 2010). The ACA accomplishes this through a combination of individual and employer insurance requirements and adjustments to public health programs. As a result, the vision of *equitable* health care in the United States becomes more realistic.

National legislation and public demand have raised the bar on what quality health care means. To meet the new standards, DNPs and other health professionals must provide health care that is effective, efficient, equitable, safe, patient centered, and timely (Institute of Medicine, 2001). These attributes were derived from the structure–process–outcome and the effectiveness–efficiency–equity models. The models continue to offer clear blueprints for evaluating quality. There is consensus that clinical and methodological issues first identified by Donabedian and others are still valid, and that they continue to challenge health care professionals in providing quality health care. Some of these issues are discussed in the following text.

## CLINICAL CHALLENGES TO IMPROVING HEALTH CARE QUALITY

Arguably, one of the greatest challenges to health care quality in the United States is reducing overtreatment, which is defined as health care interventions "that, according to sound science and the patients' own preferences cannot possibly help them—care rooted in outmoded habits, supply driven behaviors, and ignoring science" (Berwick & Hackbarth, p. 3, 2012). Overtreatment is not only ineffective but also expensive and accounts for about 26% of medical waste. A midpoint estimate of the contribution of overtreatment to health care waste in 2011 was $192 billion ($158–$226 billion). Not including fraud and abuse, the midpoint estimate of the total cost of medical waste was $734 billion ($476–$992 billion) and, in addition to overtreatment, included failures of care delivery and care coordination, administrative complexity, and pricing (Berwick & Hackbarth, 2012; Lallemand, 2012). DNPs should be concerned with all of the categories of medical waste; however, overtreatment is particularly harmful to patients and is a challenge that DNPs can directly address.

Overtreatment is frequently the corollary of overdiagnosis, which is described as "the identification of an abnormality where detection will not benefit the patient" (Coon, Quinonez, Moyer, & Schroeder, 2014, p. 1014). These two areas of concern may result in physical injuries to patients when follow-up testing and unnecessary treatment lead to adverse events.

Emotional harm can occur when, for example, as a result of overdiagnosis, parents are told that their kindergarten child has attention deficit hyperactivity disorder (ADHD) because the student is not reading at the same level as the rest of the class. The provider and the school may suggest a barrage of tests along with special placement, which may lead parents, classmates, and teachers to view the child as impaired. The student's self-esteem decreases because of a perceived deficiency. If the student is the youngest in the class, it is quite possible that there is no actual deficit. The child is just at an earlier stage of maturation and will soon catch up with peers (Cha, 2015).

The financial harm to individuals includes not only copayments for gratuitous care, but also time lost from work to attend needless clinic appointments, undergo unwarranted laboratory and radiological tests, and purchase unnecessary medications. Overdiagnosis and overtreatment also have an opportunity cost. The money spent on ineffective and inefficient care will not be available for quality care (Coon et al., 2014; Welch, 2015).

There are a number of causes for overdiagnosis and overtreatment (Chiolero, Paccaud, Aujesky, Santschi, & Rodondi, 2015). Indiscriminant screening for disease may be the most significant cause. As discussed in Chapter 4, all tests have false-positive results and there is an inverse proportion between the incidence of a condition and the frequency of false-positive results. Universal screening for relatively rare conditions can trigger a torrent of expensive follow-up tests, clinic visits, and hospitalizations.

Another cause is increasing the sensitivity of screening and diagnostic tests, which not only results in the diagnosis of more persons who actually have the disease, but also in the identification of persons with mild cases who do not require treatment. Because of the side effects of treatment, providers may place patients at increased risk by intervening in these benign cases. As an example, some national screening programs for neuroblastoma found a previously unknown self-limiting form of the disease. In the decade before realization that some positive screens were benign, many children were managed as having the classic malignancy and exposed to adverse events associated with surgery and chemotherapy. Screening had not improved mortality from neuroblastoma (Coon et al., 2014).

Overtreatment may result from a tendency by both providers and patients to confuse the risk of a disease with the disease itself. Providers may be afraid of overlooking a treatable condition because they failed to order enough tests. They may fear the malpractice lawsuits that could follow a missed diagnosis. In addition, the fee-for-service health care system supports additional testing. Patients may encourage testing because of the barrage of unfiltered medical information from TV, radio, and social media. They may decide that even a tiny risk of disease should be addressed. Lost in the fear is the consideration that a small risk of illness needs to be measured against the risk of harm resulting from continued testing and unnecessary treatment (Chiolero et al., 2015).

Responding to overtreatment is complex and demands a coordinated team approach. There are a number of approaches that the DNP and other health professionals can adopt. First, become familiar with the evidence about the benefit and risks of screening and diagnostic tests. What is the absolute risk reduction of the test? Which tests have high false-positive rates? What tests pick up a large number of mild cases of the condition? What is the value in treating persons with a mild or slowly progressing condition and what is the possible harm (Chiolero et al., 2015; Welch, 2015)?

Second, discuss treatment options with your patients. One helpful resource, developed by the ABIM Foundation, is choosing wisely (http://www.choosing-wisely.org). This website provides information about interventions that are effective, timely, and safe. The program uses easy-to-read patient information and encourages providers and patients to engage in discussions about health care decisions. Another useful resource is the U.S. Preventive Services Task Force (USPSTF) established by AHRQ (http://www.ahrq.gov/professionals/clinicians-providers/guidelines-recommendations/uspstf/index.html). The Task Force is composed of health care professionals who volunteer their time to develop evidence-based guidelines and recommendations about clinical prevention for patients and providers.

Third, DNP curricula should contain content on health care waste, with a special focus on overtreatment. An increasing number of studies are being conducted on this topic and there is evidence that it is a major detriment to quality health care (Morgan, Wright, & Dhruva, 2015). DNPs who are familiar with the evidence, skilled in evaluating the harms and benefits of clinical interventions, and have a collaborative relationship with other health professionals are in a good position to address overtreatment. Decreasing inefficient, ineffective, and unsafe care will go a long way toward increasing the value of health care for providers, consumers, and payers.

## METHODOLOGICAL CHALLENGES TO IMPROVING HEALTH CARE QUALITY

It is essential that evaluation moves from using process indicators to mainly using outcome indicators in measuring health care quality. Process indicators are a direct approach to evaluate whether health care is in compliance with best practice standards at a particular place and time. While they are helpful in measuring quality improvement in individual hospitals and agencies, they do not provide direct evidence about the effectiveness of care across geographical settings over time. Porter (2010) observed that the overwhelming majority of performance measures used by programs such as the Healthcare Effectiveness Data and Information Set are still process indicators.

Selection of indicators is often influenced by the interests of those requesting an evaluation. Indicators that are essential to the health care marketplace and quality often differ. The marketplace is generally more interested in using process indicators and less interested in using the outcome indicators that are needed to objectively measure quality of care. For example, Lee (2010) observed that, in his practice, clinic administrators routinely notified physicians about process indicators that were necessary for reimbursement, such as the number of patient visits. They did not routinely notify physicians about outcome indicators that were necessary for evaluating effective care, such as the number of discharged patients later seen in the emergency department. In comparing the differing perspectives on quality, Bowers and Kiefe (2002) noted that compared with health care evaluators, marketplace evaluators have a keen interest in measuring patient satisfaction with the hospital environment and amenities but are less inclined to measure risk adjustment or changes in health status.

There is growing evidence that outcome indicators based on a change in patient health status are being used more frequently as a result of incentives stemming from the ACA. The challenge now is to identify and adapt valid and reliable end points that can be standardized across settings. The implication of measures such as mortality rates that are frequently used by hospitals in establishing quality care can vary from setting to setting, depending on the rigor of data collection and analysis. For example, evaluators in a certain location may fail to take into account patient risk factors or they may not reliably record data. The electronic health record (EHR) is seen as a way to address some of these issues, but data input to EHRs also varies, and evaluating their usefulness in measuring quality has just begun. Provonost and Lilford (2011) cited the problems of missing data and the use of unclear and idiosyncratic algorithms in calculating outcomes as challenges to overcome.

A challenge that continues to puzzle evaluators is that, frequently, what is thought to be a link between short-term and long-term outcomes may not, in fact, exist. As an example, a 2006 study funded by the National Institutes of Health (NIH) involving 3,400 individuals sought to decrease heart attacks and strokes by using a combination therapy that included niacin, a medication thought to increase high-density lipoproteins (HDLs). The trial was scheduled to last 6 years but was stopped in May 2011 (NIH, 2011). Researchers found that although niacin did increase HDL (a short-term outcome), it did not decrease the occurrence of heart attacks or strokes (a long-term outcome).

These challenges and others will not be easy to address, but there has been progress in working toward accurately and precisely measuring health care quality. Because of their education and experience, DNPs, in collaboration with other health care professionals, can make a significant contribution to the endeavor. Suggestions for tackling the methodological issues that obstruct the systematic and objective evaluation of health care quality follow.

DNPs can contribute to the development of standardized methods of measuring quality, including nurse-sensitive outcome indicators. Currently, the number of nurse-sensitive indicators is limited. The prevalence of pressure ulcers and frequency of falls are two measures that are frequently cited (Albanese et al., 2010; Loan, Patrician, & McCarthy, 2011). In developing methodologies, consideration should be given to the inclusion of short-term and long-term indicators, to valid and reliable data sources and data collection methods, and to transparent statistical analyses and algorithms used in calculating results. Outcomes should reflect the total patient experience and not just one intervention or the impact of one group of professionals (Porter, 2010; Provonost & Lilford, 2011).

DNPs are in an ideal position to lead the quest for a culture of quality. Albanese et al. (2010) reported on a quality improvement and performance improvement program at the Hospital of the University of Pennsylvania that was based on Donabedian's model and supported by hospital leaders from nursing, medicine, and administration. The goal of the program was to establish a culture that encouraged nursing clinicians to become invested in continuous quality improvement efforts at the hospital. Structure and interdisciplinary input were provided by the hospital's quality improvement committee. Nurse clinicians collaborated to develop outcomes and performance measures derived from data. They created quality improvement standards that were applied and evaluated annually. Interdisciplinary dashboards enabled viewing of the current status of outcomes in each nursing specialty as well as their link to overall hospital goals. The initiative provided valuable patient data and succeeded in engaging staff nurses in continuing quality improvement activities.

The issues inherent in improving health care quality are daunting. Health care is complicated and change must occur at the micro, meso, and macro levels if it is to be successful. A program may be so large, complex, and fragmented that no one assumes responsibility for evaluation. State-mandated newborn screening is an example of such a program. It is interdisciplinary, multifaceted, and involves nursing care at the individual, group, and population level. The case study in Exhibit 14.1 discusses some issues related to newborn screening quality and the role of the DNP in addressing those issues.

---

**EXHIBIT 14.1**

**State-Mandated Newborn Screening Programs**

Newborn screening started when Dr. Robert Guthrie developed a test for phenylketonuria (PKU) in 1961. PKU is a rare genetic disorder that can result in mental retardation if a baby is not treated within a short time after birth. Babies who were screened and diagnosed with the disorder were given a modified diet that successfully prevented retardation. The benefit was clear, and over the years, PKU testing has helped thousands of children (Guthrie, 1992). Screening was strongly backed by politicians and consumer groups. Over time, other disorders were slowly added to the panel as testing became feasible. By the early 1990s, most states screened for about five or six conditions. And then, mass spectrometry was developed. This new method allowed technicians to screen for many more disorders using the same amount of blood as previously. Today, a majority of the screening tests are analyzed by tandem mass spectrometry. States are now able to screen for almost 60 conditions (National Newborn Screening and Genetics Resource Center, 2014).

Newborn screening is mandated by every state and the District of Columbia; as a result, approximately four million children are screened annually. But other than that mandate, screening varies widely among the states. In Vermont and Minnesota, parents may refuse screening for any reason, while in Texas parents can only refuse on religious grounds. In many states, they cannot refuse. Maryland asks parents to sign a consent form before screening. Some states require that each newborn have one complete screening panel, some require two, and others require one panel but recommend a second panel. The number of tests in a screening panel also varies widely, with some states choosing to provide about 30 tests and others choosing to provide almost twice that amount. Each state decides how to finance its own screening program and how much it will charge (National Newborn Screening and Genetics Resource Center, 2014). Recently, there has been controversy around the issue of destroying or keeping for research the filter paper used in the collection of the blood specimen (Rothwell et al., 2011; The President's Council on Bioethics, 2008).

*(continued)*

---

**EXHIBIT 14.1**

**State-Mandated Newborn Screening Programs (*continued*)**

---

Although wide variation exists among the states, there is agreement that states need to follow general guidelines in administering screening programs, including education, proper testing, follow-up, diagnosis, and evaluation (The President's Council on Bioethics, 2008). There is consensus that parents should be informed about what disorders are involved, how the tests will be done, what they should do if the tests are positive, and where they can go for follow-up and treatment. Everyone agrees that there should be an established process for pricking the infant's heel to collect the blood, for placing the blood on filter paper, and for sending the filter paper to a laboratory for analysis. There should be a plan for analyzing the blood and for establishing the cut-off point that separates a positive from a negative result. There should be guidelines about where to send the results if the test is positive and who will be responsible for making sure that parents know where to take their baby for follow-up. If a baby is diagnosed with a disorder, there should be an effective treatment. Finally, all states should have a way of evaluating programs.

Nursing has an essential and continuing role in newborn screening. In the hospital, nurses provide information about the program to new parents and are usually designated to collect the blood specimen. Nurses are often the coordinators of the State Health Department Newborn Screening Programs. As coordinators, they respond to questions from families and act as liaisons between the health department and other health professionals. Nurses frequently provide and coordinate care in the pediatric clinics to which the results are reported. Public health nurses may make home visits to determine why parents have not responded to notification about an abnormal screen. Finally, nurses collaborate with other health care professionals in providing long-term care to children diagnosed with a disorder.

Evaluating a complex and fragmented program like newborn screening may be overwhelming, but at each point of patient contact, nurses have an opportunity and a responsibility to become involved in evaluation activities. Examples of evaluation activities are described in the following list.

1. A DNP coordinating maternal–child units in a large hospital assumes responsibility for evaluating the literacy level, clarity, and language of the educational materials provided to parents. The DNP analyzes how much time is spent with parents discussing the programs and the parents' understanding of what is being done. An evaluation reveals that most parents do not understand the newborn screening process because of language and literacy barriers. The DNP coordinates a team that develops new bilingual educational materials that are aimed at a ninth grade reading level.
2. A DNP practicing in a pediatric clinic observes that there is a lack of coordination in notifying parents about positive screening tests and in ensuring that parents comply with follow-up recommendations. The DNP joins other clinicians in establishing clinic protocol that standardizes notification and follow-up. Process and outcome indicators are monitored regularly.
3. A DNP employed by a state health department as coordinator of newborn screening activities observes that one of the tests has a large number of false-positive results. The DNP collaborates with members of the newborn screening team, including physicians and laboratory technicians, to evaluate the abnormal cut-off value of the screening test. The team analyzes the impact that changing the cut-off value will have on the frequency of false-positive and false-negative results. The team submits a report of their recommendations to designated administrators of the health department and clinical specialists in the state.
4. A DNP whose clinical practice involves newborn screening regularly attends national meetings on the subject. The DNP volunteers to serve on a national committee studying the storage and use of residual blood on filter paper.

Collaborating with nurses and other health care professionals in evaluating the quality of each patient contact in a large and complex program like newborn screening not only improves the quality of health care but expands nursing's influence in developing programs and policies. Are there other examples of evaluation activities that should engage the DNP?

The demand for thoughtful and systematic evaluations that can inform decision making has never been greater. An evaluation plan is normally a prerequisite before a project is approved. A substantive evaluation is required at the completion of a project to determine outcomes and value added. Health care providers have been forced to recognize that health care is a business, and that its business model includes evaluation of return on investment. This transition from a mindset of endless available resources to one of limited resources that must be wisely used and justified has shifted how health professionals must think. Making a decision is choosing one option over other options with recognition of intended and unintended consequences. It is comprehensive, valid, and reliable information from well-conceived and conducted evaluations that assists decision makers in making the best choices.

Many decisions are "high stake" choices that will have a significant impact on how and what kind of health care and health policies are implemented. Quality indicators for evaluations include comprehensiveness, contextual relevancy, focus on the information needs of the user, validity, reliability, transparency, balanced information (e.g., control of bias), and fairness. Because of the demand for evaluation of the relative effectiveness of the various diagnostics, procedures, devices, pharmaceuticals, guidelines, protocols, and other interventions in clinical practice, the DNP will be invited to participate in evaluation both as a leader and team member.

## SCOPE OF EVALUATION EXPECTATIONS FOR DNPS

DNPs are considered by the nursing profession, other professions, and society to be clinical experts by virtue of their education and experience. The expectation of evaluation has been included in graduate education at the master's level in nursing, but it has generally been underplayed and defined within the context of the individual patient for achieving very specific outcomes. The emerging and growing cadre of graduates from DNP programs increases the expectation that these clinical scholars have a deep and substantive knowledge of evaluation and can lead efforts to inform the transformation of the health care system. The scope and depth of evaluation are among the areas of professional differentiation of performance within doctoral nursing education and competency.

The following text highlights major areas for evaluation competencies in which DNPs are needed.

## Standards, Guidelines, and Protocols

DNPs must be able to evaluate standards, guidelines, and protocols. As discussed in Chapter 10, standards are broad statements that address expectations for professional performance and care. The DNP must understand applicable standards in order to evaluate current levels of performance and care in contemporary practice. A major responsibility of DNPs is to evaluate guidelines and protocols to be sure that they are aligned with current and valid evidence of best practices. Keeping up with the published scientific literature and evaluating current practices for needed updates are huge and ongoing commitments that are directly linked to quality patient outcomes. It is an expectation that DNPs will be leaders in this realm of clinical practice.

## Models of Practice and Care

Another important responsibility of the DNP is to evaluate models of practice and care based on best practices and to have an understanding of the local contextual environment in which practice occurs and care is delivered. For example, concurrent with the responsibility for providing the best care shown to lead to the best patient outcomes, the DNP must evaluate the currently used models of practice and care to determine if there are gaps and unmet needs. Much discussion centers around transitional care and niche care for selected populations, which could lead to better, more convenient, and cost-effective care. As patients move along the continuum of care, many gaps are evident. By most accounts, fragmentation of care is common, and it needs to be replaced by seamless integrated systems. For example, in an obstetrical unit in a major facility, a DNP noted that mothers and babies were not being discharged on weekends because there was no staff available to conduct newborn screening examinations. This tied up beds for an extra 2 days and was inconvenient for patients and families. There was also a substantial economic loss to the facility that was not reimbursable by insurers. By initiating a pediatric nurse practitioner weekend clinic, bed flow, cost, and convenience were addressed. The clinic did not just happen. It took an astute DNP to recognize the problem, conduct a comprehensive evaluation, propose options with risk–benefit analyses, prepare a business plan, and employ leadership skills to move an innovative solution through the organization and decision makers.

Another example of evaluation is appraising a current facility's readiness for a major shift in focus, such as to a patient–family centered model of care. What would it take for an organization to make the cultural change from its current model of a patient being directed by an interdisciplinary team to a patient–family centered model? A comprehensive evaluation would be needed to assess the multiple interrelated structural and process-driven changes that need to be addressed in order to make such a transition.

All quality care is interdisciplinary; it takes a village of health professionals representing a number of disciplines to provide comprehensive care that leads to optimal outcomes. The DNP has a huge role in evaluating teams for effectiveness. As discussed in Chapter 11, interdisciplinary collaborative teams are the fundamental pivotal hubs of care. High-performance teams are dynamic and highly interactive groups of professionals focused on mutually accepted goals. Team communications are very complex and are subject to misunderstandings and disruption. DNPs, as members of interdisciplinary teams as well as outside evaluators, can contribute to ongoing optimal group function.

## Acquisitions

Employers expect DNPs to participate in the decision making surrounding acquisition of new equipment and other resources to support health care delivery. These purchases often represent major expenditures and capital investments. The DNP must be able to determine how the item will impact care delivery and concurrent changes in practice, current equipment and workflow, patient outcomes, care provider user-friendliness (e.g., ease of use, reliability, and workflow), and patient acceptance (e.g., comfort, acceptability), as well as to assess its potential for reimbursement and cost. As a member of a team providing input on acquisitions, the DNP must base that input on a systematic and thorough evaluation of current resources and a comparison of the proposed products to determine feasibility and usefulness to the practice setting. DNPs understand the spectrum of questions that emerge throughout the product or intervention life cycle in clinical practice and can therefore ask pertinent questions that contribute to an evaluation. The emerging science of comparative effectiveness should assist the DNP in providing data-driven input related to acquisitions.

For example, the digital revolution is a reconfiguring practice and care in health care facilities. Multimillion dollar contracts for digital information systems are major capital investments that require a comprehensive evaluation of clinical and organizational practice patterns for interface with current databases and systems. Many organizations have found, to their dismay, that their current information systems do not interface with the newly purchased system. Although most DNPs do not have the technical knowledge to question how the interface might operate, they do have the expertise to raise questions from the clinician perspective. Do new orders for drugs entered into the electronic order sheet go electronically to the pharmacy, or do the orders have to be reentered into a separate pharmacy order system? Can arrangements be made to mine data from large databases so that the unit has a monthly report on admissions, lengths of stay, infections, and other items used for quality improvement purposes? Chapter 7 has addressed the role of DNPs in the evaluation of health care information systems and patient technology.

## Current Programs and Program Development

Evaluation of current and potential programs is often linked to practice-care issues and health policy. Programs are organized services that address the needs of a designated population of patients. DNPs are often requested to conduct a program evaluation. The impetus for a program evaluation might be to determine comprehensive outcomes of a program (e.g., patient outcomes, satisfaction, and cost) with possible interest in expanding, revising, or deleting a program. Of all of the focus areas of evaluation, program evaluation is the most frequently addressed.

Numerous books, articles, and websites readily offer information on program evaluation. The DNP should be familiar with these resources. An evaluation to establish the need for a new parent education program about newborn screening is an example of one type of evaluation that the DNP may conduct. Another example might be to evaluate a current program to confirm the need for expansion. A current heart failure program may be evaluated to determine if a special program should be established for women with heart failure to address their special needs. There are endless opportunities for DNPs to engage in program evaluation.

## Health Policy

One recommendation in *The Future of Nursing: Leading Change, Advancing Health* (Institute of Medicine, 2011) is that nurses should become full partners with physicians and other health professionals to redesign health care in the United States. The greatest opportunity for this recommendation to be fulfilled is in the health policy arena. Health policy is where the rules and regulations that control practice and care issues are influenced and negotiated. More than 3 million professional nurses in the United States represent the largest health care workforce compared with other health care professionals. Their voices need to be heard at the health policy table at the local, state, and national levels. It is often the DNP who is the voice for nurses and who speaks as an advocate for patients and quality care. DNPs must understand the processes involved in influencing health policy and develop the competencies to participate in the process. Several chapters in this book, including Chapters 3, 6, 12, and 13, address this critical leadership role. In order to be an effective participant, the DNP must be able to evaluate current and proposed health policies.

For example, at the local level a current organizational policy on scheduling of new patients may be creating a hardship for some patients. Perhaps in approving this policy there was no thought about the impact on patients. The DNP could assume the advocacy role for the patient. An example of health policy on the state level is the requirement for frequent physician oversight of nurse practitioners in a rural underserved area. If the closest physicians are 75 miles away from the clinic and unable to travel that distance every few weeks to review charts, the nurse practitioner may be unable to practice and patients may be left without any health care. On the national level, DNPs are often invited to serve on committees and boards that make recommendations about health policy. DNP participation is critical to providing the advocacy voice for patients and quality care.

## Big Data and Big Data Science

For the last few years, the term *big data* has had an intriguing presence in the scientific literature and is positioned to be a prominent driving force in science, business, and health care. Big data has been defined in a number of ways, often with a focus primarily on size. The National Institutes of Health "Big Data to Knowledge" (2014) describes big data as that which exceeds the capacity of unaided human cognition and strains the computer process units, bandwidth, and storage capabilities of modern information processing. However, it is now recognized that big data is not just based on size, but also on the characteristics of data coming from sensors, novel research techniques, and a variety of information technologies (Brennan & Bakken, 2015).

Brennan and Bakken (2015) described big data science as both a philosophical approach to knowledge generation and a unique set of techniques. The evaluator uses shared routines to explore and analyze data that are openly accessible, distributed across multiple locations, and fraught with uncertainty. This approach allows the harmonizing of data to answer questions that were previously unanswerable with existing methodologies. The National Consortium for Data Science has defined *data science* as the systematic study of the organization and use of digital data in order to accelerate discovery, improve critical decision-making processes, and enable a data-driven economy (Ahalt et al., 2014). One might reserve judgment on the importance of big data and big data science as a trend in health care. What is apparent to teams of investigators and practitioners is that this methodology is a paradigm shift, and that it is moving science into new and uncharted directions of exploration and knowledge development. The convergence of huge amounts of multiple and varied data sources will be used to influence the health of individuals and populations as the science develops.

## Peer and Self-Evaluation

Finally, evaluation of self and peers to determine performance and to develop an individualized development plan is a professional responsibility. The American Nurses Association (2010) has outlined both the expectation and process for peer and self-evaluation as tools for professional growth and development to support high-quality patient care and outcomes.

## DEVELOPING AND MAINTAINING COMPETENCY IN EVALUATION

The increased expectation and future role for DNPs to be experts in evaluation raises the question of how to develop and maintain evaluation expertise. DNPs need to recognize their important and expanding role in evaluation and to embrace it. An evaluation provides an opportunity to inform and influence data-driven decision making that is based on a systematic process. The following lists recommendations for the DNP to develop and maintain expertise in evaluation:

1. Learn all you can about evaluation through academic course work, continuing education programs, and reading.
2. Work with others who have expertise in evaluation for mentoring experiences.
3. Conduct your own competency analysis and achievement of objectives; set a timeline and review and update periodically.
4. Include evaluation as a focus in your individualized development plan and monitor your progress.

In the future, with the higher expectation of evaluation expertise for DNPs, job retention and promotion will be tied, in part, to expertise in evaluation. Therefore, career planning should include attention to competency development, as well as maintenance in many forms of evaluation.

Selected online resources to help DNPs expand their knowledge of evaluation are noted in the following list.

## ONLINE RESOURCES

Agency for Healthcare Research and Quality (http://www.ahrq.gov/)
A federal agency that provides funding, clinical information, and guidelines for health care quality.

American Evaluation Association (http://www.eval.org)
An international professional organization that offers literature, courses, and meetings focused on program and other types of evaluation.

Center for Health Care Evaluation (http://www.chce.research.va.gov/)
Part of the U.S. Department of Veteran Affairs, CHCE provides information to improve health care quality for veterans and the entire population.

Commonwealth Fund (http://www.commonwealthfund.org/)
Provides information on health care reform, health system performance measures, and health care quality including state report cards.

Institute for Healthcare Improvement (http://www.ihi.org/ihi)
Provides information on increasing effectiveness and efficiency in the health care system, and describes key indicators and protocols for bringing about change.
National Quality Forum (http://www.qualityforum.org/Home.aspx)
Offers instruction on measuring health care quality, including the use of dashboards to present evaluation results.
National Quality Measures Clearinghouse (www.qualitymeasures.ahrq.gov)
Supported by AHRQ and the U.S. Department of Health and Human Services. It provides a website for information, including tutorials, and an extensive database of quality measures.
Robert Wood Johnson Foundation. (2004). (http://www.rwjf.org/pr/product.jsp?cd=18657)
A guide to evaluation primers. Provides a critique of the strengths and weaknesses of 11 frequently cited primers on evaluation.
USPSTF (http://www.ahrq.gov/professionals/clinicians-providers/guidelines-recommendations/uspstf/index.html)
The Task Force is composed of health care professionals who volunteer their time to develop evidence-based guidelines and recommendations about clinical prevention for patients and providers.
W. K. Kellogg Foundation (http://www.wkkf.org)
Supports evaluation activities and tools, including an evaluation handbook.

## REFERENCES

Ahalt, S., Bizon, C., Evans, J., Erlich, Y., Ginsberg, G., Krishnamurthy, A., & Wilhelmsen, K. (2014). *Data to discovery: Genomes to health. A white paper from the National Consortium for Data Science.* Chapel Hill, NC: Renaissance Computing Institute. Retrieved from http://data2discovery.org/dev/wp-content /uploads/2014/02/NCDS-Summit-2013.pdf

Albanese, M. P., Evans, D. A., Schantz, C. A., Bowen, M., Piesieski, P., & Polomano, R. C. (2010). Engaging clinical nurses in quality and performance improvement activities. *Nursing Administration Quarterly, 34*(3), 226–245.

American Nurses Association. (2010). *Scope and standards of practice* (2nd ed.). Silver Spring, MD: Author.

Berwick, D. M., & Hackbarth, A. D. (2012). Eliminating waste in US health care. *JAMA, 307*(14), 1513–1516.

Bowers, M. R., & Kiefe, C. I. (2002). Measuring health care quality: Comparing and contrasting the medical and the marketing approaches. *American Journal of Medical Quality, 17*(4), 136–144.

Brennan, P. F., & Bakken, S. (2015). Nursing needs big data and big data needs nursing. *Journal of Nursing Scholarship, 47*(5), 477–484.

Cha, A. E. (2015). CDC blames ADHD spike on bad diagnoses. *Houston Chronicle,* p. A25.

Chiolero, A., Paccaud, F., Aujesky, D., Santschi, V., & Rodondi, N. (2015). How to prevent overdiagnosis. *Swiss Medical Weekly,* pp. 1–7. doi:10.4414/smw.2015.14060

Coon, E. R., Quinonez, R. A., Moyer, V. A., & Schroeder, A. R. (2014). Overdiagnosis: How our compulsion for diagnosis may be harming children. *Pediatrics, 134*(5), 1013–1023.

Ebner, A. L. (2010). What nurses need to know about health care reform. *Nursing Economics, 28*(3), 191–194.

Guthrie, R. (1992). The origin of newborn screening. *Screening, 1,* 5–15.

Institute of Medicine. (2001). *Crossing the quality chasm: A new health system for the 21st century.* Washington, DC: The National Academies Press.

Institute of Medicine. (2011). *The future of nursing: Leading change, advancing health.* Washington, DC: The National Academies Press.

Kaiser Family Foundation. (2013). *Focus on health reform. Summary of the Affordable Care Act* (Publication number 8061–02). Kaiser Family Foundation. Retrieved from www.kff.org

Kocher, R., & Sahni, N. R. (2010). Physicians versus hospitals as leaders of accountable care organizations. *New England Journal of Medicine, 363*(27), 2579–2582.

Lallemand, N. C. (2012). Health policy brief: Reducing waste in health care. *Health Affairs,* 1–5. Retrieved from www.healthaffairs.org

Lee, T. H. (2010). Putting the value framework to work. *New England Journal of Medicine, 363*(26), 2481–2483.

Loan, L. A., Patrician, P. A., & McCarthy, M. (2011). Participation in a national nursing outcomes database: Monitoring outcomes over time. *Nursing Administration Quarterly, 35*(1), 72–81.

Morgan, D. J., Wright, S. M., & Dhruva, S. (2015). Update on medical overuse. *JAMA Internal Medicine, 175*(1), 120–124.

National Institutes of Health. (2011). NIH stops clinical trial on combination cholesterol treatment. The National Heart, Lung, and Blood Institutes. Retrieved from http://public.nhlbi.nih.gov/newsroom/home/GetPressRelease.aspx?id=2792

National Institutes of Health Big Data to Knowledge. (2014). *Workshop on enhancing training for biomedical big data.* Retrieved from http://bd2k.nih.gov/pdf/bd2k_training_workshop_report.pdf

National Newborn Screening and Genetics Resource Center. (2014, November). Retrieved from https://genes-r-us.uthscsa.edu/sites/genes-r-us/files/nbsdisorders.pdf

Oberlander, J. (2010). Beyond repeal—the future of health care reform. *New England Journal of Medicine, 363*(24), 2277–2279.

Porter, M. E. (2010). What is value in health care? *New England Journal of Medicine, 363*(26), 2477–2481.

Provonost, P. J., & Lilford, R. (2011). A road map for improving the performance of performance measures. *Health Affairs, 30*(4), 569–573.

Rothwell, E. W., Anderson, R. A., Burbank, M. J., Goldenberg, A. J., Lewis, M. H., Stark, L., & Botkin, J. R. (2010). Concerns of newborn blood screening advisory committee members regarding storage and use of residual newborn screening blood spots. *American Journal of Public Health, 101*(11), 2111–2116.

The President's Council on Bioethics. (2008). *The changing moral focus of newborn screening: An ethical analysis by the President's Council on Bioethics.* Retrieved from https://bioethicsarchive.georgetown.edu/pcbe/reports/newborn_screening/

Welch, H. G. (2015). *Less medicine, more health.* Boston, MA: Beacon Press.

# INDEX